T0239637

NEURODEGENERATIVE DISEASE and MICRONUTRIENTS

Prevention and Treatment

NEURODEGENERATIVE DISEASE and MICRONUTRIENTS

Prevention and Treatment

KEDAR N. PRASAD, PhD

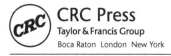

CRC Press
Taylor & Francis Group
Boca Raton London New York

CRC Press is an imprint of the
Taylor & Francis Group, an **informa** business

CRC Press
Taylor & Francis Group
6000 Broken Sound Parkway NW, Suite 300
Boca Raton, FL 33487-2742

First issued in paperback 2016

© 2015 by Taylor & Francis Group, LLC
CRC Press is an imprint of Taylor & Francis Group, an Informa business

No claim to original U.S. Government works

Version Date: 20140425

ISBN 13: 978-1-138-03414-3 (pbk)
ISBN 13: 978-1-4822-1047-7 (hbk)

This book contains information obtained from authentic and highly regarded sources. Reasonable efforts have been made to publish reliable data and information, but the author and publisher cannot assume responsibility for the validity of all materials or the consequences of their use. The authors and publishers have attempted to trace the copyright holders of all material reproduced in this publication and apologize to copyright holders if permission to publish in this form has not been obtained. If any copyright material has not been acknowledged please write and let us know so we may rectify in any future reprint.

Except as permitted under U.S. Copyright Law, no part of this book may be reprinted, reproduced, transmitted, or utilized in any form by any electronic, mechanical, or other means, now known or hereafter invented, including photocopying, microfilming, and recording, or in any information storage or retrieval system, without written permission from the publishers.

For permission to photocopy or use material electronically from this work, please access www.copyright.com (http://www.copyright.com/) or contact the Copyright Clearance Center, Inc. (CCC), 222 Rosewood Drive, Danvers, MA 01923, 978-750-8400. CCC is a not-for-profit organization that provides licenses and registration for a variety of users. For organizations that have been granted a photocopy license by the CCC, a separate system of payment has been arranged.

Trademark Notice: Product or corporate names may be trademarks or registered trademarks, and are used only for identification and explanation without intent to infringe.

Library of Congress Cataloging-in-Publication Data

Prasad, Kedar N., author.
   Neurodegenerative disease and micronutrients : prevention and treatment / Kedar N. Prasad.
      p. ; cm.
      Includes bibliographical references and index.
      ISBN 978-1-4822-1047-7 (hardcover : alk. paper)
      I. Title.
      [DNLM: 1. Neurodegenerative Diseases--etiology. 2. Neurodegenerative
Diseases--therapy. 3. Micronutrients--therapeutic use. 4. Neurodegenerative
Diseases--prevention & control. 5. Nutrition Therapy--methods. WL 358.5]

RC376.5
616.8'3--dc23   2014015958

**Visit the Taylor & Francis Web site at
http://www.taylorandfrancis.com**

**and the CRC Press Web site at
http://www.crcpress.com**

This book is dedicated to my family for their support.

Contents

Preface

According to Medline Plus, there are more than 600 neurological diseases. This book includes major neurodegenerative diseases such as Alzheimer's disease (AD), Parkinson's disease (PD), and Huntington's disease (HD), and certain neurological disorders such as posttraumatic stress disorder (PTSD), traumatic brain injury (TBI), concussive injury, and cerebrovascular insufficiency. HD is caused by a mutation in the Huntington gene. Most neurodegenerative diseases, such as AD and PD, are acquired, although a small percentage of them are due to mutations in the gene specific to each disease. Some neurological diseases such as PTSD, TBI, concussions, and cerebrovascular insufficiency are induced by external agents.

Among individuals 65 years or older, AD and PD remain a major medical concern. Since the number of people in this age group is expected to increase from 33 million to 51 million by the year 2025, these neurodegenerative diseases will create huge medical problems and associated cost of their management. Among veterans of foreign wars, increased rates of detection of PTSD and other mental disorders among survivors of acute and mild TBI have become major concerns for the US military. In addition, concussive injuries are being detected at increased rates among high school, college, and professional athletes, especially football players. At present, there are no adequate strategies for the prevention of neurodegenerative diseases. Treatments of AD, PD, PTSD, and TBI remain unsatisfactory. Except for the physical protection of the skull, there are no biological strategies to protect the brain tissue against concussive injury.

In this book, a unified hypothesis is proposed that increased oxidative stress, chronic inflammation, and glutamate release are primarily responsible for the initiation and progression of neurodegenerative and neurological diseases. HD is a familial disease with mutation in the Huntington gene. Increased oxidative stress, chronic inflammation, and glutamate release also play an important role in the progression of this disease. Therefore, attenuation of oxidative stress, chronic inflammation, and release of glutamate and its toxicity appears to be one of the rational choices for the prevention and progression of these chronic diseases. In order to achieve this goal, it is essential to elevate the levels of all antioxidant enzymes and all dietary and endogenous antioxidants. This goal cannot be realized by the use of one or two antioxidants that have been used in most clinical studies on neurological diseases.

It is necessary to activate a nuclear transcription factor-2 (Nrf2) in order to increase the levels of antioxidant enzymes, and supplementation is required in order to increase the levels of dietary and endogenous antioxidants levels. Normally, in response to reactive oxygen species (ROS), Nrf2 dissociates itself from the inhibitor Nrf2I and migrates to the nucleus where it binds with the antioxidant response element (ARE), which increases the expression of antioxidant genes. This normal response of Nrf2 is impaired in the neurodegenerative diseases. This is evidenced by the fact that increased oxidative stress is found in patients with these diseases. Certain antioxidants and polyphenolic compounds activate Nrf2 by a mechanism that does not require ROS. Therefore, I have proposed the use of a preparation of micronutrients containing multiple dietary and endogenous antioxidants, vitamin D, B vitamins with high doses of vitamin B_3, and certain polyphenolic compounds (curcumin and resveratrol) for prevention, and, in combination with standard therapy, for improved management of neurodegenerative diseases. The proposed preparation of micronutrients would decrease oxidative stress, chronic inflammation, and release of glutamate and its toxicity by activating the Nrf2/ARE pathway and increasing the levels of dietary and endogenous antioxidants.

At present, there are no strategies to prevent or delay the onset of symptoms of a genetic basis of neurological diseases. Individuals carrying a gene mutation wait until the symptoms of the disease appear and then receive treatment to improve the symptoms. Increased oxidative stress and chronic inflammation also play an important role in the development of symptoms of a genetic basis of the disease. Laboratory data suggest that supplementation with a preparation of multiple dietary and endogenous antioxidants prevents the development of a genetic basis of the disease.

Most neurologists believe that micronutrients including antioxidants have no significant role in the prevention or improved management of neurodegenerative diseases. These beliefs are primarily based on a few clinical studies in which supplementation with a single antioxidant, such as vitamin E in AD and coenzyme Q_{10} in PD, produced modest beneficial effects; however, vitamin E alone was ineffective in reducing the progression of PD. Patients with neurodegenerative diseases may have a high-oxidative environment in the brain. Administration of a single antioxidant is not expected to produce any significant beneficial effect. This is due to the fact that an individual antioxidant in the presence of a high-oxidative environment may be oxidized and then acts as a pro-oxidant rather than as an antioxidant. The levels of the oxidized form of antioxidant may increase after prolonged consumption and damage brain neurons. In addition, the use of a single antioxidant in a clinical study is unlikely to increase the levels of all antioxidant enzymes as well as all dietary and endogenous antioxidants. Published results on clinical studies on the effect of antioxidants in neurodegenerative diseases confirm this view.

The author has published a few reviews in peer-reviewed journals challenging the current trends of using single antioxidants in prevention or improved management of neurodegenerative diseases in high-risk populations. Nevertheless, the use of one or two micronutrients continues to dominate clinical study designs; consequently, inconsistent results are being published, adding to the current controversies regarding the value of micronutrients in the prevention and improved management of neurodegenerative diseases.

Some books on neurodegenerative diseases and their causes and symptoms are available; however, none of them have critically analyzed the published data on antioxidant and neurodegenerative diseases, and they never questioned whether the experimental designs of the study on which the conclusions are based are scientifically valid, whether the results obtained from the use of a single antioxidant in a high-risk population can be extrapolated to the effect of the same antioxidant in a multiple antioxidant preparation for the same population, and whether they could be extrapolated to normal populations. In this book, the author briefly discusses the incidence, cost, and causes of each neurodegenerative disease; critically examines the experimental designs and data on the effectiveness of antioxidants in reducing the progression of neurodegenerative diseases; points out the flaws of experimental designs; and proposes ideas on how to resolve the current controversies with respect to the use of antioxidants.

Furthermore, a preparation of micronutrients containing multiple dietary and endogenous antioxidants, vitamin D, and B vitamins with high doses of vitamin B_3 for the prevention or, in combination with standard therapy, for the improved management of neurodegenerative diseases has never been proposed. The author proposes this in this book.

The author hopes that this book will arouse enough passion for and against taking multiple micronutrient supplements to lead to randomized, double-blind, and placebo-controlled clinical studies in high-risk populations such as those with early-phase AD or PD to test the efficacy of proposed micronutrients in reducing the risk of developing these diseases. A similar study can be initiated in combination with standard therapy to establish whether the proposed micronutrients can improve the efficacy of standard therapy in reducing the progression and improving the management of these diseases.

The author hopes that this book will serve as a reference book for graduate students in neurobiology, instructors teaching courses in nutrition and neurological diseases, and researchers involved in the prevention and improved management of neurodegenerative diseases, using micronutrients. Primary care and academic and practicing neurologists interested in complementary medicine may find this book as a useful resource for recommending micronutrient supplements to their patients.

Author

Dr. Kedar N. Prasad earned a MS in zoology from the University of Bihar in India and a PhD in radiation biology from the University of Iowa, Iowa City. He then went to the Brookhaven National Laboratory for post-doctoral training. Dr. Prasad joined the Department of Radiology at the University of Colorado Health Sciences Center where he became a professor in 1980. Later, he was appointed the director for the Center for Vitamins and Cancer Research. He has published over 200 papers in peer-reviewed journals, including *Nature, Science,* and *Proceedings of the National Academy of Sciences (PNAS)*. He has written several book chapters and abstracts as well as authored or edited 19 books on radiobiology, radiation protection, and nutrition and cancer. He is a member of several professional organizations and serves as an ad hoc member of various study sections of the National Institutes of Health (NIH). He is a frequently invited speaker at national and international meetings on nutrition and cancer. In 1982, he was invited by the Nobel Prize Committee to nominate a candidate for the Nobel Prize in Medicine. He was selected to deliver the 1999 Harold Harper Lecture at the meeting of the American College of Advancement of Medicine. He is a former president of the International Society for Nutrition and Cancer. Dr. Prasad has consistently obtained NIH grants for his research. His current interests are in the areas of radiation protection, nutrition and cancer, and nutrition and neurological diseases, particularly Alzheimer's disease and Parkinson's disease. Since 2005, he has been a chief scientific officer of the Premier Micronutrient Corporation.

1 Evolution, Sources, and Functions of Antioxidant Systems

INTRODUCTION

Antioxidant systems in humans consist of antioxidant enzymes and dietary and endogenous antioxidant chemicals. Although all micronutrients are essential for growth and development, antioxidants have been the subject of extensive laboratory research and clinical studies because of their potential importance in reducing oxidative stress and inflammation that contribute to the initiation and progression of chronic diseases. Before discussing the role of antioxidant systems in reducing the risk of developing chronic diseases, it is essential to understand certain basic facts about them. Some dietary and endogenous antioxidant chemicals and certain polyphonic compounds reduce oxidative stress by directly scavenging free radicals as well as by increasing antioxidant enzymes through the activation of a transcriptional factor-2 (Nrf2)/ARE (antioxidant response element) pathway. Therefore, a combination of dietary and endogenous antioxidant chemicals and certain polyphenolic compounds would reduce oxidative stress and chronic inflammation optimally.

This chapter briefly describes the evolution of antioxidant systems, the historical perspective of some antioxidants, and the sources, distribution, and function of antioxidant systems. In addition, this chapter discusses current controversies about antioxidants for health and disease prevention, and misuse of antioxidants in clinical studies for the prevention of chronic diseases. There are several books on this topic; however, only a few of them are referenced at the end of this chapter.[1–11]

EVOLUTION OF ANTIOXIDANT SYSTEMS

Antioxidants are essential for the growth and survival of all organisms, including humans, who depend on oxygen. In the beginning, Earth's atmosphere had no oxygen. Anaerobic organisms, which can live without oxygen, thrived in the oceans and rivers. About 2.5 billion years ago, blue-green algae in the ocean acquired the ability to split water (H_2O) into hydrogen (H) and oxygen (O_2). This chemical reaction initiated the release of oxygen into the atmosphere, leading to the extinction of many anaerobic organisms due to the oxygen's toxicity. Those organisms that developed antioxidant defense systems that can protect against oxygen's toxicity survived—an important biological event that led to the rapid evolution of multicellular organisms, including humans. Today, the amount of oxygen in dry air is about 21%, and in water, it is about 34%.

ANTIOXIDANT SYSTEMS

Antioxidant systems in humans consist of two separate components: (1) antioxidant enzymes, which include glutathione peroxidase, catalase, and superoxide dismutase (SOD), and (2) dietary and endogenous antioxidant chemicals, which include vitamin A, carotenoids, vitamin C, vitamin E, glutathione, alpha-lipoic acid coenzyme Q_{10}, L-carnitine, and polyphenolic compounds derived from plants, fruits, and vegetables. Antioxidant enzymes destroy free radicals by catalysis, whereas antioxidant chemicals destroy free radicals by directly scavenging them. Therefore, elevated levels of both components of the antioxidant system are essential for reducing oxidative stress optimally.

BRIEF HISTORY OF DISCOVERY OF SOME MICRONUTRIENTS

VITAMIN A

The night blindness that we know now to be caused by vitamin A deficiency existed for centuries before the discovery of vitamin A. As early as about 1500 B.C., Egyptians knew how to cure this disease. Roman soldiers suffering from night blindness used to go to Egypt, where they would receive liver extract for the treatment. Now, it is well established that the liver is the richest source of vitamin A. The treatment of night blindness with the liver extract was not used outside Egypt for centuries; medical establishments during that period must not have accepted this treatment. It was not until 1912 when Dr. McCollum of the University of Wisconsin discovered vitamin A from butter, and therefore, it was initially called as "fat-soluble A." The structure of vitamin A was determined in 1930, and this vitamin was synthesized in the laboratory in 1947. It should be pointed out that the medical establishment of that period delayed the cure of night blindness for centuries.

CAROTENOIDS

In 1919, carotenoid pigments were isolated from yellow plants, and in 1930, it was found that some of the ingested carotene was converted to vitamin A. This carotene was referred to as beta-carotene.

VITAMIN C

The scurvy that we know today is caused by vitamin C deficiency. The symptoms of this disease were known to the Egyptians as early as 1500 B.C., but Hippocrates in the fifth century described the symptoms of scurvy that included bleeding gums, hemorrhaging, and death. Native American Indians knew the cure for this disease, but its value in treatment of diseases remained limited to this population. During the sea voyage of European explorers that occurred between the twelfth and sixteenth centuries, the epidemic of scurvy among sailors forced some to land in Canada, where Native Indians gave them extracts of pine bark and needles (prepared like tea). This treatment totally cured scurvy in these sailors. In 1536, Jacques Cartier, a French explorer, brought this formulation for curing scurvy to France, but the medical establishment rejected it as a fraud because it came from Native Indians from Canada whom they used to call savages. It was not until 1593 that Sir Richard Hawkins recommended taking sour oranges and lemons to his sailors. It was not until 1770 that the British Navy began recommending that ships carry sufficient lime juice for all personnel aboard. In 1928, Albert Szent-Gyorgyi, a Hungarian scientist, isolated a substance from the adrenal gland that was called hexuronic acid. This substance was vitamin C, and in 1932, it was the first vitamin to be synthesized in the laboratory. It should be pointed out that the medical establishment of that period delayed the cure of scurvy for centuries.

Vitamin D

Although a bone disease, rickets might have existed in human population for centuries. It was not until 1645 that Dr. Daniel Whistler described the symptoms of rickets, which we now know to be due to vitamin D deficiency. In 1922, Sir Edward Mellanby, while working on the cure for rickets, discovered vitamin D. This vitamin was later found to require sunlight for its formation. The chemical structure of vitamin D was determined by a German scientist, Dr. Windaus, in 1930. Vitamin D_3 was chemically characterized in 1936 and was considered a steroid that was effective in the treatment of rickets.

Vitamin E

In 1922, Dr. Herbert Evans from the University of California, Berkeley, observed that rats that were reared exclusively on whole milk grew normally but were not fertile. The fertility was restored when they were additionally fed with wheat germ. However, it took another 14 years (1936) before the active substance responsible for restoring fertility was isolated. Dr. Evans named it *tocopherol*, from the Greek word meaning "to bear offspring" and with the ending "ol" signifying its chemical status as an alcohol.

B Vitamins

All B vitamins were discovered during 1912–1934. In 1912, the Polish-born biochemist Dr. Casimir Funk isolated the active substances from the rice husks of the unpolished rice that prevented the disease beriberi. He named this substance "vitamines," because he thought they were "amines" that are derived from ammonia. In 1920, the "e" was dropped when it was found out that not all vitamins were "amines."

SOURCES AND FORMS OF VITAMINS

Vitamin A

The richest source of vitamin A is the liver (6.5 mg per 100 g liver) from beef, pork, chicken, turkey and fish, carrot (0.8 mg per 100 g), broccoli leaves (0.8 mg per

100 g), sweet potato (0.7 mg per 100 g), kale (0.7 mg per 100 g), butter (0.7 mg per 100 g), spinach (0.5 mg per 100 g), and pumpkin (0.4 mg per 100 g). Other minor sources include cantaloupe melon, eggs, apricot, papaya, and mango (40–170 μg per 100 g). Fruits and vegetables (yellow and red) are a very rich source of beta-carotene. One molecule of beta-carotene is converted to two molecules of retinol in the intestinal tract.

Vitamin A exists as retinyl palmitate or retinyl acetate that is converted into retinol form in the body. Vitamin A can also exist as a retinoic acid in the cells. It was determined that 1 IU (international unit) equals 0.3 μg of retinol or 0.6 μg of beta-carotene. The activity of vitamin A is also expressed as retinol activity equivalent (RAE). It was determined that 1 μg of RAE corresponds to 1 μg of retinol and 2 μg of beta-carotene in oil. Vitamin A, beta-carotene, and the synthetic retinoids are also available commercially.

CAROTENOIDS

The richest sources of carotenoids are sweet potato, carrot, spinach, mango, cantaloupe, apricot, kale, broccoli, parsley, cilantro, pumpkin, winter squash, and fresh thyme. There are two main forms of carotenoids found in nature, alpha-carotene and beta-carotene. Beta-carotene is one of the more than 600 carotenoids found in fruits, vegetables, and plants, and it represents the more common form of carotenoids. Other carotenes include lutein and lycopene.

VITAMIN C

The richest sources of vitamin C are fruits and vegetables. They include rose hip (2000 mg per 100 g of rose hip), red pepper (2000 mg per 100 g of red pepper), parsley (2000 mg per 100 g of parsley), guava (2000 mg per 100 g of guava), kiwi fruit (2000 mg per 100 g of kiwi fruit), broccoli (2000 mg per 100 g of broccoli), lychee (2000 mg per 100 g of lychee), papaya (2000 mg per 100 g of papaya), and strawberry (2000 mg per 100 g of strawberry). Other sources of vitamin C include orange, lemon, melon, garlic, cauliflower, grapefruit, raspberry, tangerine, passion fruit, spinach, and lime and contain about 30–50 mg per 100 g of fruits and vegetables. Vitamin C is sold commercially as L-ascorbic acid, calcium ascorbate, sodium ascorbate, or potassium ascorbate.

VITAMIN E

The richest sources of vitamin E include wheat germ oil (215 mg per 100 g of oil), sunflower oil (56 mg per 100 g of oil), olive oil (12 mg per 100 g of oil), almond oil (39 mg per 100 g of oil), hazelnut oil (26 mg per 100 g of oil), walnut oil (20 mg per 100 g of oil), and peanut oil (17 mg per 100 g of oil). The sources for small amounts of vitamin E (0.1 to 2 mg per 100 g) include kiwifruit, fish, leafy vegetables and whole grains. In the United States, the fortified breakfast cereals are an important source of vitamin E. At present, most of the natural form of vitamin E is extracted from vegetable oils, primarily soybean oil.

Vitamin E exists in eight different forms, four tocopherols (alpha-, beta-, gamma-, and delta-tocopherol) and four tocotrienols (alpha-, beta-, gamma-, and delta-tocotrienol). Alpha-tocopherol has the most biological activity. Vitamin E can exist in the natural form commonly indicated as "D," whereas the synthetic form is referred to as "DL." The stable esterified form of vitamin E is available as alpha-tocopheryl acetate (alpha-TA), alpha-tocopheryl succinate (alpha-TS), and alpha-tocopheryl nicotinate. The activity of vitamin E is generally expressed in international units (IU). It is determined that 1 IU equals 0.66 mg of D-alpha-tocopherol, and 1 IU of racemic mixture (DL form) equals 0.45 mg of D-tocopherol.

GLUTATHIONE

Glutathione is synthesized from three amino acids, L-cysteine, L-glutamic acid, and L-glycine, and is present in all cells; however, the liver contains the highest amount, up to 5 mmol. Glutathione exists in the cells in reduced or oxidized form. In healthy cells, more than 90% of glutathione is present in the reduced form. The oxidized form of glutathione can be converted to a reduced form by an enzyme glutathione reductase. The reduced form of glutathione acts as an antioxidant.

COENZYME Q_{10}

In 1957, Dr. Fredrick Crane isolated coenzyme Q_{10}, and Dr. Wolf working under Dr. Karl Folkers determined the structure of coenzyme Q_{10} in 1958.

L-CARNITINE

L-Carnitine is synthesized from amino acids lysine and methionine and was originally found as a growth factor for mealworms. It is primarily synthesized in the liver and kidney. Vitamin C is necessary for the synthesis of L-carnitine. It exists as L-carnitine, a biologically active form, and as D-carnitine, a biologically inactive form.

POLYPHENOLS

Polyphenols are a group of compounds found in herbs, fruits, vegetables, and plants. They include tannins, lignins, and flavonoids. The best-studied polyphenols are flavonoids, which include resveratrol (in grape skin and seed), curcumin (in spices such as turmeric), ginseng extract, cinnamon extract, and garlic extract, quercetin, epicatechin, and oligomeric proanthocyanidins. The major sources of flavonoids include all citrus fruits, berries, ginkgo biloba, onions, parsley, tea, red wine, and dark chocolate. Over 5000 naturally occurring flavonoids have been characterized from various plants.

SOLUBILITY OF ANTIOXIDANTS AND POLYPHENOLS

The lipid-soluble antioxidants include vitamin A, vitamin E, carotenoids, coenzyme Q_{10}, and L-carnitine, and the water-soluble antioxidants include vitamin C, glutathione, and alpha-lipoic acid. Polyphenols are generally fat soluble. Fat-soluble vitamins and polyphenols should be taken with meals, so that they are more readily absorbed.

DISTRIBUTION OF ANTIOXIDANTS IN THE BODY

CAROTENOIDS

Beta-carotene is one of more than 600 carotenoids found in fruits and vegetables and plants. It is commercially available in natural or synthetic form. The natural form of beta-carotene is more effective than the synthetic form. Preparations of natural carotenoids contain primarily beta-carotene; however, the other type of carotenoids is also present. A portion of ingested beta-carotene is converted to retinol (vitamin A) in the intestinal tract before absorption, and the remainder is distributed in the blood and tissues of the body. One molecule of beta-carotene forms two molecules of vitamin A. In humans, the conversion of beta-carotene to vitamin A does not occur if the body already has sufficient amounts of vitamin A. Beta-carotene is primarily stored in the eyes and fatty tissues. Other carotenoids, such as lycopene, accumulated in the prostate more than in other organs, whereas lutein accumulated in the eyes more than any other organs.

VITAMIN A

Vitamin A is commercially sold as retinyl palmitate, retinyl acetate, and retinoic acid and its analogues. Retinyl acetate or retinyl palmitate is converted to retinol in the intestine before absorption. Retinol is converted to retinoic acid in the cells. Retinoic acid performs all functions of vitamin A except for maintaining good vision. Retinol is stored in the liver as retinyl palmitate. Vitamin A exists as a protein-bound molecule. The level of retinol can be determined in plasma.

VITAMIN C

Vitamin C is commercially sold as ascorbic acid, sodium ascorbate, magnesium ascorbate, calcium ascorbate, and time-release capsules containing ascorbic acid and vitamin C-ester. It is present in all cells. Ascorbic acid is converted to dehydroascorbic acid that can be reduced to form vitamin C. It is interesting to note that dehydroascorbic acid can cross the blood–brain barrier, but vitamin C cannot. All mammals make vitamin C, except guinea pigs. An adult goat makes about 13 g of vitamin C every day. The plasma levels of vitamin C may not reflect the tissue levels of vitamin C, but in humans, it is difficult to obtain tissues for determining vitamin C. Vitamin C can recycle oxidized vitamin E to a reduced form that acts as an antioxidant.

VITAMIN E

Among vitamin E isomers, alpha-tocopherol is biologically more active than others. In recent years, the research on tocotrienols has also revealed some important biological functions. Vitamin E is commercially sold as D- or DL-tocopherol, alpha-TA, or alpha-TS. The esterified forms of vitamin E (alpha-TA and alpha-TS) are more stable than alpha-tocopherol. Alpha-TA has been widely used in the basic research and clinical studies. It has been presumed that alpha-TA or alpha-TS is converted to alpha-tocopherol before absorption. This assumption may be true as long as the stores of alpha-tocopherol in the body are not saturated; however, if the body stores of alpha-tocopherol are saturated, alpha-TS can be absorbed as alpha-TS. Alpha-TS enters the cells more easily than alpha-tocopherol because of its greater solubility. Alpha-TS has some unique functions that cannot be produced by alpha-T. Alpha-TS is now considered the most effective form of vitamin E, but it cannot act as an antioxidant until converted to alpha-T. Alpha-T is located primarily in the membranous structures of the cells. The level of vitamin E can be determined in the plasma.

GLUTATHIONE AND ALPHA-LIPOIC ACID

Glutathione is the most important antioxidant within the cells. It is sold commercially for an oral consumption; however, this is destroyed totally in the intestine. Therefore, an oral administration of glutathione does not increase the cellular level of glutathione. N-acetylcysteine (NAC) increases the cellular levels of glutathione. In the body, N-acetyl is removed from NAC by the enzyme esterase, and then cysteine is used to synthesize glutathione. Alpha-lipoic acid also increases the cellular levels of glutathione by a mechanism that is different from NAC, and it is present in all cells.

COENZYME Q_{10}

About 95% of energy is generated from the use of coenzyme Q_{10} by the mitochondria. Therefore, organs, such as the heart and the liver, that require high energy have the highest concentrations of coenzyme Q_{10}. Other organelles inside the cells that contain coenzyme Q_{10} include endoplasmic reticulum, peroxisomes, lysosomes, and Golgi apparatus.

L-CARNITINE

L-Carnitine is made in our body, but we can also obtain it from our diet. The highest concentration of L-carnitine is found in red meat (95 mg per 3.0 oz. of meat). In contrast, chicken breast has only 3.9 mg per 3.5 oz. It is present in all cells of our body.

NICOTINAMIDE (VITAMIN B_3) AND NICOTINAMIDE ADENINE DINUCLEOTIDE DEHYDROGENASE (NADH)

Nicotinamide adenine dinucleotide (NAD+) and NADH (reduced form of NAD) are present in all cells of our body. NAD+ is an oxidizing agent; therefore, it can act as a pro-oxidant, whereas NADH can act as an antioxidant. NAD+ accepts electron from other molecules and is reduced to form NADH. NADH can recycle oxidized vitamin E into a reduced form that can act as an antioxidant. NADH is essential for mitochondria to generate energy.

POLYPHENOLS

Flavonoids are poorly absorbed by the intestinal tract in humans. All of them possess varying degrees of antioxidants and anti-inflammation activities.

MELATONIN

Melatonin is a naturally occurring hormone produced primarily by the pineal gland in the brain. It is also produced by the retina, lens, and gastrointestinal tract. Melatonin is synthesized from the amino acid tryptophan. It is also produced by various plants, such as rice. It is readily absorbed from the intestinal tract; however, 50% of it is removed from the plasma in 35 to 50 min. It has several biological functions, including antioxidant and anti-inflammation activities. Melatonin is necessary for the sleep.

STORING OF ANTIOXIDANTS

CAROTENOIDS

Most commercially sold carotenoids in solid form can be stored at room temperature away from light for a few years. Beta-carotene in solution, however, degrades within a few days even in cold and when stored away from light.

VITAMIN A

Crystal forms of retinol, retinoic acid, retinyl acetate, and retinal palmitate can be stored at 4°C for several months. A solution of retinoic acid is stable at 4°C, stored away from light, for several weeks.

VITAMIN C

Vitamin C should not be stored in solution form, because it is easily destroyed within a few days. Crystal or tablet forms of vitamin C can be kept at room temperature, away from light, for a few years.

VITAMIN E

Alpha-tocopherol is relatively unstable at room temperature in comparison to alpha-TA or alpha-TS. Alpha-tocopherol can be stored at 4°C for several weeks, but alpha-TA or alpha-TS can be stored at room temperature for a few years. A solution of alpha-TS is stable for several months at 4°C, if kept away from the light.

GLUTATHIONE, NAC, AND ALPHA-LIPOIC ACID

Solid forms of glutathione, NAC, and alpha-lipoic acid are stable at room temperature away from light, for a few years. The solutions of these antioxidants are stable at 4°C away from the light for several months.

COENZYME Q_{10} AND NADH

These antioxidants in solid forms are stable at room temperature, away from the light, for a few years. The solutions of these antioxidants are stable at 4°C away from the light for several months.

POLYPHENOLS

They are very stable at room temperature, away from light, for a few years.

MELATONIN

The powder form of melatonin is stable at 4°C for a year or more.

CAN ANTIOXIDANTS BE DESTROYED DURING COOKING?

CAROTENOIDS

Most carotenes, especially lutein and lycopene, are not destroyed during cooking. In fact, their bioavailability improves when they are derived from a cooked or extracted preparation, for example, lycopene from the tomato sauce.

VITAMIN A

Routine cooking does not destroy vitamin A, but slow heating for a long period of time may reduce its potency. Canning and prolonged cold storage also may diminish the activity of vitamin A. The vitamin A content of fortified milk powder substantially declines after 2 years.

VITAMIN E

Food processing, frying, and freezing destroy vitamin E. The vitamin E content of fortified milk powder is unaffected over a 2-year period.

GLUTATHIONE, NAC, AND ALPHA-LIPOIC ACID

They can be partially destroyed during cooking.

POLYPHENOLS

They are not destroyed during cooking.

COENZYME Q_{10} AND NADH

They can be partially degraded during cooking.

ABSORPTION OF ANTIOXIDANT AND ITS SIGNIFICANCE

Antioxidants are absorbed from the intestinal tract and then distributed to various organs of the body. The highest levels of vitamins A, C, and E are present in the liver, and the lowest levels of these antioxidants are in the brain. The heart and the liver have the highest levels of coenzyme Q_{10}. Only about 10% of ingested water-soluble or fat-soluble antioxidants are absorbed from the intestinal tract. It has been argued by some that 90% of antioxidants are therefore wasted. This argument has no scientific merit. During digestion processes, many toxic substances, including mutagens and carcinogens, are formed. Meat eaters form such toxic substances more than the vegetarians. The consumption of organic food will make no difference in amounts of toxins formed during digestion of food. A portion of these toxins is absorbed from the gut and could increase the risk of chronic diseases over a long period of time. The presence of excessive amounts of antioxidants markedly reduces the levels of toxins formed during digestion and thereby reduces the risk of these toxins on health and the incidence of chronic diseases. Thus, unabsorbed antioxidants perform a very useful function in reducing the levels of mutagens and carcinogens during the digestion of food.

FUNCTIONS OF INDIVIDUAL ANTIOXIDANTS

The functions of antioxidants are varied and complex. Most believe that antioxidants have only one function, i.e., neutralize free radicals. In view of recent advances in antioxidant research, this belief alone is incorrect. In addition to neutralizing free radicals, they reduce inflammation, stimulate immune function, act as cofactors for several biological reactions, and regulate expressions of genes involved in proliferation, growth, differentiation, and immune function. Each antioxidant has some unique function that cannot be produced by others.

VITAMIN A

In addition to quenching free radicals, vitamin A plays an important role in maintaining vision, stimulating immune function, regulating gene activity, embryonic development and reproduction, bone metabolism, inhibiting precancer and cancer cell proliferation, and skin health.

CAROTENOIDS

Beta-carotene is a precursor of vitamin A. Carotenes are also known to protect against ultraviolet light-induced damage. Beta-carotene increases the expression of connexin gene that codes for gap junction protein, which holds two normal cells together, whereas vitamin A cannot produce such an effect. Beta-carotene is a more effective quencher of free radicals in high atmospheric pressure than vitamin A or vitamin E.

Vitamin D₃

It is essential for bone formation and regulates calcium and phosphorus levels in the blood. Vitamin D_3 inhibits parathyroid hormone secretion from the parathyroid glands. It stimulates immune function by promoting phagocytosis. It also exhibits antitumor activity.

Vitamin C

It acts as an antioxidant and participates as a cofactor of enzymes that participates in the formation of many vital compounds in our body. It helps in the formation of collagen, and it also takes part in formation of interferon, a naturally occurring antiviral agent. It regenerates oxidized vitamin E.

Vitamin E

It acts as an antioxidant and regulates gene expression and translocation of certain protein from one compartment to another. It helps to maintain good skin texture, reduces scarring, and acts as an anticoagulant. Vitamin E reduces inflammation and stimulates immune function. Its derivative, vitamin E succinate, exhibits a potent anticancer activity.

Alpha-Lipoic Acid

Alpha-lipoic acid is a more potent antioxidant than vitamin C or vitamin E because it is easily oxidized or reduced. It is soluble in both water and lipid; therefore, it protects cellular membranes as well as water-soluble compounds. It regenerates the tissue levels of vitamin C and vitamin E and markedly elevates the glutathione level in the cells. Alpha-lipoic acid acts as a cofactor for multienzyme dehydrogenase complexes.

N-Acetylcysteine

It increases the glutathione levels within the cells. This function is important because orally administered glutathione is totally destroyed in the small intestine. At high doses, NAC binds with the metals and removes them from the body.

Glutathione

Glutathione is one of the most important antioxidants that protect cellular components inside the cells. It is needed for detoxification of toxins that are produced as by-products of normal metabolism or certain exogenous toxins. Glutathione also acts as a substrate for several enzymes. It reduces inflammation.

COENZYME Q_{10}

This is a weak antioxidant, but it recycles vitamin E. Coenzyme Q_{10} is essential to generate energy by the mitochondria.

NICOTINAMIDE (VITAMIN B_3)

Nicotinamide (vitamin B_3), a precursor of NAD^+, is a competitive inhibitor of Class III NAD^+-dependent histone deacetylase activity. Treatment with nicotinamide restores memory deficits in transgenic mice with Alzheimer's disease (AD),[12] and attenuates glutamate-induced toxicity and preserves cellular levels of NAD+ to support the activity of SIRT-1.[13] Treatment with nicotinamide reduces oxidative stress-induced mitochondrial dysfunction and increases survival of neurons in culture. A reduced form of NAD (NADH) acts as an antioxidant and is essential for generating energy by the mitochondria. Thus, addition of nicotinamide to a preparation of micronutrient may be necessary in order to prevent and/or reduce the progression of chronic diseases in an effective manner.

POLYPHENOLS

They exhibit antioxidant activity and reduce inflammation. They also regulate expression of certain genes. Some polyphenols such as resveratrol and curcumin increase the levels of antioxidant enzymes by activating a nuclear transcriptional factor Nrf2.

MELATONIN

Melatonin is important in regulating circadian rhythms through its receptor. It also acts as an antioxidant and reduces inflammation. Unlike other antioxidants, the oxidation of melatonin is irreversible and thus cannot be regenerated by other antioxidants. It also stimulates immune function.

CURRENT CONTROVERSIES ABOUT ANTIOXIDANTS IN PREVENTION OF CHRONIC DISEASES

Despite the fact that antioxidants are so essential for our growth and survival, they remain the most misunderstood and misused molecules by most public and health professionals. The reasons for this include inaccurate claims by many in the nutrition industry, inconsistent human data (stemming from epidemiologic studies), and the results of poorly designed clinical studies in which one or sometimes two or more dietary antioxidants in high-risk populations for developing chronic diseases were administered.

We consume some antioxidants such as vitamin A, carotenoids, vitamin C, and vitamin E from the diet, whereas we make ourselves some antioxidants such as glutathione, alpha-lipoic acid, coenzyme Q_{10}, and L-carnitine. Despite basic scientific evidence for the importance of multiple antioxidants in disease prevention and improvement in the management of chronic diseases, when they are used in combination with standard therapy, the medical establishments are not convinced. This is not the first time that the medical establishments have resisted the application of novel agents in the treatment of diseases. As a matter of fact, the history of the discovery of vitamin A and vitamin C illustrates that the cure for night blindness and scurvy was delayed by centuries because of the resistance of the medical establishment.

MISUSE OF ANTIOXIDANTS IN CLINICAL STUDIES FOR PREVENTION OF CHRONIC DISEASES

Humans need dietary antioxidants (vitamins A, C, and E; carotenoids; and mineral selenium) as well as endogenous antioxidants made by the body, such as antioxidant enzymes, glutathione, coenzyme Q_{10}, R-alpha-lipoic acid, L-carnitine, reduced NAD^+ (NADH), B vitamins, and certain minerals for growth and survival. The distribution of these antioxidants markedly varies from one organ to another, and even within the same cell. Their subcellular distribution markedly differs from one cellular compartment to another within the same cell.

The human body generates different types of inorganic and organic free radicals derived from oxygen and nitrogen in response to the utilization of oxygen. The exposure to various environmental stressors, such as ozone, dust particles, smoke, toxic fumes, toxic chemicals, and ionizing radiation (x-rays or gamma rays), also produces excessive amounts of free radicals. Excessive amounts of free radicals are also produced during the normal aging process and during the initiation and progression of certain chronic diseases. Both dietary and endogenous antioxidants neutralize free radicals by directly scavenging them, but their affinities to specific types of free radicals differ and their efficacy in reducing oxidative damage may also differ. Some antioxidants also reduce the levels of chronic inflammation and reduce glutamate release and its toxicity. Increased oxidative damage, chronic inflammation, and glutamate release are associated with acute and chronic neurodegenerative diseases. These observations make it clear that supplementation with one or two dietary or endogenous antioxidants may not be useful in reducing progression of damage in patients with acute or chronic neurodegenerative diseases. I have proposed that supplementation with a preparation of micronutrients containing dietary and endogenous antioxidants, B vitamins, vitamin D, selenium, and certain herbs (curcumin and resveratrol) may be essential for reducing the progression of damage in patients with acute or chronic neurodegenerative diseases. Additional rationales are described in Chapters 3–9, discussing individual neurodegenerative diseases. Unfortunately, nearly all previous clinical studies have utilized just one or two dietary antioxidants in high-risk populations of developing certain chronic diseases, yielding inconsistent results.

In addition to the above considerations, selection of the type of antioxidants is equally important for any human clinical studies. For example, it has been reported that natural beta-carotene prevented x-ray–induced transformation of normal-like murine fibroblasts in culture, whereas synthetic beta-carotene did not. An animal study showed that various organs accumulated the natural form of vitamin E (D-alpha-tocopherol) more than the synthetic form (DL-alpha-tocopherol). Furthermore, it has been reported that vitamin E in the form of D-alpha-TS is more effective than other forms of vitamin E. The published human studies with antioxidants have not taken into consideration these important issues in the design of experiments; therefore, the results regarding the efficacy of antioxidants have been contradictory.

The doses of antioxidants are very important in order to produce optimal health benefits or disease prevention. Low doses (around recommended dietary allowance [RDA] values) may be useful in reducing some oxidative damage and preventing deficiency; however, they may not be sufficient in reducing inflammation or optimizing immune function. The differences in changes in the expression of gene profiles between low and high doses of an antioxidant are very marked. In commercially sold multivitamin preparations, the doses of antioxidants and other micronutrients markedly vary. The selection of appropriate doses of various micronutrients, including dietary and endogenous antioxidants that are safe and standardized, is essential for health benefits and disease prevention.

The dose schedule of antioxidant micronutrients is very critical for achieving the desired health benefits. Most people take micronutrient supplements once a day, which may not produce optimal health benefits. This is due to a high degree of fluctuation in the levels of antioxidants in the body because of variation in the plasma half-lives of various micronutrients. In addition, the expression gene profiles of cells markedly differ depending upon the level of antioxidants in the body, and therefore, cells have to readjust their genetic activity all the time, which can stress cells over a long period of time. It is interesting to note that all previous human studies with antioxidants have utilized the once-a-day schedule in spite of scientific evidence to the contrary.

In all human studies with antioxidants, the selection of the target population and the statistical analysis have been appropriate, but the selection of antioxidants and their doses and dose schedule have been without any scientific rationale. This can be demonstrated by a few widely publicized results on antioxidant studies in humans. In one clinical study, the synthetic form of beta-carotene was administered orally once a day to male heavy tobacco smokers in order to reduce the incidence of lung cancer. The results showed that the incidence of lung cancer in beta-carotene–treated smokers increased by about 17%. Federal agencies then promoted the idea that supplementation with beta-carotene may be harmful to your health and recommended that consumers not take beta-carotene in any form or in any other multiple vitamin preparations. These erroneous conclusions and recommendations were without any scientific merit for the following reasons.

It had been known before the start of the above human studies that individual antioxidants such as beta-carotene can be oxidized in a high-oxidative environment to become a pro-oxidant. Heavy tobacco smokers have a high internal oxidative environment. Therefore, when beta-carotene is administered to smokers, it is oxidized and acts as a pro-oxidant rather than as an antioxidant. This would then expect to increase the incidence of cancer in tobacco smokers.

Knowing the above facts about beta-carotene and heavy tobacco smokers, one could have predicted that beta-carotene would increase the risk of lung cancer in smokers. Indeed, the results of the trials confirmed this prediction. In contrast to the adverse effects of beta-carotene in heavy tobacco smokers, the same dose and type of beta-carotene did not increase the risk of cancer among doctors and nurses who were nonsmokers during a 5-year follow-up. Again, this result was also expected because populations of nonsmokers do not have a high internal oxidative environment.

The synthetic form of vitamin E has produced inconsistent results in patients with a high risk of cardiovascular disease who have increased internal oxidative environment. Some studies showed beneficial effects, whereas others showed no effect or even adverse effects in some cases. Harmful effects of vitamin E alone on cardiovascular disease can be attributed to the same biological events as those observed with beta-carotene. At this time, cardiologists do not recommend vitamin E to their patients. There are no human data (intervention studies) to show that the same dose of vitamin E or beta-carotene, when present in appropriately prepared multiple micronutrients, produces adverse health effects among normal or high-risk populations.

The human studies featuring a single antioxidant have also produced inconsistent results in neurological diseases such as Parkinson's disease (PD) and AD. In both studies, high doses of the synthetic form of vitamin E at doses of 800 IU per day in PD and 2000 IU per day in AD were used. No beneficial effects of vitamin E were observed in PD, but some beneficial effects were observed in AD. These studies were started without careful consideration of the biochemical factors involved in the disease processes and antioxidant status in the patients. It has been reported that deficiency of the antioxidant glutathione rather than vitamin E is found in both AD and PD patients. In addition, dysfunction of the mitochondria is consistently observed in autopsied samples of brains of patients with PD or AD. Furthermore, evidence of high-oxidative damage and chronic inflammation is also found in these brains. Therefore, the idea of supplementation with a combination of multiple anti-oxidants, some of which would reduce oxidative stress by directly scavenging free radicals while others may reduce oxidative stress by enhancing antioxidant enzymes through Nrf2/ARE pathway as well as by directly scavenging free radicals for the prevention and reduction in the rate of progression of chronic disease, is a very good one. Indeed, two recent studies showed that supplementation with multiple vitamin preparations reduced cancer incidence by 10% in men[14] and improved clinical outcomes in patients with HIV/AIDS who were not taking medication.[15]

It is very unfortunate that the harmful results obtained with the use of primarily one antioxidant in high-risk populations are often extrapolated to the effects of multiple antioxidant preparation on high-risk or normal risk populations. This erroneous extrapolation of data regarding the harmful effects of beta-carotene or vitamin E alone is further propagated by the publication of meta-analysis of published data on the same vitamins with the same conclusion. A meta-analysis publication is often misinterpreted as an original study. In my opinion, a meta-analysis should critically examine an experiment's design instead of just summarizing the results of previous studies. These kinds of experiments and extrapolations have created a wide disconnect between the public and most health professionals—especially physicians—regarding the health benefits of micronutrients. In order to avoid these problems, the subsequent chapters in this book discuss the scientific basis for using multiple micronutrients, including dietary and endogenous antioxidants, in reducing the risk of neurodegenerative diseases. In addition, the role of these micronutrients in improving the efficacy of standard therapy for various chronic neurological diseases is also discussed.

ANTIOXIDANT DEFENSE SYSTEMS

What are antioxidants? Generally speaking, antioxidants are defined as chemical substances that donate an electron to a free radical and convert it into a harmless molecule. The antioxidant defense system in humans can be divided into three groups.

GROUP 1 ANTIOXIDANTS

These refer to antioxidant chemicals not made in the body and consumed principally through the diet. They include vitamin A, carotenoids, vitamin C, vitamin E, selenium, and certain polyphenolic compounds. Some of them reduce oxidative stress by directly scavenging free radicals, while others inhibit oxidative stress by enhancing antioxidant enzymes through the Nrf2/ARE pathway as well as by directly scavenging free radicals.

GROUP 2 ANTIOXIDANTS

These are antioxidant chemicals primarily made in the body but also consumed through the diet (primarily through meat and eggs) or in the form of supplements. They include glutathione, coenzyme Q_{10}, reduced NAD^+ (NADH), alpha-lipoic acid, and L-carnitine. Some of them reduce oxidative stress by directly scavenging free radicals, while others inhibit oxidative stress by enhancing antioxidant enzymes through the Nrf2/ARE pathway as well as by directly scavenging free radicals.

GROUP 3 ANTIOXIDANTS

These point to antioxidant enzymes made in the body, such as SOD, catalase, and glutathione peroxidase. SOD requires manganese (Mn) or copper (Cu)–zinc SOD for its biological activity. Mn-SOD is present in the mitochondria, whereas Cu–Zn SOD is present in the cytoplasm. They can destroy free radicals and hydrogen peroxide. Catalase requires iron (Fe) for its biological activity; it, too, destroys hydrogen peroxide in the cell. Glutathione peroxidase requires selenium for its biological activity. The levels of antioxidant enzymes can be increased by activating free radical–dependent and free radical-independent Nrf2.

KNOWN FUNCTIONS OF ANTIOXIDANTS AND POLYPHENOLIC COMPOUNDS

1. Scavenge free radicals
2. Decrease markers of proinflammatory cytokines
3. Alter gene expression profiles

4. Alter protein kinase activity
5. Prevent release and toxicity of excessive amounts of glutamate
6. Act as cofactors for several biological reactions
7. Induce cell differentiation and apoptosis in cancer cells
8. Induce cell differentiation in normal cells, but not apoptosis
9. Increase immune function
10. Activate nuclear transcriptional factor Nrf2 by translocating it to the nucleus, where it binds with ARE to increase antioxidant enzymes levels

CONCLUSIONS

Antioxidant systems in humans consist of antioxidant enzymes and dietary and endogenous antioxidant chemicals that protect the body against increased oxidative stress and chronic inflammation. Antioxidant enzymes include glutathione peroxidase, catalase, and SOD. Dietary antioxidant chemicals include vitamin A, carotenoids, vitamin C, vitamin E, selenium, and certain polyphenolic compounds, whereas endogenous antioxidants include glutathione, coenzyme Q_{10}, reduced NAD^+ (NADH), alpha-lipoic acid, and L-carnitine. Some of them reduce oxidative stress by directly scavenging free radicals, while others inhibit oxidative stress by enhancing antioxidant enzymes through the Nrf2/ARE pathway as well as by directly scavenging free radicals. Therefore, both groups of antioxidants at appropriate doses are necessary to reduce oxidative stress and chronic inflammation optimally for the prevention and, in combination with standard therapy, for the improved management of neurodegenerative diseases. Therefore, the use of a single antioxidant to reduce oxidative stress in high-risk populations has no scientific merit with respect to the prevention or improved management of these chronic neurological diseases. Unfortunately, clinical studies of antioxidants in a high-risk population of developing chronic diseases have utilized only a single antioxidant. The results of these studies have been inconsistent.

REFERENCES

1. Sen CKP, Baeuerle PA. *Antioxidants and Redox Regulation of Genes*. New York: Academic Press; 1999.
2. Prasad KN. *Micronutrients in Health and Disease*. Boca Raton, FL: CRC Press; 2011.
3. Shils ME, Shike M, Ross AC, Caballero B, Cousins RJ. *Modern Nutrition in Health and Disease*, 10th Edition. Philadelphia, PA: Lippincott Williams & Wilkins; 2005.
4. Anderson JJB, Root M, Garner SC. *Nutrition and Health: An Introduction*. Durham, NC: Carolina Academic Press; 2005.
5. Agarwal B, Bhendwal S, Halmos B, Moss SF, Ramey WG, Holt PR. Lovastatin augments apoptosis induced by chemotherapeutic agents in colon cancer cells [comment]. *Clini Cancer Res.* 1999; 5(8): 2223–2229.
6. National Research Council. *The Development of DRIs 1994–2004: Lessons Learned and New Challenges: Workshop Summary*. Washington, DC: The National Academies Press; 2008.
7. Packer L, Hiramitsu M, Yoshikawa T. *Antioxidants Food Supplements in Human Health*. New York: Academic Press; 1999.

8. Combs GF. *The Vitamins: Fundamental Aspects in Nutrition and Health*, 2nd Edition. San Diego: Academic Press; 1998.

9. Caballero B, Allen L, Prentice A. *Encyclopedia of Human Nutrition*. New York: Academic Press; 2005.

10. Cadenas E, Packer L. *Handbook of Antioxidants*. New York: Marcel Dekker, Inc; 1996.

11. Frei B. *Natural Antioxidants in Human Health and Disease*. New York: Academic Press; 1994.

12. Green KN, Steffan JS, Martinez-Coria H et al. Nicotinamide restores cognition in Alzheimer's disease transgenic mice via a mechanism involving sirtuin inhibition and selective reduction of Thr231-phosphotau. *J Neurosci*. Nov 5 2008; 28(45): 11500–11510.

13. Liu D, Pitta M, Mattson MP. Preventing NAD(+) depletion protects neurons against excitotoxicity: Bioenergetic effects of mild mitochondrial uncoupling and caloric restriction. *Ann N Y Acad Sci*. Dec 2008; 1147: 275–282.

14. Gaziano JM, Sesso HD, Christen WG et al. Multivitamins in the prevention of cancer in men: The Physicians' Health Study II randomized controlled trial. *JAMA*. Nov 14 2012; 308(18): 1871–1880.

15. Baum MK, Campa A, Lai S et al. Effect of micronutrient supplementation on disease progression in asymptomatic, antiretroviral-naive, HIV-infected adults in Botswana: A randomized clinical trial. *JAMA*. Nov 27 2013; 310(20): 2154–2163.

2 Oxidative Stress and Inflammation
Their Reduction by Micronutrients

INTRODUCTION

Increased oxidative stress due to the production of excessive amounts of free radicals derived from oxygen and nitrogen plays an important role in the initiation and progression of damage in neurodegenerative diseases, and during acute and chronic phases of cerebral injury; therefore, the basic understanding of these biological processes is essential for developing any preventive and improved management strategies. The mechanisms of generating different types of free radicals in the brain are very complex; therefore, they are discussed in general terms. Most free radicals are produced by the mitochondria, but some are also produced in the cytoplasm. The importance of increased oxidative stress in neurodegenerative diseases and acute and chronic cerebral injuries is discussed in Chapters 3 through 9.

The cellular damage, infection with pathogenic organisms or antigens, initiates an important biological event called inflammation, which is considered as a protective response. Acute inflammation is considered as a double-edged sword. It is needed to kill invading pathogenic organisms and for the removal of cellular debris in order to facilitate the recovery process. However, it can also damage normal tissues by releasing a number of toxic chemicals, such as reactive oxygen species (ROS), proinflammatory cytokines, prostaglandins, adhesion molecules, and complements. During acute inflammation, anti-inflammatory cytokines, which participate in the repair processes, are also released. The chronic inflammatory responses produce predominantly proinflammatory cytokines, ROS, prostaglandins, adhesion molecules, and complements; therefore, they are more relevant to neurodegenerative diseases than acute inflammatory reactions. Inflammation is a highly complex biological response that is tightly regulated and is turned off when the invading organisms are killed or the injured tissues are healed. Chronic inflammation in response to chronic cellular injury or chronic infection is not turned off; therefore, it is one of the major factors that contribute to the progression of neurodegenerative diseases by releasing the toxic products. In the brain, immune cells are represented primarily by microglia cells; although activated astrocytes, macrophages are present at the site of brain injury. Activated microglia cells release proinflammatory cytokines.

This chapter describes briefly the basic concepts of oxidative stress and the complexity of inflammation; therefore, they are described in simple and general terms. Some of the references and books that have been used to prepare for this chapter are listed.[1–10] Since increased oxidative stress and chronic inflammation are involved in most chronic diseases in human, this chapter also discusses how to reduce these biological processes optimally in order to prevent and reduce the progression of these diseases.

OXIDATIVE STRESS

Increased oxidative stress occurs when the endogenous antioxidant systems (antioxidant enzymes and dietary and endogenous antioxidants made by the body) are overwhelmed by excessive production of free radicals derived from oxygen and nitrogen. Increased oxidative stress plays an important role in the initiation and progression of some chronic diseases in human, including neurodegenerative diseases and neurological abnormalities among the survivors of ischemia/reperfusion injury.

WHAT ARE FREE RADICALS?

The radicals also referred to as free radicals are atoms, molecules, or ions with unpaired electrons. These unpaired electrons are highly reactive and play an important role in several chemical reactions such as combustion, atmospheric chemistry, and polymerization. In living organisms including humans, they play an important role in several biochemical reactions and gene expressions. In 1900, the first organic free radical, triphenylmethyl radical, was identified by Moses Gomberg of the University of Michigan in the USA. Free radicals can be derived from oxygen or nitrogen. Free radicals are symbolized by a dot "•."

TYPES OF FREE RADICALS

There are several types of free radicals derived from oxygen and nitrogen that are generated in the body. The oxygen-derived free radicals include hydroxyl radical ($OH^{\bullet}$), peroxyl radical ($ROO^{\bullet}$), alkoxyl radical ($RO^{\bullet}$), phenoxyl and semiquinone radicals ($ArO^{\bullet}$, $HO\text{-}Ar\text{-}O^{\bullet}$), and superoxide radical ($O^{\bullet-}2$). The nitrogen-derived free radicals include $NO^{\bullet}$, $ONOO^-$ (peroxynitrite), and $NO_2^{\bullet}$.

FORMATION OF FREE RADICALS DERIVED FROM OXYGEN AND NITROGEN

The formation of some of the ROS is described in the following. When molecular oxygen (O_2) acquires an electron, the superoxide anion ($O_2^{\bullet-}$) is formed when $O_2 + e^- = O_2^{\bullet-}$.

Superoxide dismutase (SOD) and H^+ can react with $O_2^{\bullet-}$ to form hydrogen peroxide, H_2O_2:

$$2O_2^{\cdot-} + 2H^+ \text{ plus SOD} \rightarrow H_2O_2 + O_2$$

$$O_2^{\cdot-} + H^+ \rightarrow HO_2^{\cdot}(\text{hydroperoxy radical})$$

$$2HO_2^{\cdot} \rightarrow H_2O_2 + O_2$$

Ferric and ferrous forms of iron can react with superoxide anion and hydrogen peroxide to produce molecular oxygen and hydroxyl radical (OH$^{\cdot}$), respectively:

$$Fe^{3+} + O_2^{\cdot-} \rightarrow Fe^{2+} + O_2$$

$$Fe^{2+} + H_2O_2 \rightarrow Fe^{3+} + OH^{\cdot} + OH^- (\text{Fenton reaction})$$

Hydroxyl radical can also be formed from superoxide anion by the Haber–Weiss reaction:

$$O_2^{\cdot-} + H_2O_2 \rightarrow O_2 + OH^- + OH^{\cdot}$$

Both the Fenton and Haber–Weiss reactions require a transition metal such as copper or iron. Among ROS, OH$^{\cdot}$ is the most damaging free radical and is very short lived.

Hydroxyl radical is very reactive with a variety of organic compounds, leading to the production of more radical compounds:

$$RH(\text{organic compound}) + OH^{\cdot} \rightarrow R^{\cdot}(\text{organic radical}) + H_2O$$

$$R^{\cdot} + O_2 \rightarrow RO_2^{\cdot}(\text{peroxyl radical})$$

For example, the DNA radical can be generated by a reaction with a hydroxyl radical, and this can lead to strand lesions.

Catalase detoxifies hydrogen peroxide to form water and molecular oxygen:

$$H_2O_2 + \text{catalase} \rightarrow H_2O \text{ and } O_2$$

Reactive nitrogen species (RNS) are represented by nitric oxide (NO$^{\cdot}$). NO is synthesized by the enzyme nitric oxide synthase from L-arginine. NO$^{\cdot}$ can combine with superoxide anion to form peroxynitrite, a powerful oxidant.

$$NO^{\cdot} + O_2^{\cdot-} \rightarrow ONOO^-(\text{peroxynitrite})$$

When protonated (likely at physiological pH), peroxynitrite spontaneously decomposes to reactive nitric dioxide and hydroxyl radicals:

$$ONOO^- + H^+ \rightarrow NO_2^\cdot + OH^\cdot$$

SOD can also enhance the peroxynitrite-mediated nitration of tyrosine residues on critical proteins, presumably via species similar to the nitronium cation (NO_2^+):

$$ONOO^- \text{ plus SOD} \rightarrow NO_2^+ \rightarrow \text{nitration of tyrosine}$$

In addition to free radicals, there are several oxidizing agents that are formed in the body.

Many other radical species can be formed by biological reactions in the body. For example, phenolic and other aromatic species can be formed during the metabolism of xenobiotic agents. Furthermore, any antioxidants when oxidized can act as free radicals.

Free radicals can damage DNA (deoxyribonucleic acid), RNA (ribonucleic acid), proteins, carbohydrates, and membranes. The half-lives of various free radicals vary from 10^{-9} s to days. This means that most radicals are quickly destroyed after causing damage. For example, the half-life of hydroxyl free radicals is 10^{-9} s, superoxide anion 10^{-5} s, lipid peroxyl free radical 7 s, semiquinone free radical days, nitric oxide about 1 s, and hydrogen peroxide minutes. Some organic free radicals can remain active for several days. ROS also participates in cell signaling systems that regulate growth, differentiation, and apoptosis of cells during the development and growth of organisms.

Normally, free radicals are generated in the body during the use of oxygen in the metabolism of certain compounds. Mitochondria use oxygen to produce energy. They are elongated membranous structures present in all cells in varying numbers. During the process of generating energy, superoxide anions, hydroxyl radicals, and hydrogen peroxide are produced as by-products. It is estimated that about 2% of the oxygen consumed by mitochondria remains partially used, and this unused oxygen is the leak out of the mitochondria, making about 20 billion molecules of superoxide anions and hydrogen peroxide per cell per day.

During bacterial or viral infection, phagocytic cells are activated, which generate high levels of nitric oxide, superoxide anions, and hydrogen peroxide within the infected cells in order to kill infective agents. Excessive production of free radicals by phagocytes can also damage normal cells and thereby can increase the risk of acute and/or chronic diseases. During the oxidative metabolism of fatty acids and other molecules in the body, free radicals are produced. Certain habits such as tobacco smoking, and some trace minerals such as free iron, copper, and manganese, can also increase the rate of production of free radicals in the body. Thus, the human body is exposed daily to different types and varying levels of free radicals.

OXIDATION AND REDUCTION PROCESSES

To understand the role of free radicals and antioxidants in the human body, it is important to grasp the relationship between oxidation and reduction processes, which constantly taking place in the body. Oxidation is a process in which an atom or molecule gains oxygen, or loses hydrogen or an electron. For example, carbon gains oxygen during oxidation and becomes carbon dioxide. A superoxide radical loses an electron during oxidation and becomes oxygen. Thus, an oxidizing agent is a molecule or atom that changes another chemical by adding oxygen to it or by removing electron or hydrogen from it. Examples of oxidizing agents are free radicals, ozone, and ionizing radiation.

Reduction is a process in which an atom or molecule loses oxygen, gains hydrogen, or gains an electron. For example, carbon dioxide loses oxygen and becomes carbon monoxide, carbon gains hydrogen and becomes methane, and oxygen gains an electron and becomes superoxide anion. Thus, a reducing agent is a molecule or atom that changes another chemical by removing oxygen from it or by adding electron or hydrogen to it. All antioxidants can be considered as reducing agents. Increased reduction processes over oxidation processes maintain cells in a healthy state; however, increased oxidation processes over reduction processes can lead to cellular injury and eventually to chronic neurodegenerative diseases or cell death.

HOW TO REDUCE OXIDATIVE STRESS OPTIMALLY

Oxidative stress in the body occurs when the antioxidant system fails to provide adequate protection against damage produced by free radicals (reactive oxygen species and reactive nitrogen species). Increased oxidative stress in the body can be most effectively reduced by up-regulating antioxidant enzymes as well as by existing levels of dietary and endogenous antioxidant chemicals, because they work by different mechanisms. For example, antioxidant enzymes reduce free radicals by catalysis, whereas dietary and endogenous antioxidant chemicals reduce free radicals by directly scavenging them. In response to ROS, a nuclear transcriptional factor, Nrf2 (nuclear factor-erythroid 2-related factor 2), is translocated from the cytoplasm to the nucleus, where it binds with ARE (antioxidant response element), which increases the levels of antioxidant enzymes (gamma-glutamylcysteine ligase, glutathione peroxidase, glutathione reductase, and heme oxygenase-1) and phase 2 detoxifying enzymes (NAD(P)H): quinine oxidoreductase 1 and glutathione-S-transferase, in order to reduce oxidative damage.[11–13] In response to increased oxidative stress, existing levels of dietary and endogenous antioxidant chemical levels cannot be elevated without supplementation.

FACTORS REGULATING RESPONSE OF Nrf2

Several studies suggest that antioxidant enzymes are elevated by Nrf2 activation, which depends upon ROS-dependent and -independent mechanisms. In addition, the levels of antioxidant enzymes are also dependent upon the binding ability of Nrf2 with ARE in the nucleus. These studies are described here.

ROS-DEPENDENT REGULATION OF NRF2

Normally, Nrf2 is associated with Kelch-like ECH associated protein 1 (Keap1) protein, which acts as an inhibitor of Nrf2 (INrf2).[14] INrf2 protein serves as an adaptor to link Nrf2 to the ubiquitin ligase Cul-Rbx1 complex for degradation by proteasomes and maintains the steady levels of Nrf2 in the cytoplasm. INrf2 acts as a sensor for ROS/electrophilic stress. In response to increased ROS, Nrf2 dissociates itself from INrf2-CuI-Rbx1 complex and translocates into the nucleus, where it binds with ARE that increases the levels of antioxidant enzymes and detoxifying enzymes. It has been demonstrated that Nrf2 regulates INrf2 levels by controlling its transcription, whereas INrf2 regulates Nrf2 levels by controlling its degradation by proteasome.[15]

ROS-INDEPENDENT REGULATION OF NRF2

Antioxidants such as vitamin E; genistein (a flavonoid)[16]; allicin, a major organo-sulfur compound found in garlic[17]; sulforaphane, an organosulfur compound found in cruciferous vegetables[18]; kavalactones (methysticin, kavain, and yangonin)[19]; and dietary restriction[20] activate Nrf2 without stimulation by ROS.

REDUCED BINDING OF NRF2 WITH ARE

Age-related decline in antioxidant enzymes in the liver of older rats compared to that in younger rats was due to the reduction in the binding ability of Nrf2 with ARE; however, treatment with alpha-lipoic acid restored this defect, increased the levels of antioxidant enzymes, and restored the loss of glutathione from the liver of old rats.[21]

DIFFERENTIAL RESPONSE OF Nrf2 TO ROS STIMULATION DURING ACUTE AND CHRONIC OXIDATIVE STRESS

It appears that Nrf2 responds to ROS stimulation during acute and chronic oxidative stresses differently. For example, excessive amounts of ROS are generated during acute oxidative stress, observed during strenuous exercise. In response to ROS during acute oxidative stress, Nrf2 translocates from the cytoplasm to the nucleus, where it binds with ARE to up-regulate antioxidant genes. Excessive amounts ROS are also present during chronic oxidative stress, commonly observed in older individual and neurodegenerative diseases, such as Parkinson disease and Alzheimer's disease, suggesting that Nrf2/ARE pathway has become unresponsive to ROS. A reduction in the binding ability of Nrf2 with ARE was demonstrated in older rats.[21] The reasons Nrf2/ARE pathway become unresponsive to ROS during chronic oxidative stress are unknown.

INTERPRETATION OF INHIBITION OF EXERCISE-INDUCED Nrf2 ACTIVATION BY INDIVIDUAL ANTIOXIDANT

It is well established that exercise induces acute transient oxidative stress by generating excessive amounts of ROS. Indeed, in wild-type mice, exercise activated Nrf2, which enhanced antioxidant enzymes through ARE and reduced oxidative stress; however, in Nrf2 knockout mice (Nrf2−/− mice), exercise failed to increase antioxidant enzymes and reduce oxidative stress.[22] This suggests that Nrf2/ARE pathway was responsive to ROS in reducing oxidative stress. Supplementation with single antioxidants during sprint training/training exercise reduced some of the beneficial effects of sprint training.[23] This could be due to the fact that administered single antioxidants in the presence of high oxidative environment would be oxidized, and oxidized antioxidants act as pro-oxidants that are toxic.

Pretreatment of rats with N-acetylcysteine (NAC) blocked thyroxin (a ROS donor)-induced activation of Nrf2 in the liver.[24,25] This was interpreted to mean that supplementation with individual antioxidants may impair the normal Nrf2 response to ROS in reducing oxidative stress. We interpret these results differently. In response to ROS, such as observed after treatment with thyroxin or during strenuous exercise, NAC treatment may scavenge directly all ROS; thus, ROS stimulation was not available to cells for activating Nrf2. We interpret that NAC treatment protected the normal Nrf2 response to ROS in the rat liver.

The following groups of agents in combination may be useful in reducing oxidative stress optimally:

1. Agents that can reduce oxidative stress by directly scavenging free radicals: Some examples are dietary antioxidants, such as vitamin A, beta-carotene, vitamin C, and vitamin E, and endogenous antioxidants, such as glutathione, alpha-lipoic acid, and coenzyme Q_{10}.

2. Agents that can reduce oxidative stress by activating Nrf2-regulated antioxidant genes without ROS stimulation: Some examples are organosulfur compound sulforaphane, found in cruciferous vegetables; kavalactones, found in Kava shrubs; and Puerarin, a major flavonoid from the root of *Pueraria lobata*,[18,19,26] genistein, and vitamin E[16] and coenzyme Q_{10},[27] which activate Nrf2 without ROS stimulation.

3. Agents that can reduce oxidative stress directly by scavenging free radicals as well as indirectly by activating Nrf2/ARE pathway: Some examples are vitamin E,[16] alpha-lipoic acid,[21] curcumin,[28] resveratrol,[29,30] omega-3 fatty acids,[31,32] and NAC.[33]

4. Agents that can reduce oxidative stress by ROS-dependent mechanism: They include L-carnitine which generates transient ROS.[34]

A study on the aged mouse hippocampus revealed that supplementation with allicin, a major organosulfur compound found in garlic, which has an electrophilic center (electron deficient), prevented age-related decline in cognitive function. This effect of allicin was due to the enhancement of antioxidant enzymes via Nrf2-ARE pathway.[17] This study suggests that INrf2/Nrf2 complex and the binding of Nrf2 with ARE remain responsive to allicin. Repeated administration of another organosulfur compound sulforaphane found in cruciferous vegetables simulated Nrf2-dependent increase of *Nqo1* gene, which codes for NAD(P)H:quinone oxidoreductase, an antioxidant detoxifying enzyme, and *Hmox1* gene, which codes for *HO*-1 enzyme in astrocytes in culture, and reduced oxidative damage.[18] It is also possible that sulforaphane-induced activation of Nrf2 does not require ROS. Indeed, kavalactones (methysticin, kavain, and yangonin)-induced activation of Nrf2 is not dependent upon ROS stimulation in neuronal cells and astroglia cells in culture.[19]

NAC-EFFECTS ON MURINE ALVEOLAR CELLS IN CULTURE

In one study on murine alveolar cells in culture, NAC, which directly scavenge free radicals via increasing intracellular glutathione levels, requires the presence of Nrf2 for an optimal reduction in oxidative stress.[35] For example, cigarette smoking produces greater damage in alveolar cells obtained from Nrf2-deleted mice (Nrf2–/–) than in cells obtained from wild-type mice.[35] Pretreatment of alveolar cells with NAC reduced cigarette smoke-induced damage more in cells obtained from the wild-type mice more than in cells obtained from Nrf2-deleted mice. In other studies on rat liver, pretreatment with NAC prevents the ROS-induced activation of Nrf2.[24] If NAC scavenges all ROS, then ROS was not available for activating Nrf2/ARE pathway.

ACTIVATION OF Nrf2 BY DIET RESTRICTION

A review has revealed that dietary restriction also reduces oxidative stress by activating Nrf2-ARE pathways.[20] It appears that dietary restriction-induced Nrf2 activation does not require ROS stimulation. Dietary restriction-induced reduction in oxidative stress would be difficult to implement for a long period of time. Prolonged activation of Nrf2 by dietary restriction can produce unacceptable serious side effects.[36] Therefore, dietary restriction may not be suitable for reducing oxidative stress for prevention or improved management of neurodegenerative diseases.

EFFECT OF RESVERATROL ON EXERCISE-INDUCED CARDIOVASCULAR HEALTH

A randomized, placebo clinical study on 27 healthy, physically inactive aged men (about 65 years) showed that daily supplementation with resveratrol concomitant with high-intensity exercise training blocked the beneficial effects of exercise on cardiovascular health parameters.[37] Since resveratrol exhibits antioxidant and anti-inflammation activity, it was interpreted to mean that supplementation with resveratrol during exercise is harmful. This conclusion was challenged by another study in which supplementation with resveratrol during exercise produced beneficial effects.[38] It is also possible that administered resveratrol is rapidly oxidized in the presence of high-oxidative environment and that oxidized products of resveratrol could be toxic. This potential effect of resveratrol could be avoided if it is combined with other antioxidants, which would prevent the oxidation of resveratrol. Resveratrol can cross the blood brain barrier in mice, rats, and gerbils.[39–41]

INFLAMMATION

Inflammation in Latin is referred to as *inflammation* that means a setting on fire. The primary features of inflammation at the affected sites include redness, swelling, warm when touched, and varying degrees of pain. These characteristics of inflammation were first recognized by a Roman physician Dr. Cornelius, who lived from about 30 BC to 45 AD. Inflammation is the complex biological response by which the body removes infective agents such as bacteria, viruses, and damaged cells caused by physical agents (such as ionizing radiation or traumatic bodily injuries or chemical or biological agents). The inflammatory reactions involve the movement of plasma and white blood cells (leukocytes, macrophages, monocytes, lymphocytes, and plasma cells) from the blood to the injured sites. It is a protective response by which the body removes the injurious infective microorganisms as well as initiates the healing process in the damaged tissue. During the healing process, the injured tissue is replaced by the regeneration of native parenchymal cells, by filling of the injured site with fibroblastic tissue (scarring), or most commonly by a combination of both processes. During inflammation, toxic chemicals are also released that can damage cells.

TYPES OF INFLAMMATION

Inflammation is divided into two categories: acute inflammation and chronic inflammation. Acute inflammation occurs following cellular injury or infection with microorganisms. The period of acute inflammation is relatively short, lasting from a few minutes to a few days. The main features of acute inflammations are edema (accumulation of exudation of fluid and plasma in extracellular spaces) and the migration of leukocytes, primarily neutrophils, to the site of injury. Chronic inflammation also occurs following persistent cellular injury or infection. The period of chronic inflammation is relatively long and can last as long as the injury or infection exists. The main features of chronic inflammation are the presence of lymphocytes and macrophages and the proliferation of blood vessels, fibrosis, and tissue necrosis.

ACUTE INFLAMMATION

Acute inflammation causes marked alterations in the blood vessels that allow plasma protein and leukocytes to leave the circulation. Subsequently, the leukocytes migrate to the site of injury by a process called chemotaxis. Leukocytes engulf pathogenic organisms by phagocytosis and kill them by generating bursts of reactive oxygen species and other toxins. They can also engulf cellular debris and foreign antigens by a similar process and then degrade them by lysosomal proteolytic enzymes. On the other hand, leukocytes may release excessive amounts of ROS, proinflammatory cytokines, prostaglandins, adhesion molecules, and complement proteins that can damage normal tissues. An acute inflammatory reaction is tightly regulated and turned off soon after the injured sites are healed or invading microbes are removed. It is absolutely an important process for removing both pathogens and cellular debris from the damaged site, thus allowing healing to occur.

Acute inflammation is effective only when the injurious stimuli are relatively mild. If the tissue damage is extensive, or the levels of infective organisms are high, acute inflammatory reactions are not turned off, and consequently, the toxic products of these reactions can enhance the rate of progression of damage that may cause organ failure and eventually even death.

CHRONIC INFLAMMATION

The persistence of low-grade cellular injury, exposure to exogenous agents such as particulate silica, or infection, can initiate chronic inflammation. Chronic inflammation is often associated with most human neurodegenerative diseases such as Alzheimer's disease, Parkinson disease, and acute and chronic cerebral injuries. In contrast to acute inflammation, which is characterized by vascular changes, edema, and primarily neutrophil infiltration, chronic inflammation is characterized by the presence of mononuclear cells, which include macrophages, lymphocytes, and plasma cells. In the brain, microglia cells become activated and migrate to the site of injury. During chronic inflammation, the presence of angiogenesis and fibrosis can be observed at the site of injury.

PRODUCTS OF INFLAMMATORY REACTIONS

During inflammation, several highly reactive agents are released. Among highly reactive agents include cytokines, complement proteins, arachidonic acid (AA) metabolites, ROS, and endothelial/leukocyte adhesion molecules. They are briefly described in the following.

CYTOKINES

Cytokines are proteins released during both acute and chronic inflammation. They are produced by many cell types, primarily by activated lymphocytes and macrophages, but also by endothelium, epithelium, and connective tissue cells. In the brain, they are produced primarily by microglia cells and some by neurons. Proinflammatory cytokines include interleukin-6 (IL-6), IL-17, IL-18, IL-23, and tumor necrosis factor-alpha (TNF-alpha) that are toxic to the cells, whereas anti-inflammatory cytokines include IL-1, IL-4, IL-10, IL-11, and IL-13 that help in the repair at the site of injury. If the tissue damage is severe, the proinflammatory cytokines may overcome the repair function of anti-inflammatory cytokines and participate in the progression of damage. Some proinflammatory cytokines such as IL-6 can also act as a neurotrophic factor. It acts as a proinflammatory cytokine during the acute phase of injury and as a neurotrophic factor between subacute and chronic phase of injury.

Cytokines play an important role in modulating the function of many other cell types. They are multifunctional, and individual cytokines may have both positive and negative regulatory actions. Cytokines mediate their action by binding to specific receptors on target cells. These receptors are regulated by exogenous and endogenous signals. Cytokines that regulate lymphocyte activation, growth, and differentiation include IL-2 and IL-4 (favors growth), as well as IL-10 and transforming growth factor-beta (TGF-beta) that are negative regulators of immune responses. Cytokines involved with natural immunity include inflammatory cytokines, TNF-alpha, IL-1-beta, type I interferons (IFN-alpha and IFN-beta), and IL-6. Cytokines that activate inflammatory cells such as macrophages include IFN-gamma, TNF-alpha, TNF-beta, IL-5, IL-10, and IL-12. Cytokines that stimulate hematopoiesis (growth and differentiation of immature leukocytes) include IL-3, IL-7, c-kit ligand, granulocyte-macrophage colony-stimulating factor (G-M-CSF), macrophage colony-stimulating factor (M-CSF), granulocyte CSF, and stem cell factor.

Chemokines are also cytokines that stimulate leukocyte movement and direct them to the site of injury during inflammation. Many classical growth factors may also act as cytokines, and conversely, many cytokines exhibit activities of growth factors.

COMPLEMENT PROTEINS

During inflammation, 20 complement proteins including their cleavaged products are released into the plasma, and when activated, they can cause cell lysis and can exhibit proteolytic activity. They participate in both innate and adaptive immunities for protection against pathogenic organisms. Complement proteins are numbered C1 through C9, each of which has complex mechanisms of action on cells. Some of the complement proteins are also neurotoxic.

AA METABOLITES

Arachidonic acid is a 20-carbon fatty acid that is derived from the dietary sources or is formed from the essential fatty acid linoleic acid. During inflammation, AA metabolites, also called eicosanoids, are released. These eicosanoids have diverse biological actions, depending upon the cell type. The eicosanoids are synthesized by two major classes of enzymes: cyclooxygenase (COX) for the synthesis of prostaglandins and thromboxanes and lipooxygenase for the synthesis of leukotrienes and lipoxins. There are two isoforms of cyclooxygenase, COX1 and COX2.

ENDOTHELIAL/LEUKOCYTE ADHESION MOLECULES

The immunoglobulin family molecules include two endothelial adhesion molecules: intracellular adhesion molecule-1 (ICAM-1) and vascular adhesion molecule-1 (VCAM-1). These adhesion molecules bind with leukocyte receptor integrins. They are induced by IL-1 and TNF-alpha. Both ICAM-1 and VCAM-1 are released during inflammatory reactions and have diverse mechanisms of action on cells.

HOW TO REDUCE CHRONIC INFLAMMATION OPTIMALLY

The combination of dietary and endogenous antioxidants and certain polyphenolic compounds (curcumin and resveratrol), which can activate NRF2/ARE pathway without ROS stimulation as well as inhibit the levels of proinflammatory cytokines, would be effective in reducing chronic inflammation. The antioxidants and polyphenolic compounds are listed in the section titled "How to Reduce Oxidative Stress Optimally." A low-dose aspirin (80 mg/day) may further enhance the reduction in chronic inflammation.

CONCLUSIONS

Increased oxidative stress caused by excessive production of free radicals derived from oxygen and nitrogen causes damage to cells and tissues and plays an important role in the initiation and progression of some chronic diseases in human. The cellular damage or infection with pathogenic organisms, or exposure to antigens, initiates an important biological event, called inflammation, which is considered as a protective response. There are two types of inflammation: acute inflammation and chronic inflammation. Acute inflammation occurs following cellular injury or infection with microorganisms. During acute inflammation, proinflammatory and anti-inflammatory cytokines are released, which are toxic to the cells. An acute inflammatory reaction is tightly regulated and turned off soon after the injured sites are healed or invading microbes are removed. The period of acute inflammation is relatively short. Chronic inflammation occurs following persistent cellular injury or infection. The period of chronic inflammation is relatively long and can last as long as the injury or infection exists. During chronic inflammation, proinflammatory cytokines are primarily released, which are toxic to the cells.

The reduction of oxidative stress and chronic inflammation may reduce the risk of developing chronic diseases and, in combination with standard therapy, may improve the management of these diseases. Oxidative stress can be maximally reduced by enhancing the levels of antioxidant enzymes through activating a nuclear transcriptional factor (Nrf2)/ARE (antioxidant response element) pathway as well as by increasing the levels of dietary and endogenous antioxidant compounds through supplementation. Antioxidant enzymes destroy free radicals by catalysis, whereas antioxidant chemicals destroy free radicals by directly scavenging them. Normally, the activation of Nrf2/ARE pathway requires stimulation by ROS; however, during chronic oxidative stress, this response appears to be impaired. Therefore, a combination of dietary and endogenous antioxidants and certain polyphenolic compounds (curcumin and resveratrol) which activate Nrf2/ARE pathway without ROS stimulation and which directly scavenge free radicals would be most effective in reducing oxidative stress optimally. The above combination of agents together with a low-dose aspirin would be most effective in reducing chronic inflammation optimally.

REFERENCES

1. Cotran RSK, Kumar V, Collins T. Disease of immunity. In: *Pathologic Basis of Disease.* New York: W. B. Saunders Company; 1999.
2. Ryter A. Relationship between ultrastructure and specific functions of macrophages. *Comp Immunol Microbiol Infect Dis.* 1985; 8(2): 119–133.
3. Langermans JA, Hazenbos WL, van Furth R. Antimicrobial functions of mononuclear phagocytes. *J Immunol Methods.* Sep 14 1994; 174(1–2): 185–194.
4. Holtmeier W, Kabelitz D. gammadelta T cells link innate and adaptive immune responses. *Chem Immunol Allergy.* 2005; 86: 151–183.
5. Sproul TW, Cheng PC, Dykstra ML, Pierce SK. A role for MHC class II antigen processing in B cell development. *Int Rev Immunol.* 2000; 19(2–3): 139–155.
6. Kehry MR, Hodgkin PD. B-cell activation by helper T-cell membranes. *Crit Rev Immunol.* 1994; 14(3–4): 221–238.
7. Asmus K-D, Bonifacio M. Free radical chemistry. In: Sen CK, Packer L, Hanninen O, eds. *Excercise and Oxygen Toxicity.* New York: Elsevier; 1994.
8. Vaillancourt F, Fahmi H, Shi Q et al. 4-Hydroxynonenal induces apoptosis in human osteoarthritic chondrocytes: The protective role of glutathione-S-transferase. *Arthritis Res Ther.* 2008; 10(5): R107.
9. Pryor WA. Oxidants and antioxidants. In: Frei B, ed. *Natural Antioxidants in Human Health and Disease.* New York: Academy Press, Inc; 1994.

10. Kehrer JP, Smith CV. Free radicals in biology: Sources, reactives, and roles in the etiology of human diseases. In: Frei B, ed. *Natural Antioxidants in Human Health and Disease*. New York: Academic Press, Inc; 1994.

11. Itoh K, Chiba T, Takahashi S et al. An Nrf2/small Maf heterodimer mediates the induction of phase II detoxifying enzyme genes through antioxidant response elements. *Biochem Biophys Res Commun*. Jul 18 1997; 236(2): 313–322.

12. Hayes JD, Chanas SA, Henderson CJ et al. The Nrf2 transcription factor contributes both to the basal expression of glutathione S-transferases in mouse liver and to their induction by the chemopreventive synthetic antioxidants, butylated hydroxyanisole and ethoxyquin. *Biochem Soc Trans*. Feb 2000; 28(2): 33–41.

13. Chan K, Han XD, Kan YW. An important function of Nrf2 in combating oxidative stress: Detoxification of acetaminophen. *Proc Natl Acad Sci U S A*. Apr 10 2001; 98(8): 4611–4616.

14. Williamson TP, Johnson DA, Johnson JA. Activation of the Nrf2-ARE pathway by siRNA knockdown of Keap1 reduces oxidative stress and provides partial protection from MPTP-mediated neurotoxicity. *Neurotoxicology*. Jun 2012; 33(3): 272–279.

15. Niture SK, Kaspar JW, Shen J, Jaiswal AK. Nrf2 signaling and cell survival. *Toxicol Appl Pharmacol*. Apr 1 2010; 244(1): 37–42.

16. Xi YD, Yu HL, Ding J et al. Flavonoids protect cerebrovascular endothelial cells through Nrf2 and PI3K from beta-amyloid peptide-induced oxidative damage. *Curr Neurovasc Res*. Feb 2012; 9(1): 32–41.

17. Li XH, Li CY, Lu JM, Tian RB, Wei J. Allicin ameliorates cognitive deficits ageing-induced learning and memory deficits through enhancing of Nrf2 antioxidant signaling pathways. *Neurosci Lett*. Apr 11 2012; 514(1): 46–50.

18. Bergstrom P, Andersson HC, Gao Y et al. Repeated transient sulforaphane stimulation in astrocytes leads to prolonged Nrf2-mediated gene expression and protection from superoxide-induced damage. *Neuropharmacology*. Feb–Mar 2011; 60(2–3): 343–353.

19. Wruck CJ, Gotz ME, Herdegen T, Varoga D, Brandenburg LO, Pufe T. Kavalactones protect neural cells against amyloid beta peptide-induced neurotoxicity via extracellular signal-regulated kinase 1/2-dependent nuclear factor erythroid 2-related factor 2 activation. *Mol Pharmacol*. Jun 2008; 73(6): 1785–1795.

20. Hine CM, Mitchell JR. Nrf2 and the phase II response in acute stress resistance induced by dietary restriction. *J Clin Exp Pathol*. Jun 19 2012; S4(4).

21. Suh JH, Shenvi SV, Dixon BM et al. Decline in transcriptional activity of Nrf2 causes age-related loss of glutathione synthesis, which is reversible with lipoic acid. *Proc Natl Acad Sci U S A*. Mar 9 2004; 101(10): 3381–3386.

22. Muthusamy VR, Kannan S, Sadhaasivam K et al. Acute exercise stress activates Nrf2/ARE signaling and promotes antioxidant mechanisms in the myocardium. *Free Radic Biol Med*. Jan 15 2012; 52(2): 366–376.

23. Morales-Alamo D, Calbet JA. Free radicals and sprint exercise in humans. *Free Radic Res*. Oct 7 2013.

24. Romanque P, Cornejo P, Valdes S, Videla LA. Thyroid hormone administration induces rat liver Nrf2 activation: Suppression by N-acetylcysteine pretreatment. *Thyroid*. Jun 2011; 21(6): 655–662.

25. Fernandez V, Tapia G, Varela P, Cornejo P, Videla LA. Upregulation of liver inducible nitric oxide synthase following thyroid hormone preconditioning: Suppression by N-acetylcysteine. *Biol Res*. 2009; 42(4): 487–495.

26. Zou Y, Hong B, Fan L et al. Protective effect of puerarin against beta-amyloid-induced oxidative stress in neuronal cultures from rat hippocampus: Involvement of the GSK-3beta/Nrf2 signaling pathway. *Free Radic Res*. Jan 2013; 47(1): 55–63.

27. Choi HK, Pokharel YR, Lim SC et al. Inhibition of liver fibrosis by solubilized coenzyme Q_{10}: Role of Nrf2 activation in inhibiting transforming growth factor-beta1 expression. *Toxicol Appl Pharmacol*. Nov 1 2009; 240(3): 377–384.

28. Trujillo J, Chirino YI, Molina-Jijon E, Anderica-Romero AC, Tapia E, Pedraza-Chaverri J. Renoprotective effect of the antioxidant curcumin: Recent findings. *Redox Biol.* 2013; 1(1): 448–456.

29. Steele ML, Fuller S, Patel M, Kersaitis C, Ooi L, Munch G. Effect of Nrf2 activators on release of glutathione, cysteinylglycine and homocysteine by human U373 astroglial cells. *Redox Biol.* 2013; 1(1): 441–445.

30. Kode A, Rajendrasozhan S, Caito S, Yang SR, Megson IL, Rahman I. Resveratrol induces glutathione synthesis by activation of Nrf2 and protects against cigarette smoke-mediated oxidative stress in human lung epithelial cells. *Am J Physiol.* Mar 2008; 294(3): L478–L488.

31. Gao L, Wang J, Sekhar KR et al. Novel n-3 fatty acid oxidation products activate Nrf2 by destabilizing the association between Keap1 and Cullin3. *J Biol Chem.* Jan 26 2007; 282(4): 2529–2537.

32. Saw CL, Yang AY, Guo Y, Kong AN. Astaxanthin and omega-3 fatty acids individually and in combination protect against oxidative stress via the Nrf2-ARE pathway. *Food Chem Toxicol.* Dec 2013; 62: 869–875.

33. Ji L, Liu R, Zhang XD et al. N-acetylcysteine attenuates phosgene-induced acute lung injury via up-regulation of Nrf2 expression. *Inhalation Toxicol.* Jun 2010; 22(7): 535–542.

34. Zambrano S, Blanca AJ, Ruiz-Armenta MV et al. The renoprotective effect of L-carnitine in hypertensive rats is mediated by modulation of oxidative stress-related gene expression. *Eur J Nutri.* Sep 2013; 52(6): 1649–1659.

35. Messier EM, Day BJ, Bahmed K et al. N-acetylcysteine protects murine alveolar type II cells from cigarette smoke injury in a nuclear erythroid 2-related factor-2-independent manner. *Am J Respir Cell Mol Biol.* May 2013; 48(5): 559–567.

36. Wakabayashi N, Itoh K, Wakabayashi J et al. Keap1-null mutation leads to postnatal lethality due to constitutive Nrf2 activation. *Nat Genet.* Nov 2003; 35(3): 238–245.

37. Gliemann L, Schmidt JF, Olesen J et al. Resveratrol blunts the positive effects of exercise training on cardiovascular health in aged men. *J Physiol.* Oct 15 2013; 591(Pt 20): 5047–5059.

38. Smoliga JM, Blanchard OL. Recent data do not provide evidence that resveratrol causes 'mainly negative' or 'adverse' effects on exercise training in humans. *J Physiol.* Oct 15 2013; 591(Pt 20): 5251–5252.

39. Saha A, Sarkar C, Singh SP et al. The blood–brain barrier is disrupted in a mouse model of infantile neuronal ceroid lipofuscinosis: Amelioration by resveratrol. *Human Mol Genet.* May 15 2012; 21(10): 2233–2244.

40. Mokni M, Elkahoui S, Limam F, Amri M, Aouani E. Effect of resveratrol on antioxidant enzyme activities in the brain of healthy rat. *Neurochem Res.* Jun 2007; 32(6): 981–987.

41. Wang Q, Xu J, Rottinghaus GE et al. Resveratrol protects against global cerebral ischemic injury in gerbils. *Brain Res.* Dec 27 2002; 958(2): 439–447.

3 Etiology of Alzheimer's Disease

Prevention and Improved Management by Micronutrients

INTRODUCTION

Alzheimer's disease (AD) is characterized by degeneration and death of cerebral cortex neurons and is the major cause of dementia. Individuals, who are 65 years or older, have high risk of developing this neurodegenerative disease. Progressive loss of cognitive functions occurs in this disease. Over 90% of AD is acquired and only about 5–10% is inherited from parents. This disease is the fifth leading cause of death among people aged 65 years or older. Despite extensive research on the causes of AD, it has not been possible to reduce the incidence or the rate of progression of AD. During the last few decades, several biochemical and genetic defects that contribute to degeneration and death of neurons have been identified in AD. They include: (a) increased oxidative stress, (b) mitochondrial dysfunction, (c) chronic inflammation, (d) Aβ1–42 peptides generated from the cleavage of amyloid precursor protein (APP), (e) proteasome inhibition, (f) high cholesterol levels, and (g) heritable mutations in APP, presenilin-1, and presenilin-2 genes.

Despite these advances in our understanding of this disease, no evidence-based strategy has been proposed to reduce the risk of AD or to improve the efficacy of drug therapy in the management of AD. Current drug therapies are based on the symptoms rather than on the causes of the disease. For example, acetylcholinesterase inhibitors are used to improve the symptoms of dementia by increasing acetylcholine in surviving cholinergic neurons and an antagonist of glutamate receptor N-methyl-D-aspartate (NMDA) to reduce the anxiety and fear associated with AD. These drugs produce modest beneficial effects on these symptoms; however, they also produce unpleasant side effects. None of these drugs have any effect on increased oxidative stress or chronic inflammation which plays a key role in the development and progression of AD.

Antioxidants neutralize free radicals and reduce chronic inflammation. Therefore, improving the levels of antioxidant systems (antioxidant enzymes and dietary and endogenous antioxidants) may reduce the risk of AD in high-risk populations, such as older individuals and individuals with a family history of AD. The above strategy in combination with standard therapy may improve the management of this disease more than that produced by standard therapy alone. We have published a review in which the importance of a micronutrient preparation containing dietary and endogenous antioxidants, vitamin D, B-vitamins, and certain minerals in reducing the risk of AD and in improving the effectiveness of standard therapy in the management of AD has been emphasized.[1]

This chapter discusses briefly (a) incidence, prevalence, and cost; (b) neuropathology; and (c) biochemical and genetic causes of AD. In addition, this chapter presents evidence in support of a hypothesis that (a) increased chronic oxidative stress is one of the earliest biochemical defects which initiate neurodegeneration and that other defects, such as mitochondrial dysfunction, chronic inflammation, generation of Aβ1–42, and proteasome inhibition occur subsequent to increased oxidative stress. Increased chronic oxidative stress together with other biochemical defects participates in the progression and final stage of neuronal death in AD. This chapter also provides rationale and scientific evidence for using a combination of preparation of multiple dietary and endogenous antioxidants and certain polyphenolics for prevention, and in combination with standard therapy, for improved management of AD.

PREVALENCE, INCIDENCE, AND COST OF AD

It is estimated that 5 million (3.2 million women and 1.8 million men) people aged 65 years or older and 200,000 people under the age of 65 years have AD in the USA (Alzheimer's disease: Facts and Figures [Alzheimer's Association, 2013]).

The incidence of AD and other dementia doubles every 5 years beyond the age of 65, and about 50% of the US population who are 85 years or older have symptoms of AD.[2]

Age (Years)	New Cases/Year/1000 People
65–74	53
75–84	173
85 or older	231

From Alzheimer's disease: Facts and Figures (Alzheimer's Association, 2013).

It is estimated that 11% of people age 65 years or older have AD, whereas about 32% of people aged 71 years or older have AD. About 16% of women aged 65 years or older have AD and other dementia compared to only 11% of men of the same age group. This suggests that women may be more sensitive to develop AD than men.

Only about 5–10% of AD is due to hereditary factors and appears at an early age; the remaining cases are considered to be idiopathic or sporadic and appear at a late age. It has been predicted that the number of Americans of age 65 and older would increase from about 33 million to 51 million by the year 2025.[2] The incidence and prevalence of AD and non-AD dementia is likely to increase during the above period. Thus, Alzheimer's disease remains a major medical concern now as well in the future. It is important to develop an effective preventive strategy that is based on the causes of the disease in order to minimize the risk of developing AD now and in the future.

COST OF AD

The annual economic cost of AD health care expenses and lost wages (for both AD patients and their caregivers) is estimated to be $80–100 billion in 1997.[2] In 2013, the Alzheimer's Association estimated the annual cost to be 203 billion as presented here.

COST OF HEALTH AND LONG-TERM CARE SERVICES

Medicare	$107 billion
Medicaid	$35 billion
Out-of-pocket cost	$34 billion
Other sources (health maintenance organizations, private insurance, managed care organizations, and uncompensated care)	$27 billion
Total	$203 billion

TYPES OF DEMENTIA

Alzheimer's disease represents the major form of dementia. Other types of dementia include vascular dementia, mixed dementia, dementia with Lewy bodies, Parkinson's disease with dementia, frontotemporal dementia and alcoholic dementia. Most dementia including AD is idiopathic, and only a small percentage of them are familial type.

NEUROPATHOLOGY OF AD

The diagnosis of AD is made by postmortem analysis of the brains of patients with dementia. The presence of intracellular neurofibrillary tangles (NFT) containing hyperphosphorylated tau protein and apolipoprotein E,[3,4] and extracellular senile plaques containing several proteins, including alpha-synuclein, beta-amyloids, ubiquitin, apolipoprotein E, presenilins, and alpha antichymotrypsin, are considered hallmarks of AD.[5–7] Neurofibrillary tangles are insoluble and are difficult to degrade by proteolytic enzymes. They are commonly found in cortical neurons. Senile plaques are focal and spherical, and their size ranges from 20 to 200 microns in diameter. Microglia and reactive astrocytes are present at their periphery. Interestingly, a study has shown that Lewy bodies are present in the brains of about 60% of AD cases.[8] The mechanisms of formation and dissolution of these cytoplasmic inclusions are under extensive investigation in order to develop novel drugs for the treatment of AD.

CAUSES OF AD

The agents which can increase the risk of developing AD may include external (environment-, diet-, and lifestyle-related factors) and internal factors (increased oxidative stress, mitochondrial dysfunction, chronic inflammation, and generation of Aβ1–42 peptides from APP, increased cholesterol levels, and proteasome inhibition. In addition, mutations in APP, presenilin-1, and presenilin-2 genes cause increased production of Aβ1–42 peptides that induce neurodegeneration by producing free radicals.

EXTERNAL RISK FACTORS FOR THE DEVELOPMENT OF AD

ENVIRONMENT, DIET, AND LIFESTYLE

Studies on the environment-, dietary-, and lifestyle-related factors that increase the risk of AD are important in order to identify targets that can be used for reducing the incidence of AD. Among environmental factors, high consumption of aluminum from drinking water may increase the risk of developing dementia.[9] Vitamin D deficiency appears to be associated with both AD and Parkinson's disease.[10] It has been reported that high dietary intake of vitamin C and vitamin E may reduce the risk of AD, and among current smokers, the intake of beta-carotene and flavonoids may also decrease the risk of AD.[11] It has been demonstrated that feeding high fat/high cholesterol (HFC) diet causes loss of working memory associated with increased chronic inflammation and generation of Aβ peptides in mice.[12] Feeding above diet also enhanced the levels of hyperphosphorylated tau (P-tau) and reduced the levels of postsynaptic protein, PSD95, and dendritic spine-specific protein, drebrin, which would reduce synaptic plasticity.[13] HFC diet-induced increased production of Aβ peptides could be due to increased activity of beta-secretase. It has been demonstrated that increased levels of beta-secretase were correlated with increased levels of total tau and P-tau in the cerebrospinal fluid (CSF) of patients with AD.[14]

CIGARETTE SMOKING

Cigarette smoking is considered a risk factor for developing AD. A study showed that exposure to cigarette smoke increased the levels of oxidative stress in the hippocampus region of rats compared to those which were not exposed to cigarette.[15] Exposure to smoke also reduced synaptic activity by decreasing the levels of presynaptic proteins including synaptophysin and synapsin-1. In addition, exposure to cigarette smoke decreased the levels of acetylated tubulin and increased the levels of phosphorylated tau protein in the hippocampus. Dentate gyrus is considered the site for continued neurogenesis in the adult brain. Cornu Ammonis-3 (CA3) region of hippocampus receives projection of nerve fibers from dentate gyrus and sends back to dentate gyrus. Exposure to cigarette smoke also increased the rate of generation and accumulation beta-amyloid fragments in CA3 and dentate gyrus region. Exposure to cigarette smoke also increased markers of oxidative stress and proinflammatory cytokines in the brain of Lewis rats compared to control animals.[16]

EXERCISE

Intracerebroventricular injection of Aβ1–40 caused cognitive dysfunction, increased oxidative stress, and chronic inflammation in male Swiss albino mice; however, exercise prevented cognitive decline, oxidative stress, and inflammation in these mice.[17]

EXPOSURE TO ELECTROMAGNETIC FIELD

Growing use of electromagnetic field (EMF) technology has raised concerns regarding long-term health consequences of this technology. Electromagnetic pulse (EMP) is one type of widely used EMF. Exposure of healthy male rats to 100, 1000, and 10,000 EMP (field strength 50 kV/m, repetition rate 100 Hz) induced cognitive dysfunction, increased the levels of Aβ peptides as well as Aβ oligomer and APP, and decreased superoxide dismutase (SOD) activity and glutathione levels. These results suggest that exposure to EMP induces cognitive dysfunction by increasing oxidative stress.[18] Exposure of male mice to EMP (field strength 400 kV/m, rise time 10 ns, pulse width 350 ns, O.5 Hz, total 200 pulses) increased lipid peroxidation, but reduced the activities of antioxidant enzymes (SOD, glutathione peroxidase, and catalase), and the levels of glutathione. These results suggest that exposure to EMP increases oxidative stress in mice. Exposure to EMP also decreased learning ability of mice.[19] In contrast to the effect of EMP, long-term exposure of AD transgenic (Tg) old mice to EMF (pulse-mediated GSM [global system for mobile communication], 918 MHz, and W/kg) improved cognitive function in very old transgenic mice and normal mice, and reversed advanced Aβ-induced neurodegenerative changes in transgenic mice.[20] These studies suggest that at least in transgenic AD model mice, exposure to high EMF improved cognitive functions. The relevance of these observations in humans remains uncertain.

EXPOSURE TO CHRONIC NOISE

Chronic noise exposure (100 dB 4 h per day for 14 days) increased the levels of P-tau in the hippocampus and the prefrontal cortex of male Wistar rats.[21] Phosphorylation of tau persisted 7 to 14 days after the cessation of noise exposure. The presence of NFT was observed 14 days after cessation of noise exposure. These data suggest that exposure to chronic noise may induce AD-related pathology in the brain as shown by the increased P-tau and NFT in the hippocampus and prefrontal cortex of rats. This is not surprising because chronic noise produced increased amounts of free radicals.[22,23]

INTERNAL RISK FACTORS FOR DEVELOPMENT AND PROGRESSION OF AD

The major internal risk factors that increase the risk of development and progression of AD include increased oxidative stress, mitochondrial dysfunction, chronic inflammation, and generation of Aβ1–42 peptides from APP, increased levels of cholesterol, proteasome inhibition, and mutations in APP, presenilins, and other genes. Among these internal risk factors, increased oxidative stress appears to be one of the earliest biochemical defects that initiate damage to the nerve cells in the brain of patients with AD. Increased oxidative stress together with other biochemical defects participate in the progression of AD. These risk factors provide useful targets to develop a rational strategy for prevention and improved management of AD.

INCREASED OXIDATIVE STRESS

Before discussing the role of oxidative stress in the development of AD, it is important to describe the sources and the type of free radicals in the normal brain. Generally, mitochondria are the major source of free radicals; however, some free radicals are also produced outside the mitochondria. Damaged mitochondria produce more free radicals.

Sources of Free Radicals in Normal Brain

The brain utilizes about 25% of respired oxygen even though it represents only 5% of the body weight. Free radicals are generated in the brain during the normal intake of oxygen, during infection, and during normal oxidative metabolism of certain substrates. During normal aerobic respiration, the mitochondria of one rat nerve cell will process about 10^{12} oxygen molecules and reduce them to water. During this process, superoxide anion ($O_2^{-\bullet}$), hydrogen peroxide (H_2O_2), and hydroxyl free radicals ($OH^\bullet$) are produced. In addition, partially reduced oxygen, which represents about 2% of consumed oxygen, leaks out from the mitochondria and generates about 20 billion molecules of superoxide anion $O_2^{-\bullet}$ and H_2O_2 per cell per day.[24] During bacterial or viral infection, phagocytic cells (primarily microglia cells) generate high levels of nitric oxide (NO), $O_2^{-\bullet}$, and H_2O_2 in order to kill infective agents; however, these radicals can also damage normal cells.[25] During degradation of fatty acids and other molecules by peroxisomes, H_2O_2 is produced as a byproduct. During oxidative metabolism of ingested toxins, free radicals are also generated.

Some brain enzymes such as monoamine oxidase (MAO), tyrosine hydroxylase, and L-amino acid oxidase produce H_2O_2 as a normal byproduct of their activities.[26] Furthermore, auto-oxidation of ascorbate and catecholamines generates free radicals and H_2O_2.[27] Oxidative stress can also be generated by Ca^{2+}-mediated activation of glutamate receptors. The Ca^{2+}-dependent activation of phospholipase A_2 by NMDA releases arachidonic acid, which then liberates $O_2^{-\bullet}$ during the biosynthesis of eicosanoids.[28] Another radical, NO, is formed by nitric oxide synthase stimulated by Ca^{2+}. NO can react with $O_2^{-\bullet}$ to form peroxynitrite that can form $OH^\bullet$, the highly reactive hydroxyl radical. NMDA receptor stimulation produces marked elevations in $O_2^{-\bullet}$ and $OH^\bullet$ levels.[29] Some enzymes such as xanthine oxidase and flavoprotein oxidase (e.g., aldehyde oxidase) also form superoxide anions during metabolism of their respective substrates. Oxidation of hydroquinone and thiols and synthesis of uric acid from purines form superoxide anions.

Certain external agents can increase oxidative stress. For example, cigarette smoking increases the level of NO[30,31] and depletes antioxidant levels.[32,33] Free iron and copper can increase the levels of free radicals.[34] Some plants contain large amounts of phenolic compounds, such as chlorogenic and caffeic acid, which can be oxidized to form radicals.[35] These studies suggest that the brain generates high levels of reactive oxygen species (ROS) and reactive nitrogen species (RNS) every day. In addition, the brain has the highest levels of unsaturated fatty acids which are easily oxidizable by free radicals. Paradoxically, the brain is least prepared to handle this excessive load of free radicals. It has low levels of both antioxidant enzymes and dietary and endogenous antioxidant chemicals. These inherent biological features make brains very vulnerable to increased oxidative stress. Despite this, the risk of idiopathic AD becomes significant only after the age of 65 or more. This is due to the fact that neurons exhibit a high degree of plasticity in maintaining normal brain functions. The fact that clinical symptoms of neurological diseases including AD appear only when a significant number of neurons are lost supports the value of plasticity of the neurons in maintaining normal brain function.

Types of Free Radicals Derived from Oxygen and Nitrogen

The brain utilizes 3.5 mL oxygen/100 g of brain tissue/min.[36] About 2% of the partially used oxygen produces increased levels of ROS in the brain. The formation of some of these ROS is described in the following.

When molecular oxygen (O_2) acquires an electron, the superoxide anion

$$\left(O_2^{\cdot-}\right) \text{ is formed: } O_2 + e^- = O_2^{\cdot-}$$

SOD and H^+ can react with $O_2^{\cdot-}$ to form hydrogen peroxide, H_2O_2:

$$2O_2^{\cdot-} + 2H^+ + SOD \rightarrow H_2O_2 + O_2$$

$$O_2^{\cdot-} + H^+ \rightarrow HO_2^{\cdot} \text{ (hydroperoxy radical)}$$

$$2HO_2^{\cdot} \rightarrow H_2O_2 + O_2$$

Ferric and ferrous forms of iron can react with superoxide anion and hydrogen peroxide to produce molecular oxygen and hydroxyl radical ($OH^{\cdot}$), respectively:

$$Fe^{3+} + O_2^{\cdot-} \rightarrow Fe^{2+} + O_2$$

$$Fe^{2+} + H_2O_2 \rightarrow Fe^{3+} + OH^{\cdot} + OH^- \text{ (Fenton reaction)}$$

Hydroxyl radical can also be formed from superoxide anion by the Haber–Weiss reaction:

$$O_2^{\cdot-} + H_2O_2 \rightarrow O_2 + OH^- + OH^{\cdot}$$

Both the Fenton and Haber–Weiss reactions require a transition metal such as copper or iron. Among ROS, $OH^{\cdot}$ is the most damaging free radical and is very short lived. Hydroxyl radical is very reactive with a variety of organic compounds, leading to production of more radical compounds:

$$RH \text{ (organic compound)} + OH^{\cdot} \rightarrow R^{\cdot} \text{ (organic radical)} + H_2O$$

$$R^{\cdot} + O_2 \rightarrow RO_2^{\cdot} \text{ (peroxy radical)}$$

Catalase detoxifies hydrogen peroxide to form water and molecular oxygen:

$$H_2O_2 + catalase \rightarrow H_2O \text{ and } O_2$$

RNS are represented by nitric oxide (NO·). NO is synthesized by the enzyme nitric oxide synthase from L-arginine, and in the brain, it acts both as a neurotransmitter and, in excessive amounts, acts as a neurotoxin. NO· can combine with superoxide anion to form peroxynitrite, a powerful oxidant.

$$NO· + O_2^{·-} \rightarrow ONOO^- \text{ (peroxynitrite)}$$

When protonated (likely at physiological pH), peroxynitrite spontaneously decomposes to reactive nitric dioxide and hydroxyl radicals:

$$ONOO^- + H^+ \rightarrow ·NO_2 + OH·$$

SOD can also enhance the peroxynitrite-mediated nitration of tyrosine residues on critical proteins, presumably viato the nitronium cation (NO_2^+):

$$ONOO^- + SOD \rightarrow NO_2^+ \rightarrow \text{nitration of tyrosine}$$

These data reveal that several different types of free radicals are constantly formed in the brain. The levels of free radicals can be increased by enhanced turnover of catecholamines, increased levels of free iron, impaired mitochondrial functions, decreased glutathione levels, and antioxidant enzymes activities. Consumption of a diet low in antioxidants may also increase the levels of free radicals. Thus, maintenance of a balance in the favor of antioxidants is essential for the protection of brain function against oxidative damage. When this balance is shifted in favor of oxidants, the epigenetic and genetic components of neurons suffer damage which gradually initiate degeneration and eventually cause death of neurons.

EVIDENCE FOR INCREASED OXIDATIVE STRESS IN AD

Because of increased production of free radicals, reduced levels of antioxidants and high levels of unsaturated fatty acids that are easily damaged by free radicals, the brain is particularly sensitive to oxidative stress. Extensive studies on animal models of AD and autopsied brain samples from patients with AD showed that increased oxidative stress play an important role in the initiation and progression of AD. A simplified diagrammatic representation of the various pathways of increased oxidative stress in causing neuronal death in the brain of patients with AD is described in Table 3.1. Mitochondria appear to be an early target of free radicals causing mitochondrial dysfunction that further increases oxidative stress. These studies are described here.

TABLE 3.1

Simplified Diagrammatic Representation of Various Pathways of Oxidative Stress in Causing Neuronal Death in Brain of Patients with AD

Increased oxidative stress→→Beta-secretase elevation→→Gamma-secretase elevation→→APP cleavage→→Aβ1–42 peptides elevation→→Aggregation of Aβ by Cu^{2+} and Zn^{2+}→→Produce free radicals→→Death of neurons

Increased oxidative stress→→Tau hyperphosphorylation→→Formation of oligomer of phosphorylated tau→→Disrupts synaptic function→→Loss of synapses→→Death of neurons

Increased oxidative stress→→Mitochondrial dysfunction by inhibiting activities of complexes, mutation in mtDNA, and increasing cytochrome oxidase activity→→Reduce production of energy→→Produce free radicals→→Death of neurons

Increased oxidative stress→→Activate microglia cells→→Produce proinflammatory cytokines and free radicals→→Death of neurons

Increased oxidative stress→→Inhibit proteasome activity→→Accumulation misfolded proteins (hyperphosphorylated tau and APOE)→→Participate in the formation of NFT→→Death of neurons

Mutations in APP, presenilin-1, and presenilin-2→→Increase production of Aβ1–42 peptides→→Increase production of free radicals→→Death of neurons

Extracellular senile plaque contains several proteins including beta-amyloid, APOE, alpha-synuclein, and presenilins. It serves as a constant source of chronic inflammation that maintains high levels of chronic inflammation in the brain of AD patients.

ANIMAL STUDIES

Energy metabolism is essential for the synaptic plasticity and synaptic transmission. Reduced energy metabolism due to mitochondrial dysfunction may account for defects in synaptic plasticity and function in AD. Using a transgenic mouse model of AD (APP23 mice), it was demonstrated that reduced energy metabolism and increased protein oxidation occur in the cortex of asymptomatic mice, suggesting that these biochemical markers of oxidative stress occur prior to the development of other biochemical defects and amyloidogenic phenotype.[37] Using an imaging technique on the brain of transgenic mouse AD model, it was shown that oxidative stress was markedly elevated in neuritis near plaques, propagated to cell bodies, and preceded caspase activation that led to death of neurons within 24 h.[38] The results suggested that local increase in oxidative stress surrounding plaques may initiate neurodegeneration and death of neuron in that area.

Transgenic A mice (tau 3xTg) exhibited cognitive dysfunction and fear conditioning. Pretreatment with the SOD/catalase mimetic, EUK-207, prevented cognitive dysfunction and fear conditioning, and reduced the levels of Aβ42, tau and hyperphosphorylated tau, oxidized nucleic acid, and lipid peroxidation in amygdala and hippocampus.[39] The above studies on animal models of AD suggest that increased oxidative stress occur prior to other biochemical defects associated with neurodegeneration in AD. This is further supported by the fact that administration of antioxidants in these transgenic AD model mice prevented memory loss.

Cell Culture Studies

Using primary neuron cultures from new born wild-type mice and transgenic mice expressing mutated APP and mutated presenilin-1, it was demonstrated that markers of oxidative stress, such as protein carbonyl, 4-hydroxynonenal (4-HNE), and 3-nitrotyrosine (3-NT) were elevated, and the membrane potential of mitochondria was reduced in developing and mature neurons expressing mutated APP and presenilin-1 compared to those in nerve cells obtained from wild type mice.[40] This study suggested that increased oxidative stress occurs in neurons of transgenic AD mice.

Treatment of human neuroblastoma cells in culture with hydrogen peroxide (H_2O_2) significantly increased Aβ production.[41] This was due to increased expression of beta- and gamma-secretases responsible for cleavage of APP to form Aβ peptides. Thus, increased oxidative stress causes increased production of beta-amyloids. Treatment nerve cells with H_2O_2 also induced hyperacetylation of histone by downregulating histone deacetylase that causes increased expression of APP-cleaving enzymes beta- and gamma-secretases. These results suggest that increased oxidative stress produces more beta-amyloids which cause damage to nerve cells by generating free radicals.

Primary culture of neurons obtained from transgenic mice expressing both mutated APP and mutated preseninlin-1 exhibited increased oxidative stress and increased sensitivity to oxidative stress induced by Aβ1–42, H_2O_2, and kainic acid that contribute to neuronal death.[42] These results also suggest that mutation in presenilin-1 and APP may cause neurodegeneration in familial AD via increasing oxidative stress. These results suggest that increased oxidative stress continue to occur and contribute to the progression of AD.

Human Studies (Autopsied Brain Tissue)

In a review, it was shown that markers of oxidative stress, such as protein nitrotyrosine, carbonyls in proteins, lipid oxidation products, and oxidized DNA bases were elevated in the autopsied samples of brain of patients with AD.[43] A number of observations substantiate the presence of high levels of oxidative stress in patients with AD. For example, (a) higher expression of heme oxygenase-1 is found in the brains of AD patients[44]; (b) increased consumption of oxygen is found in AD patients[45]; (c) increased activity of glucose-6-phosphate dehydrogenase is found in the AD brain[46]; and (d) activation of calcium-dependent neural proteinase (calpain) is found in AD brains[47] which may trigger events leading to the formation of free radicals.[48] The increased levels of lipofuscin formation in a small number of degenerating neurons probably results in a marked progressive increase in superoxide radicals and H_2O_2 formation and reduced production of adenosine triphosphate (ATP), which overwhelms the endogenous antioxidant systems that protect nerve cells against free radical-induced damage.[49] Additional evidence for the increased oxidative stress in AD brain include the following: (a) homogenates of frontal cortex from AD brains obtained at autopsy revealed a 22% higher production of free radicals and, in the presence of iron, a 50% higher production of free radicals than those from age-matched normal controls[50]; (b) peroxynitrite also exacerbates the pathogenesis of AD[51]; (c) increased neuronal nitric oxide synthase (nNOS) expression in reactive astrocytes correlated with apoptosis in hippocampal neurons of AD brains[52]; (d) the activity of glutamine synthetase decreased in AD brains[51]; and (e) the level of glutathione transferase is decreased in ventricular CSF and in AD brains compared to that in the brains from age-matched controls.[53] Analysis of 50 patients with AD and 100 control subjects revealed that deletion of glutathione-S-transferase T1 increased the risk of AD by 2.47 times.[54] Taken together, these data strongly suggest that increased oxidative stress represents one of the major internal risk factors that play an important role in progression of AD. The persistence of high levels of markers of oxidative stress in autopsied brain samples cannot be explained by the loss of neurons in the late stage of the disease.

Biliverdin reductase-A (BVR-A) is considered a pleiotropic enzyme that plays an important role in the antioxidant defense against free radical damage. BVR-A in combination with heme oxygenase regulate cellular stress responses. In patients with AD as well as in patients with mild cognitive impairment (MCI), a significant increase in oxidized and nitrated BVR-A was found in the hippocampal region, but not in the cerebellum.[55] It was concluded that nitrosylative stress-induced modification of BVR-A in the hippocampus may be an early event in the pathogenesis of AD, since nitrated BVR-A is also present in patients with mild cognitive impairment.

HUMAN STUDIES (PERIPHERAL TISSUE)

The markers of oxidative stress were evaluated in peripheral tissue in order to establish whether or not they can be used as a diagnostic tool for prediction of the presence of AD and/or MCI. The fibroblasts obtained from familial AD patients were more sensitive to oxidative stress than those obtained from age-matched normal controls.[56] In another study using fibroblasts from patients with AD and normal subjects, it was shown that treatment with hydrogen peroxide altered the expression of 215 genes and their associated pathways that may be responsible for cell death.[57] The serum levels of vitamins A and E and beta-carotene were lowerin patients with AD (who were well nourished) than in control patients.[58] In a clinical study involving 82 patients with AD, 42 with vascular dementia and 26 healthy controls, it was shown that the concentration of serum total antioxidant status decreased; the risk of medial temporal lobe atrophy (MTA) assessment increased in both patients with AD and vascular dementia, whereas the scores of white matter hyperintensities rating were higher in patients carrying the apolipoprotein E-e4 (APOE4) allele than in healthy control.[59] Increased levels of oxidized proteins were found in the blood of both AD patients and their relatives when compared with non-AD control.[60] This particular study reveals that increased oxidative stress occur in the relatives of AD patients who have no symptoms of the disease confirming my hypothesis that increased oxidative stress is one of the earliest biochemical defects that initiate damage to the nerve cells in the brain of patients with AD.

In a clinical study involving 12 patients with AD, 13 patients with non-AD dementia, 14 age-matched subjects and 14 young adult controls, it was demonstrated that in red blood cells (RBCs), elevated levels of markers of oxidative stress (H_2O_2 and organic hydroperoxides) were associated with age-related dementia, whereas decreased activity of glutathione peroxidase was associated with AD.[61] The author suggested that decreased activity of glutathione peroxidase in RBC can be used as a new peripheral marker for AD. The analysis of serum levels of markers of oxidative stress in 101 patients with AD, 134 patients with mild cognitive impairment, suggested that increased levels of serum hydroperoxides were independently associated with the increased risk of developing mild cognitive impairment as well as AD, whereas low levels of serum total antioxidant capacity were associated with the increased risk of developing mild cognitive impairment.[62] In a clinical study involving 33 patients with mild cognitive impairment, 29 patients with probable mild AD, and 26 healthy age-matched subjects, it was demonstrated that plasma levels of malondialdehyde (MDA) were higher in patients with mild cognitive impairment and AD than in control subjects, whereas glutathione reductase activity in RBC was lower in patients with mild cognitive impairment and AD than in control subjects.[63] These results suggest that increased oxidative stress is present in patients with early stage of the disease.

In a study involving individuals carrying mutated preseninline-1 or APP or their relatives carrying no mutated genes, it was demonstrated that plasma oxidative markers, such as methionine sufoxide oxidation product of methionine, were elevated in individuals carrying a mutated gene in comparison to that in relatives with no mutated genes.[64] The results of this study provides the strongest foundation in support of my hypothesis that increased oxidative stress is one of the earliest biochemical defects that initiate damage to the nerve cells in the brain of AD patients.

MITOCHONDRIAL DYSFUNCTION

Most free radicals are produced in the mitochondria, although some are also produced in the cytoplasm. Mitochondria may be one of the most sensitive primary targets of oxidative stress in adult neurons.[65] This may be due to the fact that mitochondrial DNA (mtDNA) does not encode for any repair enzymes, and unlike nuclear DNA, it is not shielded by protective histones. In addition, mtDNA is in close proximity to the site where free radicals are generated during oxidative phosphorylation.[65] Indeed, an increased frequency of mutations in mtDNA has been found in the autopsied samples of AD brains,[66] and several studies have implicated other types of mitochondrial defects in the pathogenesis of AD.[66-68] Because the onset of AD coincides with older age, it is reasonable to suggest that damaged mtDNA, which is normally removed during mitochondrial turnover, accumulates in neurons, due to slowing down of this process in older individuals. Thus, the number of defective mitochondria may accumulate with aging, and this could lead to reduced production of ATP that could then initiate slow degenerative processes in neurons. Reduced ATP levels result in decreased energy metabolism. For example, decreased glucose uptake coupled with reduced activity of cytochrome oxidase (complex IV) leads to increased production of ROS by mitochondria.[67] Excess of free Zn is found in the autopsied brain of AD,[69] and increased free Zn can impair mitochondrial function.[70] This could then constitute a continuous cycle of production of increased levels of free radicals and enhanced mitochondrial dysfunction. A defect in energy production may also increase the sensitivity of neurons to excitatory amino acids such as glutamate.[71] Impaired mitochondria may alter metabolism of APP leading to increased generation of Aβ1–42 peptides.[72]

Alpha-ketoglutarate dehydrogenase complex (KGDHC), a mitochondrial enzyme, is decreased in brains of AD patients.[73] It is interesting to note that in AD patients who carry the APOE4 allele of the APOE gene, the clinical dementia rating (CDR) correlated better with KGDHC activity than with densities of senile plaques and neurotrophic factors (NTFs); however, in patients without APOE4 allele, the CDR correlated better with plaques and NTFs than with KGDHC activity.[73] This suggests that mitochondrial dysfunctions may be more important for the development of AD in patients who carry APOE4 allele than in those who do not.

In a review, several oxidized mitochondrial proteins in the brain were detected by using proteomics assay. In addition, decreased energy metabolism was detected in patients with AD exhibiting a mild cognitive dysfunction.[74] In another review, it was shown that decreased energy production preceded the development of clinical symptoms of AD.[75] In addition, reduced cerebral energy metabolism can lead to hyperphosphorylation of tau protein and increased production of Aβ1–42 peptides. A study has reported that peripheral lymphocytes obtained from the patients with AD as well as from the patients with mild cognitive impairment exhibited mitochondrial dysfunction as evidenced by decreased mitochondrial membrane potential and enhanced sensitivity to different inhibitors of respiratory chain complexes.[76] Further studies revealed that AD was associated with an early increase in markers of oxidative stress, such as nitric oxide synthase and nicotinamide adenine dinucleotide phosphate (NADPH), oxidases which could impair the mitochondrial function by reducing activities of chain complexes VI and V. In addition, reduction in the levels of uncoupling protein (UCP) and peroxisome proliferator-activated receptor (PPAR) which protect the neurons further aggravates oxidative stress-induced damage.[77] These results suggest that increased oxidative stress and reduced energy metabolism occur in the early phase of AD.

In a review, it was shown that vascular and mitochondrial dysfunction and reduced energy metabolism were commonly observed in patients with AD. Vascular dysfunctions included reduced cerebral blood flow and defects in blood-brain barrier that can reduce the clearance of beta-amyloids from the brain. These defects in cerebral blood flow increased deposits of beta-amyloid fragments in the brain.[78] Increased beta-amyloids contribute to the degeneration and death of neuron via free radicals. Mitochondrial dysfunction caused an elevation of ROS and deregulation of Ca^{2+} homeostasis that resulted in neuronal death. Increased levels of ROS induced chronic inflammation in the brain by increasing the transcription and release of pro-inflammatory cytokines, such as IL-1, IL-6, TNF-alpha and chemokines. The products of chronic inflammation then activated microglia and astrocytes to enhance further the levels of ROS; hence, chronic inflammation may serve as a constant source of ROS production. Increased oxidative stress can lead to increased production of Aβ peptides in the brain. The results of the above studies suggest that increased oxidative stress is one of the earliest events which induce mitochondrial dysfunction that further produce free radicals.

GENERATION AND AGGREGATION OF Aβ1–42 PEPTIDES FROM APP

Increased generation of Aβ1–42 peptides and aggregation of these peptides contribute to the death of neurons in the brain of AD patients. It is now established that

Aβ1–42 peptides (also called beta-amyloids or Aβ peptides) generated by the cleavage of APP play a central role in the pathogenesis of AD.[5,6] There are two pathways of processing of APP in neurons. The predominant pathway of APP processing consists of successive cleavages by alpha- and gamma-secretases, whereas the other pathway involves sequential cleavage of APP by beta- and gamma-secretases. It is the latter pathway that generates neurotoxic beta-amyloids. Normally, alpha-secretase cleaves inside the beta-amyloid sequence of APP, releasing the soluble N-terminal domain of APP that exhibit neurotrophic and neuroprotective properties. In patients with AD, a decrease in alpha-secretase-mediated processing of APP has been found in the autopsied brain samples.[79] This suggests that a decrease in alpha-secretase-mediated processing of APP is associated with an increase in processing of APP by beta- and gamma-secretases to beta-amyloids.

Oxidative Stress Increases Production of Aβ1–42 Peptides

Increased chronic oxidative stress may enhance intracellular accumulation of beta-amyloid in neurons.[80] In addition, studies show that membrane containing oxidized phospholipids accumulated beta-amyloids faster than membrane containing only unoxidized saturated phospholipids.[81] Using transgenic AD mouse model lacking cytoplasmic SOD-1, it was demonstrated that the rate of cleavage of APP to Aβ1–42 was increased in transgenic mice compared to those in which SOD-1 was present. These results suggested that increased in cytoplasmic oxidative stress can increase the production of Aβ1–42 peptides.[82]

Several studies have indicated that the level and activity of beta-secretase-1 were elevated in the autopsied samples of cortex of patients with AD.[83] Using primary culture of neurons, it was demonstrated that mild oxidative stress does not modify beta-secretase expression, but caused increased distribution of beta-secretase in the area rich in APP that would result into increased generation of beta-amyloids.[83]

Aggregation of Aβ1–42 Peptides

It has been shown that aggregates of beta-amyloids are toxic to neurons in culture[84,85] and can cause cell death by apoptosis[86] or necrosis.[87] Several agents can enhance the aggregation of beta-amyloids. They include excess amounts of free Zn and Cu,[88] iron, and aluminum[89] and complement proteins.[90] Cu^+ and Zn^+ interaction with Aβ40 and Aβ42 caused the deposition of amorphous aggregates; however, Fe^{3+} caused the deposition of fibrillar amyloid plaques at neutral pH.[91] It has been reported that Al–Aβ complexes caused increased production of APP and tau 181 protein.[92] It was further demonstrated that iron enhances Aβ toxicity only if iron is present throughout aggregation process.[93] The role of Fe–Aβ complexes in the development and progression of AD is supported by the fact that administration of Fe^{3+} increased the expression and phosphorylation of APP, enhanced the production and deposition of Aβ1–42 peptides, and impaired the spatial learning and memory in transgenic mouse AD model. Intranasal administration of deferoxamine, a chelator of iron, prevented iron-induced toxicity.[94] Curcumin, which exhibits antioxidant and anti-inflammation activities, binds with redox-active metals such as iron and copper more readily than with redox-inactive metal zinc. Therefore, curcumin treatment may prevent iron- and copper-induced aggregation of Aβ1–42 peptides, their deposition, and toxicity.[95] Using human neuroblastoma cells in culture and rat primary culture of hippocampal neurons, it was shown that treatment with heme inhibited the aggregation of Aβ40 in the presence of Cu^{2+} and protected nerve cells from cell death.[96]

Soluble Aβ oligomers (AβO) trigger increased levels of oxidative stress and endo-plasmic reticulum (ER) stress, and disrupts intracellular Ca^{2+} homeostasis and sig-naling leading to astrogliosis, a common neuropathological feature, in the brain of AD patients.[97] AβO interacts with GluN2B, a subunit of glutamate receptor, induces ER stress and NADPH oxidase-mediated superoxide production in mature neurons of hippocampus in culture.[98] These AβO-induced events lead to neuronal dysfunc-tion in the hippocampus. These results suggest that GluN2B plays an important role in ER stress-induced hippocampal dysfunction. The role of GluN2B in neurodegen-eration was further confirmed by the fact that ifenprodil, an antagonist of GluN2B subunit of glutamate receptor, prevented AβO-induced neurodegeneration. In mature hippocampal neurons in culture, it was demonstrate that AβO caused disassembly of microtubules and induced DNA fragmentation. AβO also has been implicated in degeneration of the synapses.[99]

The aggregated form of beta-amyloid participates in the formation of senile plaque, which can serve as a chronic source of inflammatory reactions, the products of which can enhance the progression of degeneration in nerve cells.

Aβ1–42 PEPTIDE-INDUCED FREE RADICALS

It has been proposed that one of the mechanisms of action of beta-amyloid-induced neurotoxicity is mediated by free radicals.[84,87,100] This is supported by the fact that vitamin E protects neuronal cells in culture against beta-amyloid-induced toxicity.[101] It has been shown that methionine in the 35 position of beta-amyloid may be respon-sible for generating free radicals.[102] This was confirmed by a series of studies on substitutions of amino acid[102] and by prevention of beta-amyloid-induced toxicity with vitamin E.[101] RBCs bind with Aβ peptides which can trigger increased oxida-tive stress that could impair delivery of oxygen to the brain tissue. The binding of Cu with Aβ (CuAβ) caused aggregation of Aβ peptides which generate excessive amounts of free radicals that cause increased oxidation of hemoglobin.[103] These data suggest that CuAβ promotes vascular oxidative stress that causes decrease in oxygen delivery to the brain causing neurodegeneration in AD.

CHOLESTEROL-INDUCED GENERATION OF BETA-AMYLOIDS

Epidemiologic studies have found that hypercholesterolemia may be a risk factor in the development of AD.[104,105] This was confirmed in the transgenic animal model of AD.[105] The results of study on animal AD model revealed that high dietary cho-lesterol increases beta-amyloid accumulation and thereby accelerates AD-related pathology in animals.[106] The accumulation of beta-amyloids can be reversed by removing cholesterol from the rabbit's diet.[106] Inhibitors of 3-hydroxy-3-methyl-glutaryl-coenzyme A (HMG CoA) reductase, which reduce cholesterol, decrease production of beta-amyloids in rabbit[105] and in fetal rat hippocampal neurons in culture.[107] An epidemiologic study has shown that lovastatin, an inhibitor of HMG CoA reductase, reduced the risk of AD in hypercholesterolemic patients.[108] In an epidemiologic study, the use of statins, but not of non-statin cholesterol-lowering drugs, was associated with the reduced incidence of AD in comparison to those who never took statins.[109] These results suggest that lower levels of cholesterol may reduce the risk of AD and that some of the effects of high cholesterol levels are primarily mediated via increased production of beta-amyloids which cause degeneration of neurons by increasing oxidative stress.

Statins (cholesterol-lowering drugs) can be divided into two distinct groups, those with a closed-ring structure (lovastatin, simvastatin, and mevastatin) and those with an open-ring structure (pravastatin and fluvastatin). Statins with a closed-ring structure are metabolized *in vivo* to an open-ring structure which then inhibits HMG CoA reductase activity. However, a small amount of the drug could be maintained in a closed-ring structure which can inhibit proteasome activity.[110] We have demonstrated that mevastatin with a closed-ring structure caused rapid degeneration of differentiated neuroblastoma (NB) cells in culture, whereas pravastatin with an open-ring structure did not.[111] Mevastatin inhibited proteasome activity in differentiated NB, whereas pravastatin did not. Differentiated NB cells did not convert any portion of mevastatin into an open-ring structure. This is in sharp contrast to the observation made *in vivo* where most mevastatin is converted to an open-ring structure by the liver enzyme. These results suggest that mevastatin-induced degeneration of differentiated NB cells may be related to inhibition of proteasome activity.[111] The studies discussed in this section reveal that lowering cholesterol levels could reduce the risk of AD, whereas the presence of increased amounts of unmetabolized statin with a closed-ring structure could increase the risk of AD. A careful study on the effects of statins with a closed-ring and an open-ring structure on neuroprotection and neurodegeneration should be evaluated by laboratory experiments and epidemiologic studies before their relevance in AD can be determined.

MUTATED APP, PRESENILIN-1, AND PRESENILIN-2 GENES CAUSE INCREASED PRODUCTION OF BETA-AMYLOIDS

In some familial AD, mutations (about 7) in the APP gene have been reported, all of which increase the production of beta-amyloids[112]; however, this accounts for less than 1% of all familial AD. Mutations (about 50) in presenilin-1 gene have been found in about 50% of familial AD; whereas mutations in presenilin-2 have been observed in less than 1% of familial AD. Presenilin-1 is present in senile plaques and NTFs of AD brains.

Mutations in APP and presenilin-1 increase the production of beta-amyloids that causes neuronal death via increasing oxidative stress in primary neuronal cultures obtained from knock-in mice expressing mutant human APP and presenilin-1 in comparison to those obtained from wild-type mice.[42] The levels of oxidative damage as a function of age was more pronounced in knock-in mice expressing mutant human APP and presenilin-1 genes in comparison to those observed in wild-type mice.[113] This effect was independent of dietary cholesterol.[114] It has been reported that mutations in presenilin-1 may increase neuronal sensitivity to apoptosis by decreasing the levels of beta-catenin, which is involved in regulation of apoptosis.[115] Mutation in presenilin-1 increased the activity of gamma-secretase that increases the production of beta-amyloids.[116]

Mutation in the gamma-secretase gene results in rare forms of early onset of AD due to production of increased amounts of beta-amyloids.[117] The activity of gamma-secretase increases as a function of age in female mice[117] that may in part be responsible for the relatively increased incidence of AD commonly observed in women.

These studies suggest that mutations in APP, presenilin-1, presenilin-2, and gamma-secretase genes increase the rate of production of beta-amyloids. Excessive production of beta-amyloids can generate more free radicals, inhibit proteasome activity, and contribute to the formation of senile plaques, all of which contribute to progressive neurodegeneration and finally death of neurons in AD brain.

INCREASED LEVELS OF MARKERS OF CHRONIC INFLAMMATION IN AD

Evidence of chronic inflammatory reactions in the autopsied brain samples from patients with AD was first observed by Dr. Alois Alzheimer himself. The role of chronic inflammation in AD pathogenesis is supported by the epidemiologic studies which show that rheumatoid arthritis patients, who were on high doses of non-steroidal anti-inflammatory drugs (NSAIDs), had a reduced incidence of AD.[118,119] The direct evidence came from the studies in which it was demonstrated that the products of chronic inflammatory reaction, such as cytokines,[120] complement proteins,[121,122] free radicals,[123-125] adhesion molecules,[126,127] and prostaglandins[128] were toxic in experimental models of neurons.

Increased levels of pro-inflammatory cytokines such as IL-1 beta and TNF-alpha are found in the autopsied samples of brains of AD patients.[129] There appears to be close interaction between beta-amyloids and pro-inflammatory cytokines with respect to production and levels of beta-amyloids and beta-amyloid-induced neurotoxicity. Beta-amyloid-induced inflammatory responses and vascular disruption in AD brain are mediated through TNF-alpha and IL-1 beta.[130,131] In wild-type mice, the levels of beta-amyloids can be enhanced by INF-gamma and TNF-alpha through suppression of degradation of beta-amyloids. TNF-alpha also enhanced the levels of beta-amyloids by stimulating the activity of beta-secretase, a rate-limiting enzyme in the production of beta-amyloids.[131] The combination of INF-gamma and TNF-alpha increased the production of beta-amyloids and reduced the secretion of nontoxic soluble APP fragments in human neuronal cells in culture.[132] Beta-amyloid-induced toxicity can be enhanced by IL-1beta and TNF-alpha.[130] Interferon-gamma, IL-1beta, and TNF-alpha increase the activity of gamma-secretase and production of beta-amyloids via JNK-dependent mitogen-activated protein kinase pathway.[133]

Both beta-amyloids and glutamate receptor NMDA interact with each other in causing neuronal damage. Individually, beta-amyloids and NMDA produced neuronal damage, whereas IL-6, a pro-inflammatory cytokines, did not.[134] The combination of beta-amyloids and NMDA was more effective than the individual agents in causing neuronal damage. However, the combination of three (beta-amyloids, NMDA, and IL-6) was most effective in causing damage to neurons.[134] It appears that the combination of beta-amyloids and NMDA caused the increased production of reactive oxygen species in cortical neurons through activation of NADPH oxidase,[135] suggesting the involvement of NMDA receptor subtype in the mechanisms of damage produced by beta-amyloids.

The role of inflammatory reactions in AD pathogenesis was further supported by clinical studies in which administration of NSAIDs reduced the rate of deterioration of cognitive function in moderate to advanced AD patients.[136–138] However, a clinical study with new NSAIDS (celecoxib or naproxen) in men and women aged 70 years or more with a familial history of AD revealed that these drugs did not improve cognitive function, but a detrimental effect of naproxen was observed.[139] In another clinical trial the effect of ibuprofen on sources of resting electroencephalographic (EEG) rhythms in mild AD patients was evaluated. The results showed that in the placebo group, amplitude of delta sources was globally greater at follow up than the baseline; however, the amplitude of delta sources remained stable or decreased in the majority of patients receiving ibuprofen.[140] It has been reported that NSAIDs such as ibuprofen, aspirin, indomethacin, and naproxen inhibit to a varying degree formation of beta-amyloid fibrils and destabilize preformed beta-amyloid fibrils *in vitro*.[141] Ibuprofen reduced the levels of beta-amyloids and hyperphosphorylated tau protein and improved memory deficits in AD transgenic mice.[142]

There appears to be strong evidence to suggest that increased oxidative stress and chronic inflammation play an important role in the pathogenesis of idiopathic AD; however, in familial AD, chronic inflammation may play a minor role in the initiation of AD. This is due to the fact that mutations in APP, presenilin-1, or presenilin-2 that are found in familial AD increase production of beta-amyloids which mediate its action through free radicals.[42,112,113] Most studies with NSAID on patients with idiopathic AD reported some beneficial effects.[136,137,143] However, a study with NSAID on patients with familial AD reported no beneficial effect.[139] This result may not be surprising, because in familial AD, excessive production of beta-amyloids that mediate their action through free radicals causes neurodegeneration, and inflammation may not play any significant role in the development of AD.

Prostaglandin E2 (PGE2)-induced neurotoxicity is mediated through its receptor EP3. It was demonstrated that deletion of EP3 receptor reduced pro-inflammatory gene expression, cytokine production, and oxidative stress in a model of Aβ42-induced neuroinflammation.[144] This observation was confirmed in transgenic AD mice (APPSwe-PS1ΔE9) in which deletion of EP3 receptor reduced induction of pro-inflammatory gene and protein expression and lipid peroxidation as well as Aβ peptides.

P-TAU PROTEIN IN AD

Tau is a microtubule-binding protein and a major component of NFT which is found in AD brain neurons. Increased oxidative stress causes hyperphosphorylation of tau in transgenic AD mice (Tg2576). This hyperphosphorylation of tau was prevented by high doses of antioxidants.[145] It has been shown that an increase in beta-amyloids precedes tau pathology (hyperphosphorylation of tau and formation of NTFs) in the frontal cortex.[146] It is present in axons as well as in presynaptic and postsynaptic terminals of normal human brain; however, in AD, tau becomes hyperphosphorylated and misfolded at both presynaptic and postsynaptic terminals. The accumulation of hyperphosphorylated tau oligomers at the synapses is associated with the inhibition of ubiquitin-proteasome system, and it disrupts synaptic function.[147] P-tau in aggregated and oligomer forms disrupts microtubules causing impairment of axoplasmic flow that leads to slow progressive retrograde degeneration and loss of connectivity of neurons.[148]

The activity of protein phosphatase-2A (PP-2A) is decreased in AD brain causing hyperphosphorylation of tau. Zinc (Zn) is widely distributed in the brain but accumulated in AD affected areas of brain more than in other areas. It has been reported that Zn inhibited PP-2A activity and caused hyperphosphorylation of tau protein in rat brain and in neurons in culture.[149] Chelation of Zn completely prevented Zn-induced hyperphosphorylation of tau.

It has been shown that iron interacts with hyperphosphorylated tau that contributes to the formation of NFT. Treatment with high doses of iron markedly increased the levels of phosphorylation of tau. Intranasal administration of deferoxamine (DFO), an iron chelator, abolished the above effect of iron in transgenic AD mice (APP/PS1). DFO has been shown to slow down the clinical progression of cognitive dysfunction in AD patients.[150]

Tau pathology, which requires at least two steps, hyperphosphorylation and accumulation of hyperphosphorylated tau, occurs later than increased generation of beta-amyloids. Hyperphosphorylation of tau (P-tau) can result from increased PKA activity or decreased phosphatase activity. Proteasome inhibition may also reduce degradation of hyperphosphorylated tau proteins, causing them to slowly accumulate and lead to the formation of NFTs within the cells. It has been reported that intraneuronal tau inclusions (NFT) appear decades before the deposition of Aβ plaques.[151] However, increases in Aβ peptides occur before the elevation of phosphorylated tau which becomes apparent with the progression of clinical symptoms of AD.

Several studies have shown that aggregated tau oligomers are also toxic to neurons; therefore, it was suggested that they can be targets for developing immunotherapy for AD.[152] A novel positron emission tomography (PET) imaging agent[18] (F-T807) to detect the presence of P-tau has been developed.[153] This technique would be very valuable in defining the role of P-tau in neurodegeneration and cognitive dysfunction.

White matter lesions are commonly found in the brain of patients with dementia. The follow up of 159 patients with APOE genotype for 5.7 years showed that 59 developed AD.[154] Patients without APOE4 alleles had more white matter lesions than those with at least one APOE4 allele. Furthermore, patients with MCI who had pathological levels of P-tau and parietal white matter lesions showed higher risk of developing AD than those who had one of the two pathological features. These data suggest that P-tau and white matter lesions have independent but synergic effect on the early development of AD.

In addition to hyperphosphorylation of tau, acetylation of tau at lysine residue 280 occurs. Acetylated tau is present within the neuron of hippocampus of patients with AD. The distribution pattern of acetylated tau is similar to that of P-tau, and it is present in all stages of the disease. However, it is markedly elevated at the advanced stage of the disease when levels of P-tau are also elevated.[155] Thus, it appears that acetylation of tau also participate in the progression of AD.

PROTEASOME INHIBITION-INDUCED NEURODEGENERATION IN AD

Proteasome plays an important role in regulating certain transcriptional factors by splicing inactive peptide fragments into active ones. In addition, proteasome also play a crucial role in the degradation of ubiquitin-conjugated abnormal proteins that could be toxic to neurons. Therefore, inhibition of proteasome in neurons can promote neurodegeneration. Indeed, the role of proteasome inhibition has been proposed for the degeneration of neurons in AD brain.[156,157] In our study, inhibition of proteasome by lactacystin causes rapid degeneration of neuronal cells in culture.[158] Several factors can inhibit proteasome activity. They include increased oxidative stress, defects in ubiquitin conjugate enzymes,[159] mutation in ubiquitin,[160] and APP.[156] The exact mechanisms of proteasome inhibition in AD neurons are unknown, but increased oxidative stress may be one of the earliest events in inhibition of proteasome activity.

GENETIC DEFECTS IN IDIOPATHIC AD

APOLIPOPROTEIN E

Apolipoprotein E (APOE) is present in the high-density lipoprotein-like particles in the brain and appears to be involved in various protective functions including cholesterol transport, anti-inflammation, and antioxidant. Administration of an APOE mimetic peptide (Ac-hE18A-NH2) in transgenic AD mice (human APP/PS1ΔE9) for a period of 6 weeks improved cognitive function, reduced amyloid plaque deposition, and activated microglia and astrocytes. APOE mimetic peptide also reduced oxidative stress-induced APOE secretion.[161] These results suggest that high levels of APOE in the brain could reduce the development of AD.

Several studies have suggested that persons who are homozygous for the APOE4 allele develop AD 10–20 years earlier than those who have APOE2 allele or APOE3 allele.[162,163] Even persons who are heterozygous for APOE4 allele develop AD 5–10 years earlier than those who have APOE2 allele or APOE3 allele.[164] About 40% of idiopathic AD is associated with the presence of APOE4 allele, and it is present in the senile plaque.[164] These data suggest that the presence of APOE4 allele could be an important risk factor for developing AD.

In a clinical study on 63 patients with AD, 58 patients with mild cognitive impairment and 20 nondemented subjects, the effect of APOE4 allele on the relation between cognitive decline and CSF levels of F2-isoprostanes, a marker of oxidative stress, was determined. The results showed that in patients carrying APOE4 allele, annual increase in the levels of F2-isoprostanes was greater than in APOE4 allele noncarriers. Increase in F2-isoprostane levels was associated with enhanced cognitive dysfunction compared to that in APOE4 allele noncarriers. These studies further suggest the importance of oxidative stress in initiation and progression of AD.[165] APOE4 allele also stimulated the accumulation of Aβ peptides and P-tau and reduced the levels of presynaptic glutamatergic vesicular transporter (VGlut).[166]

DEFECTS IN OTHER GENES

Some studies have identified two additional gene defects in idiopathic AD. Mutation in the ubiquitin gene and downregulation of presenilin-2 were observed in AD brains.[167] We have shown that differentiated neuronal cells in culture overexpressing human APP become sensitive to neurotoxin including oxidative stress.[168]

The genetic polymorphisms play an important role in determining the risk of AD in some populations.[169] The levels of beta-secretase, a rate-limiting enzyme in formation of beta-amyloid, were elevated in the autopsied samples of AD brain.[170] Elevated levels of beta-secretase increase generation of Aβ1–42 from APP.

Calcineurin-1(RCAN-1) gene encodes three different protein isoforms which include RCAN1-4, RCAN-1-1L, and RCAN-1-1S. The isoform RCAN-1-IL is expressed predominantly in human brain. It has been demonstrated that short-term exposure of human neuroblastoma cells in culture to elevated levels of RCAN-1-1L protected these cells against oxidative stress-induced apoptosis by inhibiting caspase-3 activity. However, long-term exposure of neuroblastoma cells to RCAN-1-1L caused oxidative stress-apoptosis by activating caspase-3.[171] In addition, elevated levels of RCAN-1-1L were present in the brains of patients with AD and Down syndrome. Thus, increased levels of RCAN-1-1L appear to be involved in pathogenesis of AD.

NEUROGLOBIN

Neuroglobin (Ngb) is O_2-binding heme protein related to hemoglobin and myoglobin. It is widely and specifically located in neurons of central and peripheral nervous system of vertebrates. It reversibly binds with oxygen with a high affinity. Overexpression of wild type of Ngb in neuronal cells in culture (PC-12 cell line) decreased H_2O_2-induced free radical accumulation and lipid peroxidation without changing the levels of antioxidant enzymes.[172] It also reduced H_2O_2-induced mitochondrial dysfunction and improved the survival of cells. It has been reported that Ngb also protected neurons against beta-amyloid-induced toxicity in PC-12 neuronal cell line[173] and in murine cortical neurons in culture.[174] Ngb also attenuates the AD phenotype of transgenic mice.[175] Using transgenic AD mouse models (Tg2576 mice and TgMAPt mice); it was shown that Ngb may decrease tau hyperphosphorylation through activating Akt signaling pathway.[176] Ngb also protects neurons by interfering with the apoptotic action of cytochrome C.[177] These studies suggest that Ngb reduces oxidative stress in neurons by acting as an antioxidant.

Age-dependent loss of Ngb was found in rat cerebral neocortex, hippocampus, caudate-putamen, and cerebellum.[178,179] It has been observed that Ngb expression is reduced with increasing age, and it is lower in women than in men.[175] The latter in part may account for the increased risk of AD in women.

NEUROPEPTIDE Y

Neuropeptide Y (NPY) is a 36-amino acid peptide widely distributed in the brain. This peptide has been implicated in regulating several functions including food intake, learning and memory, mood, and neuroprotection. It has been shown that pretreatment with NPY prevented Aβ1–40-induced depressive behavior and cognitive dysfunction by reducing oxidative stress in hippocampus without changing the activity of glutathione peroxidase or glutathione levels.[180]

PARKIN GENE

Parkin gene (Parkinson protein 2, E3 ubiquitin protein ligase) is considered neuroprotective. Mutation in this gene causes Parkinson's disease. Delivery of parkin directly into the brain prevented Aβ1–42-induced AD phenotypes and disturbance in brain metabolism.[181]

The studies discussed above strongly suggest that increased oxidative stress play a central role in the initiation and progression of damage; therefore, inhibiting oxidative stress may reduce the risk of developing AD. Because of complexity of regulation of oxidative stress in humans, it is not possible to reduce oxidative stress optimally by the use of a single antioxidant for the prevention of AD.

HOW TO REDUCE OXIDATIVE STRESS OPTIMALLY

Oxidative stress in the body occurs when the antioxidant system fails to provide adequate protection against damage produced by free radicals (reactive oxygen species and reactive nitrogen species). Increased oxidative stress in the body is reduced by upregulating antioxidant enzymes as well as by existing levels of dietary and endogenous antioxidant chemicals, because they work by different mechanisms. For example, antioxidant enzymes reduce free radicals by catalysis, whereas dietary and endogenous antioxidant chemicals reduce free radicals by directly scavenging them. In response to ROS, a nuclear transcriptional factor, Nrf2 (nuclear factor-erythroid 2-related factor 2) is translocated from the cytoplasm to the nucleus where it binds with ARE (antioxidant response element) which increases the levels of antioxidant enzymes (gamma-glutamylcysteine ligase, glutathione peroxidase, glutathione reductase, and heme oxygenase-1) and phase 2 detoxifying enzymes (NADPH) quinine oxidoreductase 1 and glutathione-S-transferase) in order to reduce oxidative damage.[182–184] In response to increased oxidative stress, existing levels of dietary and endogenous antioxidant chemicals levels cannot be elevated without supplementation.

FACTORS REGULATING RESPONSE OF NRF2

Antioxidant enzymes are elevated by activation of Nrf2 which depends upon ROS-dependent and -independent mechanisms. In addition, elevated levels of antioxidant enzymes are also dependent upon the binding ability of Nrf2 with ARE in the nucleus. These studies are described here.

ROS-Dependent Regulation of Nrf2

Normally, Nrf2 is associated with Kelch-like ECH associated protein 1 (Keap1) protein which acts as an inhibitor of Nrf2 (INrf2).[185] INrf2 protein serves as an adaptor to link Nrf2 to the ubiquitin ligase CuI-Rbx1 complex for degradation by proteasomes and maintains the steady levels of Nrf2 in the cytoplasm. INrf2 acts as a sensor for ROS/electrophilic stress. In response to increased ROS, Nrf2 dissociates itself from INrf2- CuI-Rbx1 complex and translocates into the nucleus where it binds with ARE that increases antioxidant genes. It has been demonstrated that Nrf2 regulates INrf2 levels by controlling its transcription, whereas INrf2 regulates Nrf2 levels by controlling its degradation by proteasome.[186]

ROS-Independent Regulation of Nrf2

Antioxidants such as vitamin E, genistein (a flavonoid),[187] allicin, a major organosulfur compound found in garlic,[188] sulforaphane, an organosulfur compound found in cruciferous vegetables,[189] kavalactones (methysticin, kavain, and yangonin),[190] and dietary restriction[191] activate Nrf2 without stimulation by ROS.

Reduced Binding of Nrf2 with ARE

Age-related decline in antioxidant enzymes in the liver of older rats compared to that in younger rats was due to reduction in the binding ability of Nrf2 with ARE; however, treatment with alpha-lipoic acid restored this defect, increased the levels of antioxidant enzymes, and restored the loss of glutathione from the liver of older rats.[192]

DIFFERENTIAL RESPONSE OF Nrf2 TO ROS STIMULATION DURING ACUTE AND CHRONIC OXIDATIVE STRESS

It appears that Nrf2 responds to ROS generated during acute and chronic oxidative stress differently. For example, acute oxidative stress during strenuous exercise translocates Nrf2 from the cytoplasm to the nucleus where it binds with ARE to upregulate antioxidant genes. However, during chronic oxidative stress commonly observed in older individuals and in neurodegenerative diseases, such as Parkinson's disease and Alzheimer's disease, Nrf2/ARE pathway becomes unresponsive to ROS. A reduction in the binding ability of Nrf2 with ARE was demonstrated in older rats.[192] The reasons for Nrf2/ARE pathway to become unresponsive to ROS during chronic oxidative stress are unknown.

Nrf2 IN AD

The levels of nuclear Nrf2 decreased in the hippocampal neurons in AD cases despite increased oxidative stress.[193] This suggests that Nrf2/ARE pathway in AD becomes unresponsive to ROS stimulation or that Nrf2 binding ability with ARE is impaired. It is not known whether the defect in Nrf2 pathway occurs at the cytoplasm where Nrf2 forms a complex with INrf2 or at the level of nucleus where it binds with ARE to upregulate antioxidant genes or at both levels. Treatment with tert-butylhydroquinone, a known inducer of Nrf2, or with adenoviral Nrf2 gene transfer protected neurons against Aβ-induced toxicity in transgenic AD mice.[194] Therefore, the following groups of selected nontoxic agents in combination may be useful in reducing oxidative stress optimally:

1. *Agents that can reduce oxidative stress by directly scavenging free radicals*: Some examples are dietary antioxidants, such as vitamin A, beta-carotene, vitamin C, and vitamin E, and endogenous antioxidants, such as glutathione, alpha-lipoic acid, and coenzyme Q_{10}.
2. *Agents which can reduce oxidative stress by activating Nrf2-regulated antioxidant genes without ROS stimulation*: Some examples are organosulfur compound sulforaphane found in cruciferous vegetables, kavalactones, found in Kava shrubs, and Puerarin, a major flavonoid from the root of *Pueraria lobata*,[189,190,195] genistein and vitamin E,[187] and coenzyme Q_{10}[196] activate Nrf2 without ROS stimulation.
3. *Agents which can reduce oxidative stress directly by scavenging free radicals as well as indirectly by activating Nrf2/ARE pathway*: Some examples are vitamin E,[187] alpha-lipoic acid,[192] curcumin,[197] resveratrol,[198,199] omega-3-fatty acids,[200,201] and N-acetylcysteine (NAC).[202]
4. *Agents reducing oxidative stress by ROS-dependent mechanism*: They include L-carnitine which generates transient ROS.[203]

Treatment of primary culture of hippocampal neurons with Puerarin, a major flavonoid from the root of *Pueraria lobata*, significantly reduced beta-amyloid-induced oxidative stress by activating Nrf2/ARE pathway.[195] Genistein, a flavonoid, and vitamin E reduced oxidative damage produced by beta-amyloids (Aβ25–35) in transformed cerebrovascular mouse endothelial cells in culture by activating Nrf2-regulated antioxidant genes.[187]

A study on the aged mouse hippocampus revealed that supplementation with allicin, a major organosulfur compound found in garlic, which has an electrophilic center (electron deficient), prevented age-related decline in cognitive function. This effect of allicin was due to enhancement of antioxidant enzymes via Nrf2/ARE pathway.[188] This study suggests that INrf2/Nrf2 complex and binding of Nrf2 with ARE remain responsive to allicin. Repeated administration of another organosulfur compound sulforaphane, found in cruciferous vegetables, simulated Nrf2-dependent increase of Nqo1 gene which codes for NADPH: quinone oxidoreductase, and Hmox1 gene which codes for HO-1 enzyme in astrocytes in culture, and reduced oxidative damage.[189] It is also possible that sulforaphane-induced activation of Nrf2 does not require ROS stimulation. Indeed, kavalactones (methysticin, kavain, and yangonin)-induced activation of Nrf2 is not dependent upon ROS stimulation in neuronal cells and astroglia cells in culture.[190]

In a study on murine alveolar cells in culture, NAC, which directly scavenges free radicals via increasing intracellular glutathione levels, requires the presence of Nrf2 for an optimal reduction in oxidative stress.[204] For example, cigarette smoking produces greater damage in alveolar cells obtained from Nrf2-deleted mice (Nrf2$^{-/-}$)

than in cells obtained from wild-type mice.[204] Pretreatment of alveolar cells with NAC reduced cigarette smoke-induce damage more in cells obtained from the wild-type mice than in cells from Nrf2-deleted mice. In other studies on rat liver, pretreatment with NAC prevents the ROS-induced activation of Nrf2.[205] If NAC scavenge all ROS, then ROS was not available for activating Nrf2/ARE pathway.

LABORATORY AND CLINICAL STUDIES WITH ANTIOXIDANTS IN AD

Considering the complexity involved in reducing oxidative stress in humans, it is not possible to hypothesize that use of a single antioxidant or polyphenolic compound would reduce oxidative stress optimally. Nevertheless, most laboratory and human studies have utilized a single antioxidant for reducing oxidative stress in AD. These studies are described here.

ALPHA-LIPOIC ACID

The natural form of alpha-lipoic acid (R-LA) is more effective than the synthetic form (Rac-LA); however, the salt form of alpha-lipoic acid is absorbed better than R-LA or Rac-LA.[206] The orally administered alpha-lipoic acid crosses the blood brain barrier in rats.[207]

In an open-label study involving 43 patients with mild to moderate AD receiving standard therapy and follow-up period of 48 months, it was observed that the addition of alpha-lipoic acid to the treatment protocol reduced the progression of the disease.[208] This effect was more pronounced in patients with mild AD than those with moderate AD. The fibroblasts from AD patients exhibited the highest levels of oxidative damage markers in comparison to fibroblasts from age-matched and young control; however, treatment with alpha-lipoic acid and n-acetylcysteine individually reduced the levels of markers of oxidative damage, but the combination of two was more effective than the individual agents.[209] Alpha-lipoic acid also reduced beta-amyloid-induced toxicity in neuronal cells in culture.[210]

In a mouse model of AD, administration of alpha-lipoic acid through diet reduced oxidative damage but did not improve cognitive performance or the levels of beta-amyloids.[211] Chronic administration of alpha-lipoic acid through diet reduced hippocampal-dependent memory deficits of a transgenic mice model of cerebral amyloidosis associated with AD.[212] Pretreatment of transgenic AD mice (senescence accelerated mouse prone 8 [SAMP8]) with alpha-lipoic acid improved cognitive function and learning ability by increasing glutathione levels and glutathione peroxidase activity and decreasing MDA levels.[213] Dietary supplementation with a combination of alpha-lipoic acid, acetyl-L-carnitine, glycerophosphocoline, docosahexaenoic acid, and phosphatidylserine reduced oxidative damage in murine brain and improved cognitive performance.[214] Treatment with a new conjugate molecule of ibuprofen-lipoic acid upregulated neuroglobin which decreased neuronal loss in transgenic AD model rats.[215]

The proposed mechanisms by alpha-lipoic acid include the following: (a) increasing acetylcholine production by enhancing choline acetyltransferase activity,

(b) chelating redox active transient metals, (c) scavenging free radicals, and (d) increasing glutathione levels.[216] In addition, alpha-lipoic acid also reduces the expression of proinflammatory cytokines, such as TNF-alpha and inducible nitric oxide synthase (iNOS).[217] The protective effect of alpha-lipoic acid may also be mediated through activation of protein kinase B (PKB)/Akt signaling pathway.[210] These studies suggest that treatment with alpha-lipoic acid alone produced consistent beneficial effects in animal models of AD. The effectiveness of alpha-lipoic acid in human AD has not been adequately investigated.

Coenzyme Q_{10}

Coenzyme Q_{10} reduced beta-amyloid overproduction and intracellular deposit of beta-amyloids in the cortex of the AD transgenic mice.[218] In addition, coenzyme Q_{10} treatment decreased MDA levels and enhanced the activity of superoxide dismutase in these mice. Coenzyme Q_{10} also prevented the formation of beta-amyloid fibrils and destabilized preformed beta-amyloid.[219] It decreased beta-amyloid-induced mitochondrial dysfunction *in vitro*.[220] Serum levels of coenzyme Q_{10} did not change in patients with AD.[221] It has been reported that supplementation with both coenzyme Q_{10} and alpha-tocopheryl acetate improved age-related learning deficits in mice.[222]

Melatonin

Melatonin treatment increased the levels of thiobarbituric acid reactive substances (TBARS), superoxide dismutase activity, glutathione levels, and upregulated apoptotic-related factors such as BAX, caspase-3, and prostate apoptosis response-4 (Par-4) in AD transgenic mice.[223] Long-term melatonin treatment improves cognitive function in AD transgenic mice. The mechanisms of this protection by melatonin involve preventing aggregation of beta-amyloids, reducing the levels of proinflammatory cytokines, and oxidative stress.[224] Patients with AD often exhibit both agitated behavior and poor sleep patterns. In a clinical study, supplementation with melatonin failed to affect these abnormal symptoms in AD patients compared to a placebo group.[225] However, melatonin in combination with standard therapy produced beneficial effects on cognitive function and depression tests more than that produced by standard therapy alone.[226] These studies suggest that treatment with coenzyme Q_{10} or melatonin alone does not produce consistent results in patients with AD.

Nicotinamide and Nicotinamide Adenine Dinucleotide Dehydrogenase

Histone deacetylase inhibitors increase histone acetylation and enhance memory and neuronal plasticity. Nicotinamide (vitamin B_3), a competitive inhibitor of Class III NAD$^+$-dependent histone deacetylase activity, restored memory deficits in AD transgenic mice.[227] In addition, it selectively reduced a specific phospho-species of tau protein (Thr231) that is associated with microtubule depolymerization. The overexpression of a Thr231-phospho-mimic tau in neuronal cells in culture increased clearance and decreased accumulation of tau compared with wild-type tau. Nicotinamide, a precursor of nicotinamide adenine dinucleotide (NAD$^+$), also attenuated glutamate-induced toxicity and preserved cellular levels of NAD⁺ to support the activity of silent information regulator-1 (SIRT1).[228] Treatment with nicotinamide reduced oxidative stress-induced mitochondrial dysfunction and restored defective autophagy function in neurons in culture. In addition, treatment of transgenic AD model mice (3xTg) with nicotinamide improved cognitive function and reduced the levels of Aβ peptides and hyperphosphorylated tau and their associated neurodegeneration.[229] These preclinical data suggest that oral supplementation with nicotinamide may be safe and useful in the prevention and improved treatment of AD and other taupathies. Thus, addition of nicotinamide to a preparation of micronutrient may be necessary in order to prevent and/or reduce the progression of AD in an effective manner.

It has been reported that administration of nicotinamide adenine dinucleotide dehydrogenase (NADH) (10 mg/day) improved cognitive function in AD patients.[230] In older rats, administration of NADH improved cognitive function.[231] However, further clinical studies with NADH in patients with AD did not show any improvement in cognitive function but did not allow progressive cognitive deterioration in comparison to placebo control. NADH treated patients showed significantly better performance on measures of verbal fluency, visual-constructional ability, and abstract verbal reasoning.[232] In another study, supplementation with NADH had no effect on cognitive function in patients with mild to moderate AD.[233]

VITAMIN A AND BETA-CAROTENE

Vitamin A and beta-carotene inhibited formation of beta-amyloid fibrils in a dose-dependent manner. They also destabilized preformed beta-amyloid fibrils *in vitro*.[234] Retinoic acid treatment decreased activation of microglia and astrocytes, reduced degeneration of neurons, and improved spatial learning and memory in AD transgenic mice compared with the vehicle controls.[235] It also downregulated the activity of cyclin-dependent kinase 5, a major kinase, involved in both APP and tau phosphorylation. Like vitamin A and beta-carotene, curcumin also inhibited formation of beta-amyloid fibrils and destabilized preformed beta-amyloid fibrils *in vitro* in a dose-dependent manner.[234] Vitamin E and pycnogenol protected neuronal cells in culture against beta-amyloid-induced apoptosis by attenuating caspase-3 activation, DNA fragmentation, and cleavage of poly (ADP-ribose) polymerase (PARP).[236]

VITAMIN E

Vitamin E treatment protected cortical synaptosomal membranes and hippocampal neurons[102] and other neurons[101] in culture against beta-amyloid-induced toxicity. In AD transgenic mice, it was shown that vitamin E supplementation reduced the levels and deposits of beta-amyloids in the brain; however, vitamin E supplementation was ineffective in decreasing the levels and deposits of beta-amyloids in older mice.[237]

Plasma phospholipid transfer protein (PLTP) transfers vitamin E from the plasma to the cells. Deficiency of PLTP in mice caused reduction in the levels of vitamin E in the brain. Deletion of PLTP caused increased oxidative stress, Aβ1–42 levels, and decreased synaptic function in mice. Administration of AβO (Aβ25–35) intracerebroventricularly increased cognitive dysfunction in PLTP-deleted mice. Supplementation with vitamin E through diet prevented Aβ25–35 oligomers-induced memory deficits and reduced oxidative stress and degenerative changes in the brain.[238]

An analysis of clinical studies revealed that vitamin E alone may not be useful in the prevention or improved management of AD.[239,240] However, a controlled clinical trial with *dl*-alpha-tocopherol (synthetic form; 2000 IU/day) in AD patients with moderately impaired of cognitive function showed some beneficial effects with respect to the rate of deterioration of cognitive function.[241]

VITAMIN E AND VITAMIN C

In certain counties of North Carolina, analysis of older African-American and white individuals during 1986 to 2000 revealed that the supplemental use of vitamins was low; however, supplementation with vitamin C and/or vitamin E did not delay the incidence of AD or dementia in these populations.[242] In a prospective cohort study performed by Group Health Cooperative, Seattle, Washington, it was found that supplementation with vitamin E and vitamin C individually or in combination did not reduce the risk of developing AD or overall dementia over 5.5 years of an observation period.[243] In a cross-sectional and prospective study in elderly (65 years or older) patients with dementia, it was found that use of vitamin C and vitamin E in combination was associated with reduced prevalence and incidence of AD.[244] These studies suggest that treatment with one or two dietary antioxidants alone does not produce consistent results in reducing the risk of developing AD in humans.

SELENIUM

Selenoprotein M (SelM) is highly expressed in the human brain. Treatment with sodium selenite increased the expression of this protein which acts as an antioxidant.[245] SelM and Selenoprotein P (SelP-H) inhibited Zn^{2+}–Aβ42-induced aggregation and ROS production.[246] An aggregated form of Aβ peptides is toxic to nerve cells.

EDARAVONE

Edaravone (3-methyl-1-phenyl-2-pyrazolin-5-one) is a synthetic drug widely used for the treatment of cerebral infarction in Japan and other countries. Edaravone exhibits powerful antioxidant activity. Pretreatment of rat neuroblastoma cell (PC-12) with Edaravone increased glutathione levels and SOD activity and decreased MDA levels and Aβ aggregations after treatment with Aβ25–35.[247]

SERUM AND CSF LEVELS OF DIETARY ANTIOXIDANTS

In order to determine the antioxidant status in patients with AD, serum and CSF levels of dietary antioxidants were determined. The results showed that serum levels of vitamin E and beta-carotene were lower in patients with AD and multi-infarct dementia compared to controls.[58] In another study, serum levels of beta-carotene and vitamin A were lower in AD patients compared to control; however, the level of alpha-carotene did not change.[248] The average CSF and serum level of vitamin E was lower in patients with AD than controls.[249] The plasma levels of dietary antioxidants (vitamin A, vitamin C, vitamin E, and carotenoids including beta-carotene, alpha-carotene, lutein, zeaxanthin, and lycopene) and antioxidant enzymes (SOD and glutathione peroxidase) were lower in patients with AD as well as in elderly subjects with mild cognitive impairment compared to control subjects.[250] In another study, plasma vitamin C levels were lowered in subjects with dementia compared to controls, which was not due to reduced dietary intake of vitamin C.[251]

B VITAMINS

In most studies, the serum levels of vitamin B_{12} in AD patients were significantly lower than in controls, and this may in part contribute to degeneration of neurons.[252,253] Indeed, vitamin B_{12} supplementation increased choline acetyltransferase activity in cholinergic neurons of cats[254] and improved cognitive functions in AD patients.[255] An analysis of published data revealed that there was no adequate benefit from folic acid supplementation with or without vitamin B_{12} on cognitive function or mood of healthy elderly people[256]; however, in groups of healthy elderly people with high homocysteine levels, supplementation with folic acid for a period of 3 years was associated with significant improvement in global functioning, memory storage, and information processing speed. In addition, in a pilot study, it was observed that in patients with AD, supplementation with folic acid improved the efficacy of cholinesterase inhibitor.[256] In another multicenter clinical study, supplementation with folic acid, vitamin B_6, and vitamin B_{12} did not show any beneficial effects on cognitive function decline in individuals with mild to moderate AD.[257] Supplementation with vitamin B_{12} alone did not benefit cognitive or psychiatric symptoms in a vast majority of elderly patients with dementia having low serum vitamin B_{12} levels.[258] These studies suggest that treatment with one or more B vitamins alone does not produce consistent results in patients with AD.

POLYPHENOLIC COMPOUNDS

In addition to dietary and endogenous individual antioxidants, certain polyphenolic compounds also appear to be useful in prevention and reduction in the incidence of AD primarily in animal AD models. These studies are described here.

RESVERATROL

Resveratrol, a major polyphenol in red wine, exhibits neuroprotective effects *in vitro* and in animal models. Several epidemiologic studies suggest that the moderate consumption of red wine is associated with a lower incidence of AD and dementia in the general population.[259,260] Consumption of three servings of wine daily was associated with a lower risk of AD in elderly individuals without the APOE epsilon-4-allele.[261] Resveratrol protects neuronal cells in culture against beta-amyloid-induced toxicity. This protective effect is mediated through enhancing the intracellular levels of glutathione, an important antioxidant within the cells.[262] It also lowered the intracellular levels of beta-amyloids in neuronal cell lines by increasing the degradation of beta-amyloid by proteasome.[263] This protective mechanism of resveratrol was supported by the fact that a resveratrol-induced decrease in beta-amyloids was prevented by several selective inhibitors of proteasome and by siRNA-directed silencing of proteasome subunit beta5 activity.[263]

Resveratrol treatment also upregulated SIRT1 gene, a mammalian gene homologue of yeast silent information regulator-2 (SIRT2) gene, that attenuated neuronal degeneration and death in an animal model of AD.[264,265] Resveratrol treatment of mouse astrocytes reduced lipopolysaccharide (LPS)-induced inflammation by decreasing the production of nitric oxide, TNF-alpha, IL-6, IL-1beta, and C-reactive protein (CRP).[266]

CURCUMIN

Curcumin is a natural yellow pigment of turmeric which is widely used as a spice throughout the Indian subcontinent. It exhibits antioxidant and anti-inflammation activities. Curcumin inhibits aggregation of Aβ peptides *in vitro*. In animal models of AD, it reduced aggregation of Aβ peptides, formation of AβO, and tau phosphorylation. Curcumin prevented aluminum-induced aggregation of Aβ peptides and its toxicity on rat neuronal cells in culture.[267] Preparation of curcumin-liposome was very effective in reducing the aggregation of Aβ peptides and oligomeric Aβ.[268] Two clinical studies performed in USA and China revealed no beneficial effect of curcumin on cognitive function in AD patients compared to those AD patients who received placebo.[269]

GINKGO BILOBA AND OMEGA-3 FATTY ACIDS

In a randomized, double-blind, placebo-controlled clinical trial in community volunteers aged 75 years or more with normal cognition revealed that administration of *Ginkgo biloba* was not effective in reducing the incidence of AD or overall dementia.[270] Long-term consumption of *Ginkgo biloba* extract through diet lowered human APP levels by 50% compared to controls in the cortex but not in the hippocampal regions of the brain of AD transgenic mice.[271]

In a clinical study on patients with mild to moderate AD, supplementation with omega-3 fatty acids (1.7 g of docosahexaenoic acid and 0.6 g of eicosapentaenoic acid) did not delay the rate of cognitive decline; however, beneficial effects were observed in a small group of patients with very mild AD.[272] The analysis of published observational studies and clinical trials suggest that omega-3 fatty acids may slow down cognitive decline in elderly individuals without dementia, but it was ineffective in reducing the incidence of AD or dementia.[273] In the Canadian Study of Health and Aging (CSHA), there was no association between omega-3 fatty acids and the risk of dementia.[274] In a randomized, double-blind, placebo-controlled trial, supplementation with omega-3 fatty acids showed significant improvement in Alzheimer's Disease Assessment Scale (ADAS-cog) compared to placebo control in individuals with mild cognitive impairment; however, there was no significant difference in patients with AD.[275] These studies suggest that treatment with *Ginkgo biloba* or omega-3 fatty acids alone does not produce consistent beneficial effects in patients with AD.

GREEN TEA EPIGALLOCATECHIN-3-GALLATE AND CAFFEINE

Treatment of AD transgenic mice with green tea epigallocatechin-3-gallate (EGCG) improved cognitive function and reduced the levels of beta-amyloids and phosphorylated tau isoforms.[276] Pretreatment of transgenic (Tg) AD mice with green tea catechin (GTC) improved AD phenotypes in the brain and reduced $A\beta1$–42 production.[277] Long-term caffeine treatment decreased the production of beta-amyloids and improved cognitive function in AD transgenic mice; therefore, it was suggested that daily moderate consumption of caffeine may reduce the risk of AD.[278] These studies are not sufficient to recommend either EGCG or caffeine for reduction in the risk of developing AD.

GENISTEIN

Genistein is the main active ingredient of soybean isoflavone. Treatment with genistein prevents $A\beta25$–35-induced mitochondrial DNA damage in rat glioma cells (C-6) in culture[279] and oxidative damage in rat neuroblastoma cells.[280]

The studies with individual antioxidants and polyphenolic compounds showed some consistent beneficial effects in animal models of AD, but it failed to produce such effects in human AD.

PREVENTION OF AD

Before discussing the strategies for AD prevention, it is essential to define primary and secondary prevention. The purpose of primary prevention is to protect healthy individuals from developing AD. Individuals 65 years or older and individuals with a family history of AD who have not developed any clinical symptoms of AD are suitable for primary prevention studies. The purpose of secondary prevention is to stop or slow the progression of AD. Individuals who exhibit early signs of AD, but are not taking any medication, can be included in secondary prevention studies.

PRIMARY PREVENTION

In order to develop primary prevention strategies, it is essential to identify external risk factors that increase the risk of developing AD. Some human epidemiologic and animal studies have identified environment-, diet-, and lifestyle-related risk factors that alter the risk of developing AD. Agents which may increase the risk of AD include high consumption of aluminum from drinking water,[9] high fat/high cholesterol diet,[12] vitamin D deficiency,[10] cigarette smoking,[15] exposure to electromagnetic field,[18] and exposure to chronic noise.[21] Although there are no conclusive data on the effectiveness of the above external risk factors in increasing the risk of AD in humans, I would suggest that exposure to the above risk factors should be minimized for primary prevention of AD.

Agents which may reduce the risk of developing AD include exercise.[17] In addition, daily mental exercise may also reduce the risk of AD. It has been reported that high dietary intake of vitamin C and vitamin E may reduce the risk of AD, and among current cigarette smokers, the intake of beta-carotene and flavonoids may also decrease the risk of AD.[11] Although there are no conclusive data on the effectiveness of the above external risk factors in reducing the risk of AD in humans, I would suggest that adopting exercise and sufficient intake of dietary antioxidants may be a good approach for the primary prevention of AD. Since chronic oxidative stress and chronic inflammation are involved in the initiation of AD, the above recommendations may not be sufficient to reduce oxidative stress optimally. In order to reduce oxidative stress optimally, a combination of nontoxic agents which upregulate antioxidant enzymes through activating Nrf2/ARE pathway, and which directly scavenge free radicals, may be needed.

SECONDARY PREVENTION

In order to develop secondary prevention strategies, the recommendations proposed for primary prevention should be also applicable for secondary prevention. Since increased chronic inflammation is also involved in the progression of AD, low-dose aspirin in combination with standard care may be needed for reducing chronic inflammation optimally.

PROBLEMS OF USING A SINGLE NUTRIENT IN AD

Several studies showed beneficial effects of single antioxidants, B vitamins, omega-3 fatty acids, or herbal products alone in animal and cell culture models of AD; however, supplement with above individual agents did not produce expected beneficial effects in high-risk human populations or in patients with mild to moderate AD. The fact that the high-risk populations of most chronic diseases including AD have a high internal oxidative environment suggests that administration of individual agents with antioxidant activity would result in oxidation of these agents. It is well known that an oxidized antioxidant acts as a free radical and may not produce beneficial clinical outcomes. On the contrary, oxidized antioxidant is likely to increase the risk of chronic diseases after long-term consumption. Previous studies in other chronic diseases, such as beta-carotene in male heavy smokers for reducing the risk of lung cancer, vitamin E in AD for improving cognitive function, and vitamin E in Parkinson's disease (PD) for improving the symptoms and as expected, produced inconsistent results varying from no effect as in PD,[281] to modest beneficial[241] or no effects as in AD,[240] and harmful effects as in heavy male smokers.[282] Because of the failure to obtain consistent beneficial effects with individual agents, I recommend a preparation of micronutrients containing dietary and endogenous antioxidants, vitamin D, B vitamins, certain minerals and herbs (resveratrol and curcumin), and omega-3 fatty acids for reducing the risk of AD and for improving the efficacy of standard therapy in the management of AD.

RATIONALE FOR USING MULTIPLE MICRONUTRIENTS IN AD

The references for this section are described in a review.[1] The mechanisms of action of micronutrients and herbs in the proposed formulation are in part different; their distribution in various organs and cells, their affinity to various types of free radicals, and their biological half lives are different. Beta-carotene (BC) is more effective in quenching oxygen radicals than most other antioxidants. BC can perform certain biological functions that cannot be produced by its metabolite vitamin A and vice versa. It has been reported that BC treatment enhances the expression of the connexin gene which codes for a gap junction protein in mammalian fibroblasts in culture, whereas vitamin A treatment does not produce such an effect. Vitamin A can induce differentiation in certain normal and cancer cells, whereas BC and other carotenoids do not. Thus, BC and vitamin A have, in part, different biological functions in the body. The gradient of oxygen pressure varies within cells. Some antioxidants, such as vitamin E, are more effective as quenchers of free radicals in reduced oxygen pressure, whereas BC and vitamin A are more effective in higher atmospheric pressures. Vitamin C is necessary to protect cellular components in aqueous environments, whereas carotenoids and vitamins A and E protect cellular components in lipid environments. Vitamin C also plays an important role in maintaining cellular levels of vitamin E by recycling vitamin E radical (oxidized) to the reduced (antioxidant) form.

The form of vitamin E used in a preparation of micronutrients is also important. It has been established that d-alpha-tocopheryl succinate (vitamin E succinate) is the most effective form of vitamin E both *in vitro* and *in vivo*. This form of vitamin E is more soluble than alpha-tocopherol and enters cells more readily, and therefore, it is expected that vitamin E succinate would cross the blood-brain barrier in greater amounts than alpha-tocopherol. However, this idea has not yet been tested in animals or humans. We have reported that an oral ingestion of vitamin E succinate (800 IU/day) in humans increased plasma levels of not only alpha-tocopherol but also of vitamin E succinate, suggesting that a portion of this form of vitamin E can be absorbed from the intestinal tract before hydrolysis to alpha-tocopherol, provided that the plasma pool of alpha-tocopherol is saturated. This observation is important because the conventional assumption based on the studies in rodents has been that esterified forms of vitamin E such as alpha-tocopheryl succinate, alpha-tocopheryl nicotinate, and alpha-tocopheryl acetate, can be absorbed from the intestinal tract only after they are hydrolyzed to alpha-tocopherol. Our preliminary data showed that this assumption may not be true for the absorption of vitamin E succinate in humans provided that the plasma pool of alpha-tocopherol is saturated.

An endogenous antioxidant, glutathione, is effective in catabolizing H_2O_2 and anions. However, oral supplementation with glutathione failed to significantly increase plasma levels of glutathione in human subjects, suggesting that this tripeptide is completely hydrolyzed in the GI tract. Therefore, I propose to utilize N-acetylcysteine and alpha-lipoic acid that increase the cellular levels of glutathione by different mechanisms in a multiple micronutrient preparation.

Another endogenous antioxidant, coenzyme Q_{10}, may have some potential value in prevention and improved treatment of AD. Since mitochondrial dysfunction is associated with AD and since coenzyme Q_{10} is needed for the generation of ATP by mitochondria, it is essential to add this antioxidant in multiple micronutrient preparations. A study has shown that Ubiquinol (coenzyme Q_{10}) scavenges peroxy radicals faster than alpha-tocopherol, and like vitamin C, can regenerate vitamin E in a redox cycle. However, it is a weaker antioxidant than alpha-tocopherol. Coenzyme Q_{10} administration has been shown to improve clinical symptoms in patients with mitochondrial encephalomyopathies.[283]

Nicotinamide, a precursor of NAD^+, also attenuated glutamate-induced toxicity and preserved cellular levels of NAD^+ to support the activity of SIRT1. It is also a competitive inhibitor of histone deacetylase activity and restored memory deficits in AD transgenic mice. These preclinical data suggest that oral supplementation with nicotinamide may be safe and useful in the prevention and improved treatment of AD.

Selenium is a cofactor of glutathione peroxidase, and Se-glutathione peroxidase acts as an antioxidant by increasing the intracellular level of glutathione. There may be some other mechanisms of selenium. Therefore, selenium should be added to a multiple micronutrient preparation for prevention and in combination with standard care, for improved management of AD.

In addition to dietary and endogenous antioxidants, B vitamins, especially high doses of vitamin B_3 (nicotinamide), should be added to a multiple micronutrient preparation. B vitamins are also essential for normal health. Curcumin and resveratrol were added because of their effectiveness in laboratory experiments, using transgenic AD animal models. Omega-3 fatty acids were also added because it reduced AD phenotypes in the brain of AD animal models, and most clinical studies show some benefits in patients with AD.

Two recent studies of supplementation with multiple vitamin preparations reduced cancer incidence by 10 percent in men[284] and improved clinical outcomes in patients with HIV/AIDS who were not taking medication.[285]

RATIONAL FOR USING LOW-DOSE NSAID IN AD PREVENTION

Since inflammatory reactions represent one of the major factors that initiate and promote neurodegeneration in AD brain, the use of NSAIDs in the prevention and treatment of AD appears to be one of the rationale approaches. Laboratory, epidemiological, and clinical studies support this recommendation. Laboratory data have shown that products of inflammatory reactions such as prostaglandins,[128] cytokines,[120,286] complement proteins,[121,122] adhesion molecules,[127,287] and free radicals[49,124] are neurotoxic. Epidemiological studies have revealed that rheumatoid arthritis patients, who are on high doses of NSAIDs, have a reduced incidence of AD.[119,288,289] NSAIDs also reduce the rate of deterioration of cognitive functions in AD patients.[70,137,138] However, administration of prednisone, a powerful anti-inflammatory agent, was not useful in patients with AD.[290] In another epidemiologic study, it was found that the use of NSAIDs and the salicylates without barbituates was associated with lower risk of AD and dementia from all other causes.[291]

Treatment with a mixed Cox-1/Cox-2 inhibitor and a PGE2 analog failed to produce any significant benefit on cognitive function.[292] A specific inhibitor of Cox-2 was also not useful in improving cognitive function.[293] Therefore, it was suggested that the Cox-2 enzyme may not be the appropriate target for AD treatment.[294] In contrast to Cox-2 inhibitor, treatment with a selective Cox-1 inhibitor SC-560 improved spatial learning and memory and decreased Aβ deposits and tau hyperphosphorylation in older triple transgenic AD mice (3xTg). In addition, treatment with SC560 reduced glial activation and markers of chronic inflammation.[295] Administration of indomethacin-loaded lipid-core nanocapsules blocked Aβ1–42-induced inflammation and suppressed glia and microglia activation.[296] Treatment of human neuronal cells in culture with both vitamin C and aspirin inhibited inflammatory responses more than that by aspirin alone.[297]

The potential value of nonsteroidal anti-inflammatory agents is supported by the following additional evidence: (a) the brains of nondemented elderly people taking NSAIDs had fewer activated microglia, suggesting that reduced anti-inflammatory activity[298] and chronic administration of ibuprofen reduced inflammation, dystrophic neurite formation, and beta-amyloid deposition in a transgenic AD model.[299] Thus, the use of NSAIDs for the prevention and for reducing the progression of AD remains one of the viable options.

CAN THE FAMILIAL AD BE PREVENTED OR DELAYED?

It is often believed that the familial AD cannot be prevented or delayed by any pharmacological and/or physiological means. Laboratory experiments on the genetic basis of another disease model (cancer) in *Drosophila melanogaster* (fruit fly) show that it may be possible to prevent or at least delay the onset of the familial basis of human diseases.

The gene HOP (TUM-1) is essential for the development of fruit flies. A mutation in this gene markedly increases the risk of developing a leukemia-like tumor in female flies (unpublished observation in collaboration with Dr. Bhattacharya et al. of NASA, Moffat Field, CA). Proton radiation is a powerful cancer-causing agent. Whole-body irradiation of these flies with proton radiation dramatically increased the incidence of cancer compared to that in unirradiated flies. The question arose as to whether or not a preparation of multiple antioxidants can reduce the incidence of cancer which is due to a specific gene defect. To test this possibility, a mixture of multiple dietary and endogenous antioxidants were fed to these flies through diet 7 days before proton irradiation and continued after irradiation throughout the experimental period of 7 days. The results showed that antioxidant treatment before and after irradiation totally blocked the proton radiation-induced cancer in fruit flies. This finding on fruit flies is of particular interest, because to my knowledge, this is a first demonstration in which genetic basis of a disease can be prevented by antioxidant treatment. This observation made on fruit flies cannot readily be extrapolated to humans. It is unknown whether daily supplementation with antioxidants in children of parents who had heritable mutations that increases the risk of AD can prevent or delay the onset of the disease. The results on fruit flies suggest that daily supplementation with multiple antioxidants could potentially prevent or delay the onset of familial AD in humans. A clinical study is needed to evaluate the effectiveness of multiple antioxidants in prevention of or delayed onset of AD in children of parents carrying heritable mutations in APP, presenilin-1, or presenilin-2 gene that increases the risk of developing AD.

RECOMMENDED MICRONUTRIENTS IN COMBINATION WITH LOW DOSES OF NSAID FOR PRIMARY PREVENTION OF AD

Individuals with a family history of AD and those aged 65 years or older are suitable population for primary prevention studies. These populations are very suitable to investigate the effectiveness of proposed micronutrients in combination with a low dose aspirin in prevention of AD. The selected combination of nontoxic agents include vitamin A (retinyl palmitate), vitamin E (both d-alpha-tocopherol and d-alpha-tocopheryl succinate), natural mixed carotenoids, vitamin C (calcium ascorbate), vitamin D, B vitamins with higher levels of vitamin B_3 (nicotinamide), selenium, coenzyme Q_{10}, alpha-lipoic acid, NAC, L-carnitine omega-3 fatty acids, resveratrol, and curcumin. The combination of above agents was selected because they would reduce oxidative stress and chronic inflammation optimally by activating Nrf2/ARE pathway without ROS stimulation and by directly scavenging free radicals. No iron, copper, manganese, or heavy metals (vanadium, zirconium, and molybdenum) would be added in the above preparation. The daily doses can be divided into two (half in the morning and half in the evening preferably with meal).

UNIQUENESS OF PROPOSED COMBINATION OF MICRONUTRIENTS

The proposed formulation has no iron, copper, manganese, or heavy metals (vanadium, zirconium, and molybdenum). Iron and copper are not added because they are known to interact with vitamin C and generate excessive amounts of free radicals. In addition, iron and copper are absorbed more in the presence of antioxidants than in the absence of antioxidants. Therefore, it is possible that prolonged consumption of these trace minerals in the presence of antioxidants may increase the levels of free iron or copper stores in the body, because there are no significant mechanisms of excretion of iron among men of all ages and women after menopause. Increased stores of free iron or copper may increase the risk of some human chronic diseases including AD. Heavy metals are not added because prolonged consumption of these metals may increase their levels in the body, and there is no significant mechanism for excretion of these metals from the body. High levels of these metals are considered neurotoxic. Certain herbs and classical antioxidants were added to complement the antioxidant effects of each other. The efficacy of the proposed micronutrient preparations should be tested in clinical studies.

DOSE SCHEDULE

Most clinical studies have utilized a once-a-day dose schedule. Taking vitamins and antioxidants once-a-day can create large fluctuations in their levels in the body. This is due to the fact that the biological half-lives of vitamins and antioxidants markedly vary, depending upon their lipid or water solubility. A twofold difference in the levels of vitamin E succinate can produce marked alterations in the expression profiles of several genes in neuroblastoma cells in culture. Therefore, taking a multiple vitamin preparation once-a-day may produce large fluctuations in the levels of micronutrients in the body which could potentially cause genetic stress in cells that may compromise the effectiveness of the vitamin supplementation after long-term consumption. I recommend taking a preparation of micronutrients containing multiple dietary and endogenous antioxidants twice-a-day in order to reduce fluctuations in the levels of gene expressions. Such a dose schedule may improve the effectiveness of a multiple vitamin preparation in reducing the development and progression of AD.

TOXICITY OF ANTIOXIDANTS PRESENT IN THE MICRONUTRIENT PREPARATION

Antioxidants and B vitamins used in proposed micronutrient preparation are considered safe. Antioxidants at doses higher than those that are recommended for the proposed micronutrient preparation have been consumed by the U.S. population for decades without significant toxicity. However, a few of them could produce harmful effects at certain high doses in some individuals when consumed daily for a long period of time. For example, vitamin A at doses of 10,000 IU or more per day can cause birth defects in pregnant women, and beta-carotene at doses 50 mg or more can produce bronzing of the skin that is reversible on discontinuation. Vitamin C as ascorbic acid at high doses (10 g or more per day) can cause diarrhea in some individuals. Vitamin E at high doses (2000 IU or more per day) can induce clotting defects after long-term consumption. Vitamin B_6 at high doses (50 mg or more per day) may produce peripheral neuropathy, and selenium at doses (400 mcg or more per day) can cause skin and liver toxicity after long-term consumption. Coenzyme Q_{10} has no known toxicity, and recommended daily doses are 30–400 mg. N-acetylcysteine doses of 250–1500 mg and alpha-lipoic acid doses of 600 mg are used in humans without toxicity at these doses. All ingredients present in the proposed micronutrient preparations are safe and come under the category of "Food Supplement" and therefore do not require Food and Drug Administration (FDA) approval for their use.

ASPIRIN

A low-dose aspirin is recommended because of its anti-inflammatory effect and because it, in combination with vitamin E, produced a synergistic effect on inhibition of cyclooxygenase activity[300]; therefore, the combination of two may be more effective in reducing the levels of chronic inflammation than the individual agents. Indeed, consumption of vitamin E and vitamin C together in combination with NSAIDs was associated with reduced cognitive decline over time in elderly individuals with an APOE-epsilon-4-allele.[301] The efficacy of proposed recommendation of micronutrients in combination with aspirin remains to be tested by clinical studies in high-risk populations; however, they have been used in humans for several decades, and therefore, they should be considered safe. In the meantime, the proposed recommendations can be adopted in consultation with physicians and health professionals in order to reduce the risk of AD in high-risk populations.

RECOMMENDED MICRONUTRIENTS IN COMBINATION WITH LOW DOSES OF NSAID FOR SECONDARY PREVENTION

The strategies proposed for the primary prevention may also be used in combination with standard care for secondary prevention in patients with early phase AD who are not taking any medications. Clinical studies should be initiated to test the efficacy of the proposed strategies in reducing the progression of AD.

CURRENT TREATMENTS OF AD

The purpose of treatment is to improve the symptoms of the disease. Current treatments of AD are totally unsatisfactory, because they are based on the symptoms rather than on the causes of the disease. These treatments have failed to stop the progression of the AD. Commonly prescribed drugs are cholinesterase inhibitors (donepezil, galantamine, and rivastigmine) and NMDA antagonist (memantine). The purpose of cholinesterase inhibitors is to improve cognitive function by increasing the acetylcholine levels in cholinergic neurons. The efficacy of these drugs depends upon the viability of surviving cholinergic neuron. The purpose of NMDA receptor antagonist is to stop the action of glutamate which induces fear and anxiety in patients with AD. In randomized, double-blind, parallel-group clinical trials, all acetylcholinesterase inhibitors (AChEIs) have shown varying degrees of efficacy than placebo in improving cognitive function in patients with mild to moderate AD. Among donepezil, galantamine, and rivastigmine, donepezil was found to be slightly more effective than others,[302] but others have reported no such difference between these drugs.[303] In the Hispanic population, the safety and beneficial effects of donepezil on cognitive function were similar to those found in the general population.[304] The annual cost of donepezil, galantamine, and rivastigmine was not significantly different.[305]

These drugs do not affect the level of oxidative stress or chronic inflammation primarily responsible for neurodegeneration in AD brain; therefore, their efficacy does not last for a long period of time. The progression of the disease continues to occur because of oxidative stress- and chronic inflammation-induced progressive neuronal death. The addition of agents that can reduce oxidative stress and chronic inflammation to the current therapeutic modalities may prolong the effectiveness of AChEI in improving cognitive function in AD patients. Therefore, I propose that antioxidants that neutralize free radicals and reduce inflammation and a NSAID that reduces inflammation should be utilized in combination with standard therapy in order to improve the current management of AD.

Statins are commonly used in the prevention and treatment of heart disease. Treatment with statins atorvastatin and pitavastatin reduced senile plaques and inflammation marker TNF-alpha in transgenic AD model (App-Tg) mice by reducing oxidative stress and improved insulin signaling pathways.[306] The efficacy of these statins in human AD has not been tested.

Using old transgenic AD mice (APP/swePS1ΔE9), it was shown that oral administration of memory enhancing neurotrophic molecule J147 improved cognitive function even when administered at a late stage of the disease.[307] This effect of J147 is mediated by inducing nerve growth factor (NGF) and several brain-derived neurotrophic factor (BDNF)-responsive proteins which are considered important for learning and memory. The efficacy of these growth factors in human AD has not been tested.

LIMITATIONS OF CURRENT MEDICATIONS IN AD

It has been proposed that the gradual loss of cognitive functions in AD is due to the loss of cholinergic neurons; therefore, cholinergic drugs (acetylcholinesterase inhibitors) are used to improve the function of surviving neurons in AD patients. However, these agents do not protect cholinergic neurons against the damaging effects of oxidative and nitrosylative stresses and chronic inflammation. Consequently, neurons continue to die, and the beneficial effects of cholinergic drugs do not last long.

RECOMMENDED MICRONUTRIENTS AND LOW DOSE OF NSAID IN COMBINATION WITH STANDARD THERAPY IN PATIENTS WITH DEMENTIA WITH OR WITHOUT AD

It has been proposed that the gradual loss of cognitive functions in AD is due to the progressive loss of cholinergic neurons. The presence of some viable cholinergic neurons in patients with mild to moderate dementia with or without AD allows using drugs that inhibit acetylcholinesterase activity to increase acetylcholine levels. These drugs improved cognitive function by enhancing the activity of surviving cholinergic neurons in AD patients. However, these drugs do not protect cholinergic neurons against the damaging effects of oxidative and nitrosylative stresses and chronic inflammation. Consequently, neurons continue to die despite this treatment, and thus, beneficial effects of cholinergic drugs last as long as neurons are alive. A supplement with an antagonist of glutamate receptor NMDA can be useful in reducing anxiety and fear in AD patients. This drug does not affect oxidative stress or chronic inflammation. Antioxidants reduce oxidative stress, chronic inflammation, and release and toxicity of glutamate. Aspirin enhances anti-inflammation effects of antioxidants. Therefore, addition of a multiple micronutrient preparation and a low-dose aspirin in combination with standard therapy may prolong the beneficial effects of current drugs in patients with dementia with or without AD by protecting surviving neurons from damage produced by increased oxidative stress, chronic inflammation, and glutamate. The proposed combination of micronutrients recommended for primary prevention is applicable to those who are at the various stages of AD and taking medications. The daily doses are divided into two doses (half in the morning and half in the evening preferably with meal) and are administered orally.

DIET AND LIFESTYLE RECOMMENDATIONS FOR AD

Even though there is no direct link between the diet- and lifestyle-related factors and the initiation or progression of AD, it would be beneficial to avoid exposure to aluminum and excessive consumption of iron, copper, manganese, or zinc. It is always useful to include a balanced diet that contains low fat and high fiber with plenty of fruits and vegetables. Among fruits, blueberries and raspberries are particularly important because of their protective role against oxidative injuries in brain. Lifestyle recommendations include daily moderate exercise, reduced stress, no tobacco smoking, and reduced exposure to noise and electromagnetic fields. Diet- and lifestyle-related recommendations can be adopted together with the proposed micronutrients for primary prevention, secondary prevention, and treatment strategies.

CONCLUSIONS

The results of many studies presented in this chapter suggest that increased oxidative stress is one of the earliest biochemical events which initiate neurodegeneration in AD. Other biochemical defects, such as mitochondrial dysfunction, increased levels of chronic inflammation, generation of Aβ1–42 peptides from APP, aggregation of Aβ peptides, hyperphosphorylation and acetylation of tau, inhibition of proteasome, and formation of extracellular senile plaques and intracellular NFT occur subsequent to increased oxidative stress. In addition, mutation in APP, presenilin-1, and presenilin-2 genes increased the generation of Aβ peptides which damage neurons by producing more free radicals. Increased oxidative stress together with other biochemical and genetic defects participate in the progression and final stage of neuronal death in AD.

At present, there are no effective strategies to reduce the incidence of AD. It is proposed that a combination of agents which can increase antioxidant enzymes by activating Nrf2/ARE pathway without ROS stimulation and which can directly scavenge free radicals may be necessary to reduce oxidative stress and chronic inflammation optimally in AD. Dietary and endogenous antioxidants, curcumin, resveratrol, and omega-3 fatty acids can fulfill the above requirements for reducing oxidative stress and chronic inflammation optimally. Thus, a preparation of the above antioxidants in combination with low dose NSAIDs, such as aspirin, may be useful in reducing chronic inflammation optimally. The same multiple antioxidants and phenolic compounds would also protect against glutamate induced damage to the nerve cells. All the preventive agents described here are of low toxicity, which would allow their prolonged safe usage even among high-risk populations not expressing any symptoms of AD. Clinical studies using the proposed micronutrient recommendations for primary and secondary prevention should be initiated.

The current drug treatments are based on the symptoms rather than the causes of AD and has produced transient benefits on some symptoms such as improving cognitive function; however, these drugs do not have any effect on increased oxidative stress and chronic inflammation that are responsible for neuronal degeneration. The effectiveness of cholinesterase inhibitors in improving cognitive function lasts as long as cholinergic neurons are viable. Excessive release of glutamate may induce fear and anxiety in AD patients. Glutamate is also toxic to nerve cells. Therefore, memantine, an antagonist of glutamate receptor NMDA, is used to improve these symptoms of AD. The currently used drugs have severe side effects. The micronutrient strategies recommended for primary prevention can also be used in combination with standard medications to improve the management of AD by reducing the progression of the disease and prolonging the efficacy of drugs on the symptoms. Dietary recommendations include low-fat and high-fiber diet and reduced consumption of iron, copper, and zinc. Lifestyle recommendations include stopping tobacco smoking and reducing exposure to noise and electromagnetic fields.

Clinical studies using the proposed micronutrient with a NSAID recommendations in combination with standard therapy for improved management of AD should be initiated. In the meantime, those interested in the proposed micronutrient approach in prevention or improved management of dementia with or without AD may like to adopt these recommendations in consultation with physicians or health professionals.

REFERENCES

1. Prasad KN, Cole WC, Prasad KC. Risk factors for Alzheimer's disease: Role of multiple antioxidants, nonsteroidal anti-inflammatory and cholinergic agents alone or in combination in prevention and treatment. *J Am Coll Nutr.* Dec 2002; 21(6): 506–522.
2. NIA. Progress Report on Alzheimer's disease. Bethesda: National Institute of Health; 1997.
3. Goedert M, Jakes R, Crowther RA et al. The abnormal phosphorylation of tau protein at Ser-202 in Alzheimer disease recapitulates phosphorylation during development. *Proc Natl Acad Sci U S A.* Jun 1 1993; 90(11): 5066–5070.
4. Grundke-Iqbal I, Iqbal K, Tung YC, Quinlan M, Wisniewski HM, Binder LI. Abnormal phosphorylation of the microtubule-associated protein tau (tau) in Alzheimer cytoskeletal pathology. *Proc Natl Acad Sci U S A.* Jul 1986; 83(13): 4913–4917.
5. Yankner BA, Mesulam MM. Seminars in medicine of the Beth Israel Hospital, Boston. Beta-amyloid and the pathogenesis of Alzheimer's disease. *N Engl J Med.* Dec 26 1991; 325(26): 1849–1857.
6. Selkoe DJ. Cell biology of the amyloid beta-protein precursor and the mechanism of Alzheimer's disease. *Annu Rev Cell Biol.* 1994; 10: 373–403.
7. Kudo T, Iqbal K, Ravid R, Swaab DF, Grundke-Iqbal I. Alzheimer disease: Correlation of cerebro-spinal fluid and brain ubiquitin levels. *Brain Res.* Mar 7 1994; 639(1): 1–7.
8. Hamilton RL. Lewy bodies in Alzheimer's disease: A neuropathological review of 145 cases using alpha-synuclein immunohistochemistry. *Brain Pathol.* Jul 2000; 10(3): 378–384.
9. Rondeau V, Jacqmin-Gadda H, Commenges D, Helmer C, Dartigues JF. Aluminum and silica in drinking water and the risk of Alzheimer's disease or cognitive decline: Findings from 15 year follow-up of the PAQUID cohort. *Am J Epidemiol.* Feb 15 2009; 169(4): 489–496.
10. Evatt ML, Delong MR, Khazai N, Rosen A, Triche S, Tangpricha V. Prevalence of vitamin D insufficiency in patients with Parkinson disease and Alzheimer disease. *Arch Neurol.* Oct 2008; 65(10): 1348–1352.
11. Engelhart MJ, Geerlings MI, Ruitenberg A et al. Dietary intake of antioxidants and risk of Alzheimer disease. *JAMA.* Jun 26 2002; 287(24): 3223–3229.
12. Thirumangalakudi L, Prakasam A, Zhang R et al. High cholesterol-induced neuroinflammation and amyloid precursor protein processing correlate with loss of working memory in mice. *J Neurochem.* Jul 2008; 106(1): 475–485.
13. Bhat NR, Thirumangalakudi L. Increased tau phosphorylation and impaired brain insulin/IGF signaling in mice fed a high fat/high cholesterol diet. *J Alzheimers Dis.* May 23 2013.
14. Barao S, Zhou L, Adamczuk K et al. BACE1 levels correlate with phospho-tau levels in human cerebrospinal fluid. *Curr Alzheimer Res.* Apr 8 2013.
15. Ho YS, Yang X, Yeung SC et al. Cigarette smoking accelerated brain aging and induced pre-Alzheimer-like neuropathology in rats. *PLoS One.* 2012; 7(5): e36752.
16. Khanna A, Guo M, Mehra M, Royal W, 3rd. Inflammation and oxidative stress induced by cigarette smoke in Lewis rat brains. *J Neuroimmunol.* Jan 15 2013; 254(1–2): 69–75.

17. Souza LC, Filho CB, Goes AT et al. Neuroprotective effect of physical exercise in a mouse model of Alzheimer's disease induced by beta-amyloid (1–40) peptide. *Neurotox Res.* Jan 11 2013.

18. Jiang DP, Li J, Zhang J et al. Electromagnetic pulse exposure induces overexpression of beta amyloid protein in rats. *Arch Med Res.* Apr 2013; 44(3): 178–184.

19. Chen YB, Li J, Liu JY et al. Effect of electromagnetic pulses (EMPs) on associative learning in mice and a preliminary study of mechanism. *Int J Rad Biol.* Dec 2011; 87(12): 1147–1154.

20. Arendash GW, Mori T, Dorsey M, Gonzalez R, Tajiri N, Borlongan C. Electromagnetic treatment to old Alzheimer's mice reverses beta-amyloid deposition, modifies cerebral blood flow, and provides selected cognitive benefit. *PLoS One.* 2012; 7(4): e35751.

21. Cui B, Zhu L, She X et al. Chronic noise exposure causes persistence of tau hyperphosphorylation and formation of NFT tau in the rat hippocampus and prefrontal cortex. *Exp Neurol.* Dec 2012; 238(2): 122–129.

22. Ohlemiller KK, Wright JS, Dugan LL. Early elevation of cochlear reactive oxygen species following noise exposure. *Audiol Neurootol.* Sep–Oct 1999; 4(5): 229–236.

23. Yamashita D, Jiang HY, Schacht J, Miller JM. Delayed production of free radicals following noise exposure. *Brain Res.* Sep 3 2004; 1019(1–2): 201–209.

24. Ames BN, Shigenaga MK, Hagen TM. Oxidants, antioxidants, and the degenerative diseases of aging. *Proc Natl Acad Sci U S A.* Sep 1 1993; 90(17): 7915–7922.

25. Ames BN, Durston WE, Yamasaki E, Lee FD. Carcinogens are mutagens: A simple test system combining liver homogenates for activation and bacteria for detection. *Proc Natl Acad Sci U S A.* Aug 1973; 70(8): 2281–2285.

26. Coyle JT, Puttfarcken P. Oxidative stress, glutamate, and neurodegenerative disorders. *Science.* Oct 29 1993; 262(5134): 689–695.

27. Graham DG. Oxidative pathways for catecholamines in the genesis of neuromelanin and cytotoxic quinones. *Mol Pharmacol.* Jul 1978; 14(4): 633–643.

28. Chan PH, Fishman RA. Transient formation of superoxide radicals in polyunsaturated fatty acid-induced brain swelling. *J Neurochem.* Oct 1980; 35(4): 1004–1007.

29. Lafon-Cazal M, Pietri S, Culcasi M, Bockaert J. NMDA-dependent superoxide production and neurotoxicity. *Nature.* Aug 5 1993; 364(6437): 535–537.

30. Kiyosawa H, Suko M, Okudaira H et al. Cigarette smoking induces formation of 8-hydroxydeoxyguanosine, one of the oxidative DNA damages in human peripheral leukocytes. *Free Radic Res Commun.* 1990; 11(1–3): 23–27.

31. Reznick AZ, Cross CE, Hu ML et al. Modification of plasma proteins by cigarette smoke as measured by protein carbonyl formation. *Biochem J.* Sep 1 1992; 286 (Pt 2): 607–611.

32. Schectman G, Byrd JC, Hoffmann R. Ascorbic acid requirements for smokers: Analysis of a population survey. *Am J Clin Nutr.* Jun 1991; 53(6): 1466–1470.

33. Duthie GG, Arthur JR, James WP. Effects of smoking and vitamin E on blood antioxidant status. *Am J Clin Nutr.* Apr 1991; 53(4 Suppl): 1061S–1063S.

34. Winterbourn CC. Toxicity of iron and hydrogen peroxide: The Fenton reaction. *Toxicol Lett.* Dec 1995; 82–83: 969–974.

35. Ames BN, Profet M, Gold LS. Dietary pesticides (99.99% all natural). *Proc Natl Acad Sci U S A.* Oct 1990; 87(19): 7777–7781.

36. Guyton AC. Blood flow through special areas of the body. In: Guyton AC, ed. *Textbook of Medical Physiology.* 4th ed. Philadelphia: W B Saunders Co; 1971: 367–378.

37. Hartl D, Schuldt V, Forler S, Zabel C, Klose J, Rohe M. Presymptomatic alterations in energy metabolism and oxidative stress in the APP23 mouse model of Alzheimer disease. *J Proteome Res.* May 22 2012.

38. Xie H, Hou S, Jiang J, Sekutowicz M, Kelly J, Bacskai BJ. Rapid cell death is preceded by amyloid plaque-mediated oxidative stress. *Proc Natl Acad Sci U S A.* May 7 2013; 110(19): 7904–7909.

39. Clausen A, Xu X, Bi X, Baudry M. Effects of the superoxide dismutase/catalase mimetic EUK-207 in a mouse model of Alzheimer's disease: Protection against and interruption of progression of amyloid and tau pathology and cognitive decline. *J Alzheimers Dis.* 2012; 30(1): 183–208.

40. Sompol P, Ittarat W, Tangpong J et al. A neuronal model of Alzheimer's disease: An insight into the mechanisms of oxidative stress-mediated mitochondrial injury. *Neuroscience.* Apr 22 2008; 153(1): 120–130.

41. Gu X, Sun J, Li S, Wu X, Li L. Oxidative stress induces DNA demethylation and histone acetylation in SH-SY5Y cells: Potential epigenetic mechanisms in gene transcription in Abeta production. *Neurobiol Aging.* Apr 2013; 34(4): 1069–1079.

42. Mohmmad Abdul H, Sultana R, Keller JN, St Clair DK, Markesbery WR, Butterfield DA. Mutations in amyloid precursor protein and presenilin-1 genes increase the basal oxidative stress in murine neuronal cells and lead to increased sensitivity to oxidative stress mediated by amyloid beta-peptide (1–42), HO and kainic acid: Implications for Alzheimer's disease. *J Neurochem.* Mar 2006; 96(5): 1322–1335.

43. Sultana R, Perluigi M, Butterfield DA. Protein oxidation and lipid peroxidation in brain of subjects with Alzheimer's disease: Insights into mechanism of neurodegeneration from redox proteomics. *Antioxid Redox Signal.* Nov–Dec 2006; 8(11–12): 2021–2037.

44. Schipper HM, Cisse S, Stopa EG. Expression of heme oxygenase-1 in the senescent and Alzheimer-diseased brain. *Ann Neurol.* Jun 1995; 37(6): 758–768.

45. Sims NR, Bowen DM, Neary D, Davison AN. Metabolic processes in Alzheimer's disease: Adenine nucleotide content and production of $^{14}CO_2$ from [U-^{14}C] glucose in vitro in human neocortex. *J Neurochem.* Nov 1983; 41(5): 1329–1334.

46. Martins RN, Harper CG, Stokes GB, Masters CL. Increased cerebral glucose-6-phosphate dehydrogenase activity in Alzheimer's disease may reflect oxidative stress. *J Neurochem.* Apr 1986; 46(4): 1042–1045.

47. Saito K, Elce JS, Hamos JE, Nixon RA. Widespread activation of calcium-activated neutral proteinase (calpain) in the brain in Alzheimer disease: A potential molecular basis for neuronal degeneration. *Proc Natl Acad Sci U S A.* Apr 1 1993; 90(7): 2628–2632.

48. Nixon RA, Cataldo AM. Free radicals, proteolysis, and the degeneration of neurons in Alzheimer disease: How essential is the beta-amyloid link? *Neurobiol Aging.* Jul–Aug 1994; 15(4): 463–469; discussion 473.

49. Harman D. Free radical theory of aging. *Mutat Res.* Sep 1992; 275(3–6): 257–266.

50. Zhou Y, Richardson JS, Mombourquette MJ, Weil JA. Free radical formation in autopsy samples of Alzheimer and control cortex. *Neurosci Lett.* Aug 4 1995; 195(2): 89–92.

51. Koppal T. Peroxynitrite-mediated damage to brain membrane alterations in Alzheimer's disease (AD). *Soc Neurosci.* 1998; 24: 1217a.

52. Simic G, Lucassen PJ, Krsnik Z et al. nNOS expression in reactive astrocytes correlates with increased cell death related DNA damage in the hippocampus and entorhinal cortex in Alzheimer's disease. *Exp Neurol.* Sep 2000; 165(1): 12–26.

53. Lovell MA, Xie C, Markesbery WR. Decreased glutathione transferase activity in brain and ventricular fluid in Alzheimer's disease. *Neurology.* Dec 1998; 51(6): 1562–1566.

54. Ghosh T, Mustafa M, Kumar V et al. A preliminary study on the influence of glutathione S transferase T1 (GSTT1) as a risk factor for late onset Alzheimer's disease in North Indian population. *Asian J Psych.* Jun 2012; 5(2): 160–163.

55. Barone E, Di Domenico F, Cenini G et al. Oxidative and nitrosative modifications of biliverdin reductase-A in the brain of subjects with Alzheimer's disease and amnestic mild cognitive impairment. *J Alzheimers Dis.* 2011; 25(4): 623–633.

56. Tesco G, Latorraca S, Piersanti P, Piacentini S, Amaducci L, Sorbi S. Alzheimer skin fibroblasts show increased susceptibility to free radicals. *Mech Ageing Dev.* Nov 1992; 66(2): 117–120.

57. Ramamoorthy M, Sykora P, Scheibye-Knudsen M et al. Sporadic Alzheimer's disease fibroblasts display an oxidative stress phenotype. *Free Radic Biol Med.* Sep 15 2012; 53(6): 1371–1380.

58. Zaman Z, Roche S, Fielden P, Frost PG, Niriella DC, Cayley AC. Plasma concentrations of vitamins A and E and carotenoids in Alzheimer's disease. *Age Ageing.* Mar 1992; 21(2): 91–94.

59. Zito G, Polimanti R, Panetta V et al. Antioxidant status and APOE genotype as susceptibility factors for neurodegeneration in Alzheimer's disease and vascular dementia. *Rejuv Res.* Feb 2013; 16(1): 51–56.

60. Conrad CC, Marshall PL, Talent JM, Malakowsky CA, Choi J, Gracy RW. Oxidized proteins in Alzheimer's plasma. *Biochem Biophys Res Commun.* Aug 28 2000; 275(2): 678–681.

61. Kosenko EA, Aliev G, Tikhonova LA, Li Y, Poghosyan AC, Kaminsky YG. Antioxidant status and energy state of erythrocytes in Alzheimer dementia: Probing for markers. *CNS Neurol Disord Drug Targets.* Nov 1 2012; 11(7): 926–932.

62. Cervellati C, Cremonini E, Bosi C et al. Systemic oxidative stress in older patients with mild cognitive impairment or late onset Alzheimer's disease. *Curr Alzheimer Res.* May 1 2013; 10(4): 365–372.

63. Torres LL, Quaglio NB, de Souza GT et al. Peripheral oxidative stress biomarkers in mild cognitive impairment and Alzheimer's disease. *J Alzheimers Dis.* 2011; 26(1): 59–68.

64. Ringman JM, Fithian AT, Gylys K et al. Plasma methionine sulfoxide in persons with familial Alzheimer's disease mutations. *Dement Geriatr Cogn Disord.* 2012; 33(4): 219–225.

65. Wallace DC. Mitochondrial genetics: A paradigm for aging and degenerative diseases? *Science.* May 1 1992; 256(5057): 628–632.

66. Shoffner JM, Brown MD, Torroni A et al. Mitochondrial DNA variants observed in Alzheimer disease and Parkinson disease patients. *Genomics.* Jul 1993; 17(1): 171–184.

67. Kish SJ, Bergeron C, Rajput A et al. Brain cytochrome oxidase in Alzheimer's disease. *J Neurochem.* Aug 1992; 59(2): 776–779.

68. Mutisya EM, Bowling AC, Beal MF. Cortical cytochrome oxidase activity is reduced in Alzheimer's disease. *J Neurochem.* Dec 1994; 63(6): 2179–2184.

69. Cuajungco MP, Lees GJ. Nitric oxide generators produce accumulation of chelatable zinc in hippocampal neuronal perikarya. *Brain Res.* Jul 13 1998; 799(1): 118–129.

70. Brown AM, Kristal BS, Effron MS et al. Zn^{2+} inhibits alpha-ketoglutarate-stimulated mitochondrial respiration and the isolated alpha-ketoglutarate dehydrogenase complex. *J Biol Chem.* May 5 2000; 275(18): 13441–13447.

71. Mattson MP. Calcium and neuronal injury in Alzheimer's disease. Contributions of beta-amyloid precursor protein mismetabolism, free radicals, and metabolic compromise. *Ann NY Acad Sci.* Dec 15 1994; 747: 50–76.

72. Gabuzda D, Busciglio J, Chen LB, Matsudaira P, Yankner BA. Inhibition of energy metabolism alters the processing of amyloid precursor protein and induces a potentially amyloidogenic derivative. *J Biol Chem.* May 6 1994; 269(18): 13623–13628.

73. Gibson GE, Haroutunian V, Zhang H et al. Mitochondrial damage in Alzheimer's disease varies with apolipoprotein E genotype. *Ann Neurol.* Sep 2000; 48(3): 297–303.

74. Sultana R, Butterfield DA. Oxidatively modified, mitochondria-relevant brain proteins in subjects with Alzheimer disease and mild cognitive impairment. *J Bioenerg Biomem.* Oct 2009; 41(5): 441–446.

75. Piaceri I, Rinnoci V, Bagnoli S, Failli Y, Sorbi S. Mitochondria and Alzheimer's disease. *J Neurol Sci.* Nov 15 2012; 322(1–2): 31–34.

76. Leuner K, Schulz K, Schutt T et al. Peripheral mitochondrial dysfunction in Alzheimer's disease: Focus on lymphocytes. *Mol Neurobiol.* Aug 2012; 46(1): 194–204.

77. de la Monte SM, Wands JR. Molecular indices of oxidative stress and mitochondrial dysfunction occur early and often progress with severity of Alzheimer's disease. *J Alzheimers Dis.* Jul 2006; 9(2): 167–181.

78. Sochocka MK, E.S. Gasiorowski, K. and Leszek, J. Vascular oxidative stress and mitochondrial failure in the pathobiology of Alzheimer's disease: New approach to therapy. *CNS Neurol Disord Drug Targets.* 2013.

79. Postina R. A closer look at alpha-secretase. *Curr Alzheimer Res.* Apr 2008; 5(2): 179–186.

80. Misonou H, Morishima-Kawashima M, Ihara Y. Oxidative stress induces intracellular accumulation of amyloid beta-protein (Abeta) in human neuroblastoma cells. *Biochemistry.* Jun 13 2000; 39(23): 6951–6959.

81. Koppaka V, Axelsen PH. Accelerated accumulation of amyloid beta proteins on oxidatively damaged lipid membranes. *Biochemistry.* Aug 15 2000; 39(32): 10011–10016.

82. Murakami K, Murata N, Noda Y, Irie K, Shirasawa T, Shimizu T. Stimulation of the amyloidogenic pathway by cytoplasmic superoxide radicals in an Alzheimer's disease mouse model. *Biosci Biotechnol Biochem.* 2012; 76(6): 1098–1103.

83. Tan JL, Li QX, Ciccotosto GD et al. Mild oxidative stress induces redistribution of BACE1 in nonapoptotic conditions and promotes the amyloidogenic processing of Alzheimer's disease amyloid precursor protein. *PLoS One.* 2013; 8(4): e61246.

84. Schubert D, Behl C, Lesley R et al. Amyloid peptides are toxic via a common oxidative mechanism. *Proc Natl Acad Sci U S A.* Mar 14 1995; 92(6): 1989–1993.

85. Lorenzo A, Yankner BA. Beta-amyloid neurotoxicity requires fibril formation and is inhibited by congo red. *Proc Natl Acad Sci U S A.* Dec 6 1994; 91(25): 12243–12247.

86. Loo G. Redox-sensitive mechanisms of phytochemical-mediated inhibition of cancer cell proliferation (review). *J Nutr Biochem.* Feb 2003; 14(2): 64–73.

87. Behl C, Davis JB, Lesley R, Schubert D. Hydrogen peroxide mediates amyloid beta protein toxicity. *Cell.* Jun 17 1994; 77(6): 817–827.

88. Koh JY, Suh SW, Gwag BJ, He YY, Hsu CY, Choi DW. The role of zinc in selective neuronal death after transient global cerebral ischemia. *Science.* May 17 1996; 272(5264): 1013–1016.

89. Bondy SC, Truong A. Potentiation of beta-folding of beta-amyloid peptide 25–35 by aluminum salts. *Neurosci Lett.* May 21 1999; 267(1): 25–28.

90. Eikelenboom P, Stam FC. Immunoglobulins and complement factors in senile plaques. An immunoperoxidase study. *Acta Neuropathol (Berl).* 1982; 57(2–3): 239–242.

91. Ha C, Ryu J, Park CB. Metal ions differentially influence the aggregation and deposition of Alzheimer's beta-amyloid on a solid template. *Biochemistry.* May 22 2007; 46(20): 6118–6125.

92. Bolognin S, Messori L, Drago D, Gabbiani C, Cendron L, Zatta P. Aluminum, copper, iron, and zinc differentially alter amyloid-Abeta(1–42) aggregation and toxicity. *Int J Biochem Cell Biol.* Jun 2011; 43(6): 877–885.

93. Liu B, Moloney A, Meehan S et al. Iron promotes the toxicity of amyloid beta peptide by impeding its ordered aggregation. *J Biol Chem.* Feb 11 2011; 286(6): 4248–4256.

94. Guo C, Wang T, Zheng W, Shan ZY, Teng WP, Wang ZY. Intranasal deferoxamine reverses iron-induced memory deficits and inhibits amyloidogenic APP processing in a transgenic mouse model of Alzheimer's disease. *Neurobiol Aging.* Feb 2013; 34(2): 562–575.

95. Baum L, Ng A. Curcumin interaction with copper and iron suggests one possible mechanism of action in Alzheimer's disease animal models. *J Alzheimers Dis.* Aug 2004; 6(4): 367–377; discussion 443–369.

96. Bao Q, Luo Y, Li W et al. The mechanism for heme to prevent Abeta(1–40) aggregation and its cytotoxicity. *J Biol Inorg Chem.* Jun 2011; 16(5): 809–816.

97. Alberdi E, Wyssenbach A, Alberdi M et al. Ca$^{(2+)}$-dependent endoplasmic reticulum stress correlates with astrogliosis in oligomeric amyloid beta-treated astrocytes and in a model of Alzheimer's disease. *Aging Cell.* Apr 2013; 12(2): 292–302.

98. Costa RO, Lacor PN, Ferreira IL et al. Endoplasmic reticulum stress occurs downstream of GluN2B subunit of N-methyl-D-aspartate receptor in mature hippocampal cultures treated with amyloid-beta oligomers. *Aging Cell.* Oct 2012; 11(5): 823–833.

99. Mota SI, Ferreira IL, Pereira C, Oliveira CR, Rego AC. Amyloid-beta peptide 1–42 causes microtubule deregulation through N-methyl-D-aspartate receptors in mature hippocampal cultures. *Curr Alzheimer Res.* Sep 2012; 9(7): 844–856.

100. Butterfield DA, Hensley K, Harris M, Mattson M, Carney J. Beta-amyloid peptide free radical fragments initiate synaptosomal lipoperoxidation in a sequence-specific fashion: Implications to Alzheimer's disease. *Biochem Biophys Res Commun.* Apr 29 1994; 200(2): 710–715.

101. Behl C, Davis J, Cole GM, Schubert D. Vitamin E protects nerve cells from amyloid beta protein toxicity. *Biochem Biophys Res Commun.* Jul 31 1992; 186(2): 944–950.

102. Varadarajan S, Yatin S, Kanski J, Jahanshahi F, Butterfield DA. Methionine residue 35 is important in amyloid beta-peptide-associated free radical oxidative stress. *Brain Res Bull.* Sep 15 1999; 50(2): 133–141.

103. Lucas HR, Rifkind JM. Considering the vascular hypothesis of Alzheimer's disease: Effect of copper associated amyloid on red blood cells. *Adv Exp Med Biol.* 2013; 765: 131–138.

104. Wolozin B, Kellman W, Ruosseau P, Celesia GG, Siegel G. Decreased prevalence of Alzheimer's disease associated with 3-hydroxy-3-methyglutaryl coenzyme A reductase inhibitors. *Arch Neurol.* Oct 2000; 57(10): 1439–1443.

105. Sparks DL, Martin TA, Gross DR, Hunsaker JC, 3rd. Link between heart disease, cholesterol, and Alzheimer's disease: A review. *Microsc Res Tech.* Aug 15 2000; 50(4): 287–290.

106. Refolo LM, Malester B, LaFrancois J et al. Hypercholesterolemia accelerates the Alzheimer's amyloid pathology in a transgenic mouse model. *Neurobiol Dis.* Aug 2000; 7(4): 321–331.

107. Simons M, Keller P, De Strooper B, Beyreuther K, Dotti CG, Simons K. Cholesterol depletion inhibits the generation of beta-amyloid in hippocampal neurons. *Proc Natl Acad Sci U S A.* May 26 1998; 95(11): 6460–6464.

108. Jick H, Zornberg GL, Jick SS, Seshadri S, Drachman DA. Statins and the risk of dementia. *Lancet.* Nov 11 2000; 356(9242): 1627–1631.

109. Haag MD, Hofman A, Koudstaal PJ, Stricker BH, Breteler MM. Statins are associated with a reduced risk of Alzheimer disease regardless of lipophilicity. The Rotterdam Study. *J Neurol Neurosurg Psych.* Jan 2009; 80(1): 13–17.

110. Rao S, Porter DC, Chen X, Herliczek T, Lowe M, Keyomarsi K. Lovastatin-mediated G1 arrest is through inhibition of the proteasome, independent of hydroxymethyl glutaryl-CoA reductase. *Proc Natl Acad Sci U S A.* Jul 6 1999; 96(14): 7797–7802.

111. Kumar B, Andreatta C, Koustas WT, Cole WC, Edwards-Prasad J, Prasad KN. Mevastatin induces degeneration and decreases viability of cAMP-induced differentiated neuroblastoma cells in culture by inhibiting proteasome activity, and mevalonic acid lactone prevents these effects. *J Neurosci Res.* Jun 1 2002; 68(5): 627–635.

112. Sherrington R, Rogaev EI, Liang Y et al. Cloning of a gene bearing missense mutations in early-onset familial Alzheimer's disease. *Nature.* Jun 29 1995; 375(6534): 754–760.

113. Abdul HM, Sultana R, St Clair DK, Markesbery WR, Butterfield DA. Oxidative damage in brain from human mutant APP/PS-1 double knock-in mice as a function of age. *Free Radic Biol Med.* Nov 15 2008; 45(10): 1420–1425.

114. Mohmmad Abdul H, Wenk GL, Gramling M, Hauss-Wegrzyniak B, Butterfield DA. APP and PS-1 mutations induce brain oxidative stress independent of dietary cholesterol: Implications for Alzheimer's disease. *Neurosci Lett.* Sep 23 2004; 368(2): 148–150.

115. Zhang Z, Hartmann H, Do VM et al. Destabilization of beta-catenin by mutations in presenilin-1 potentiates neuronal apoptosis. *Nature.* Oct 15 1998; 395(6703): 698–702.

116. Tabaton M, Tamagno E. The molecular link between beta- and gamma-secretase activity on the amyloid beta precursor protein. *Cell Mol Life Sci.* Sep 2007; 64(17): 2211–2218.

117. Placanica L, Tarassishin L, Yang G et al. Pen2 and presenilin-1 modulate the dynamic equilibrium of presenilin-1 and presenilin-2 gamma-secretase complexes. *J Biol Chem.* Jan 30 2009; 284(5): 2967–2977.

118. McGeer PL, Schulzer M, McGeer EG. Arthritis and anti-inflammatory agents as possible protective factors for Alzheimer's disease: A review of 17 epidemiologic studies. *Neurology.* Aug 1996; 47(2): 425–432.

119. McGeer EG, McGeer PL. The importance of inflammatory mechanisms in Alzheimer's disease. *Exp Gerontol.* Aug 1998; 33(5): 371–378.

120. Shalit F, Sredni B, Stern L, Kott E, Huberman M. Elevated interleukin-6 secretion levels by mononuclear cells of Alzheimer's patients. *Neurosci Lett.* Jun 20 1994; 174(2): 130–132.

121. Rogers J, Lue L-F, Brachova L, Webster S, Schultz J. Inflammation as a response and a cause of Alzheimer's pathophysiology. *Dementia.* 1995; 9: 133–138.

122. Webster S, O'Barr S, Rogers J. Enhanced aggregation and beta structure of amyloid beta peptide after coincubation with C1q. *J Neurosci Res.* Nov 1 1994; 39(4): 448–456.

123. Chen L, Richardson JS, Caldwell JE, Ang LC. Regional brain activity of free radical defense enzymes in autopsy samples from patients with Alzheimer's disease and from nondemented controls. *Int J Neurosci.* Mar 1994; 75(1–2): 83–90.

124. Smith MA, Sayre LM, Monnier VM, Perry G. Radical ageing in Alzheimer's disease. *Trends Neurosci.* Apr 1995; 18(4): 172–176.

125. Harman D. A hypothesis on the pathogenesis of Alzheimer's disease. *Ann NY Acad Sci.* Jun 15 1996; 786: 152–168.

126. Frohman EM, Frohman TC, Gupta S, de Fougerolles A, van den Noort S. Expression of intercellular adhesion molecule 1 (ICAM-1) in Alzheimer's disease. *J Neurol Sci.* Nov 1991; 106(1): 105–111.

127. Verbeek MM, Otte-Holler I, Westphal JR, Wesseling P, Ruiter DJ, de Waal RM. Accumulation of intercellular adhesion molecule-1 in senile plaques in brain tissue of patients with Alzheimer's disease. *Am J Pathol.* Jan 1994; 144(1): 104–116.

128. Prasad KN, Hovland AR, La Rosa FG, Hovland PG. Prostaglandins as putative neurotoxins in Alzheimer's disease. *Proc Soc Exp Biol Med.* Nov 1998; 219(2): 120–125.

129. Sutton ET, Thomas T, Bryant MW, Landon CS, Newton CA, Rhodin JA. Amyloid-beta peptide induced inflammatory reaction is mediated by the cytokines tumor necrosis factor and interleukin-1. *J Submicrosc Cytol Pathol.* Jul 1999; 31(3): 313–323.

130. Ramirez G, Rey S, von Bernhardi R. Proinflammatory stimuli are needed for induction of microglial cell-mediated AbetaPP_{244-C} and Abeta-neurotoxicity in hippocampal cultures. *J Alzheimers Dis.* Sep 2008; 15(1): 45–59.

131. Yamamoto M, Kiyota T, Horiba M et al. Interferon-gamma and tumor necrosis factor-alpha regulate amyloid-beta plaque deposition and beta-secretase expression in Swedish mutant APP transgenic mice. *Am J Pathol.* Feb 2007; 170(2): 680–692.

132. Blasko I, Marx F, Steiner E, Hartmann T, Grubeck-Loebenstein B. TNFalpha plus IFNgamma induce the production of Alzheimer beta-amyloid peptides and decrease the secretion of APPs. *FASEB J.* Jan 1999; 13(1): 63–68.

133. Liao YF, Wang BJ, Cheng HT, Kuo LH, Wolfe MS. Tumor necrosis factor-alpha, interleukin-1beta, and interferon-gamma stimulate gamma-secretase-mediated cleavage of amyloid precursor protein through a JNK-dependent MAPK pathway. *J Biol Chem.* Nov 19 2004; 279(47): 49523–49532.

134. Qiu Z, Gruol DL. Interleukin-6, beta-amyloid peptide, and NMDA interactions in rat cortical neurons. *J Neuroimmunol.* Jun 2003; 139(1–2): 51–57.

135. Shelat PB, Chalimoniuk M, Wang JH et al. Amyloid beta peptide and NMDA induce ROS from NADPH oxidase and AA release from cytosolic phospholipase A2 in cortical neurons. *J Neurochem.* Jul 2008; 106(1): 45–55.
136. Rich JB, Rasmusson DX, Folstein MF, Carson KA, Kawas C, Brandt J. Nonsteroidal anti-inflammatory drugs in Alzheimer's disease. *Neurology.* Jan 1995; 45(1): 51–55.
137. Lucca U, Tettamanti M, Forloni G, Spagnoli A. Nonsteroidal antiinflammatory drug use in Alzheimer's disease. *Biol Psychiatry.* Dec 15 1994; 36(12): 854–856.
138. Rogers J, Kirby LC, Hempelman SR et al. Clinical trial of indomethacin in Alzheimer's disease. *Neurology.* Aug 1993; 43(8): 1609–1611.
139. Martin BK, Szekely C, Brandt J et al. Cognitive function over time in the Alzheimer's disease anti-inflammatory prevention trial (ADAPT): Results of a randomized, controlled trial of naproxen and celecoxib. *Arch Neurol.* Jul 2008; 65(7): 896–905.
140. Babiloni C, Frisoni GB, Del Percio C et al. Ibuprofen treatment modifies cortical sources of EEG rhythms in mild Alzheimer's disease. *Clin Neurophysiol.* Apr 2009; 120(4): 709–718.
141. Hirohata M, Ono K, Naiki H, Yamada M. Nonsteroidal anti-inflammatory drugs have anti-amyloidogenic effects for Alzheimer's beta-amyloid fibrils *in vitro.* *Neuropharmacology.* Dec 2005; 49(7): 1088–1099.
142. McKee AC, Carreras I, Hossain L et al. Ibuprofen reduces Abeta, hyperphosphorylated tau, and memory deficits in Alzheimer mice. *Brain Res.* May 1 2008; 1207: 225–236.
143. McGeer PL, McGeer E, Rogers J, Sibley J. Anti-inflammatory drugs and Alzheimer disease. *Lancet.* Apr 28 1990; 335(8696): 1037.
144. Shi J, Wang Q, Johansson JU et al. Inflammatory prostaglandin E2 signaling in a mouse model of Alzheimer disease. *Ann Neurol.* Nov 2012; 72(5): 788–798.
145. Melov S, Adlard PA, Morten K et al. Mitochondrial oxidative stress causes hyperphosphorylation of tau. *PLoS One.* 2007; 2(6): e536.
146. Naslund J, Haroutunian V, Mohs R et al. Correlation between elevated levels of amyloid beta-peptide in the brain and cognitive decline. *JAMA.* Mar 22–29 2000; 283(12): 1571–1577.
147. Tai HC, Serrano-Pozo A, Hashimoto T, Frosch MP, Spires-Jones TL, Hyman BT. The synaptic accumulation of hyperphosphorylated tau oligomers in Alzheimer disease is associated with dysfunction of the ubiquitin-proteasome system. *Am J Pathol.* Oct 2012; 181(4): 1426–1435.
148. Iqbal K, Liu F, Gong CX, Alonso Adel C, Grundke-Iqbal I. Mechanisms of tau-induced neurodegeneration. *Acta Neuropathol.* Jul 2009; 118(1): 53–69.
149. Xiong Y, Jing XP, Zhou XW et al. Zinc induces protein phosphatase 2A inactivation and tau hyperphosphorylation through Src dependent PP2A (tyrosine 307) phosphorylation. *Neurobiol Aging.* Mar 2013; 34(3): 745–756.
150. Guo C, Wang P, Zhong ML et al. Deferoxamine inhibits iron induced hippocampal tau phosphorylation in the Alzheimer transgenic mouse brain. *Neurochem Int.* Jan 2013; 62(2): 165–172.
151. Braak H, Zetterberg H, Del Tredici K, Blennow K. Intraneuronal tau aggregation precedes diffuse plaque deposition, but amyloid-beta changes occur before increases of tau in cerebrospinal fluid. *Acta Neuropathol.* Jun 12 2013.
152. Lasagna-Reeves CA, Castillo-Carranza DL, Jackson GR, Kayed R. Tau oligomers as potential targets for immunotherapy for Alzheimer's disease and tauopathies. *Curr Alzheimer Res.* Sep 2011; 8(6): 659–665.
153. Chien DT, Bahri S, Szardenings AK et al. Early clinical PET imaging results with the novel PHF-tau radioligand [F-18]-T807. *J Alzheimers Dis.* Jan 1 2013; 34(2): 457–468.
154. Hertze J, Palmqvist S, Minthon L, Hansson O. Tau pathology and parietal white matter lesions have independent but synergistic effects on early development of Alzheimer's disease. *Dement Geriatr Cogn Disord.* Jan 2013; 3(1): 113–122.

155. Irwin DJ, Cohen TJ, Grossman M et al. Acetylated tau, a novel pathological signature in Alzheimer's disease and other tauopathies. *Brain*. Mar 2012; 135(Pt 3): 807–818.

156. Gregori L, Hainfeld JF, Simon MN, Goldgaber D. Binding of amyloid beta protein to the 20 S proteasome. *J Biol Chem*. Jan 3 1997; 272(1): 58–62.

157. Checler F, da Costa CA, Ancolio K, Chevallier N, Lopez-Perez E, Marambaud P. Role of the proteasome in Alzheimer's disease. *Biochim Biophys Acta*. Jul 26 2000; 1502(1): 133–138.

158. Nahreini P, Andreatta C, Prasad KN. Proteasome activity is critical for the cAMP-induced differentiation of neuroblastoma cells. *Cell Mol Neurobiol*. Oct 2001; 21(5): 509–521.

159. Lopez Salon M, Morelli L, Castano EM, Soto EF, Pasquini JM. Defective ubiquitination of cerebral proteins in Alzheimer's disease. *J Neurosci Res*. Oct 15 2000; 62(2): 302–310.

160. Lam YA, Pickart CM, Alban A et al. Inhibition of the ubiquitin-proteasome system in Alzheimer's disease. *Proc Natl Acad Sci U S A*. Aug 29 2000; 97(18): 9902–9906.

161. Handattu SP, Monroe CE, Nayyar G et al. In vivo and in vitro effects of an apolipoprotein E mimetic peptide on amyloid-beta pathology. *J Alzheimers Dis*. Apr 19 2013.

162. Farrer LA, Cupples LA, Haines JL et al. Effects of age, sex, and ethnicity on the association between apolipoprotein E genotype and Alzheimer disease. A meta-analysis. APOE and Alzheimer disease meta analysis consortium. *JAMA*. Oct 22–29 1997; 278(16): 1349–1356.

163. Marx J. New gene tied to common form of Alzheimer's. *Science*. Jul 24 1998; 281(5376): 507, 509.

164. McConnell LM, Koenig BA, Greely HT, Raffin TA. Genetic testing and Alzheimer disease: has the time come? Alzheimer Disease Working Group of the Stanford Program in Genomics, Ethics & Society. *Nat Med*. Jul 1998; 4(7): 757–759.

165. Duits FH, Kester MI, Scheffer PG et al. Increase in cerebrospinal fluid F2-isoprostanes is related to cognitive decline in APOE epsilon4 carriers. *J Alzheimers Dis*. Apr 29 2013.

166. Liraz O, Boehm-Cagan A, Michaelson DM. ApoE4 induces Abeta42, tau, and neuronal pathology in the hippocampus of young targeted replacement apoE4 mice. *Mol Neurodegen*. 2013; 8: 16.

167. McMillan PJ, Leverenz JB, Dorsa DM. Specific downregulation of presenilin 2 gene expression is prominent during early stages of sporadic late-onset Alzheimer's disease. *Brain Res Mol Brain Res*. May 31 2000; 78(1–2): 138–145.

168. Hanson AJ, Prasad JE, Nahreini P et al. Overexpression of amyloid precursor protein is associated with degeneration, decreased viability, and increased damage caused by neurotoxins (prostaglandins A1 and E2, hydrogen peroxide, and nitric oxide) in differentiated neuroblastoma cells. *J Neurosci Res*. Oct 1 2003; 74(1): 148–159.

169. Candore G, Balistreri CR, Grimaldi MP et al. Polymorphisms of proinflammatory genes and Alzheimer's disease risk: A pharmacogenomic approach. *Mech Ageing Dev*. Jan 2007; 128(1): 67–75.

170. Zhao J, Fu Y, Yasvoina M et al. Beta-site amyloid precursor protein cleaving enzyme 1 levels become elevated in neurons around amyloid plaques: Implications for Alzheimer's disease pathogenesis. *J Neurosci*. Apr 4 2007; 27(14): 3639–3649.

171. Wu Y, Song W. Regulation of RCAN1 translation and its role in oxidative stress-induced apoptosis. *FASEB J*. Jan 2013; 27(1): 208–221.

172. Li RC, Morris MW, Lee SK, Pouranfar F, Wang Y, Gozal D. Neuroglobin protects PC12 cells against oxidative stress. *Brain Res*. Jan 23 2008; 1190: 159–166.

173. Li RC, Pouranfar F, Lee SK, Morris MW, Wang Y, Gozal D. Neuroglobin protects PC12 cells against beta-amyloid-induced cell injury. *Neurobiol Aging*. Dec 2008; 29(12): 1815–1822.

174. Khan AA, Mao XO, Banwait S, Jin K, Greenberg DA. Neuroglobin attenuates beta-amyloid neurotoxicity in vitro and transgenic Alzheimer phenotype in vivo. *Proc Natl Acad Sci U S A.* Nov 27 2007; 104(48): 19114–19119.
175. Szymanski M, Wang R, Fallin MD, Bassett SS, Avramopoulos D. Neuroglobin and Alzheimer's dementia: Genetic association and gene expression changes. *Neurobiol Aging.* Nov 14 2008.
176. Chen LM, Xiong YS, Kong FL et al. Neuroglobin attenuates Alzheimer-like tau hyperphosphorylation by activating Akt signaling. *J Neurochem.* Jan 2012; 120(1): 157–164.
177. Brittain T, Skommer J, Raychaudhuri S, Birch N. An antiapoptotic neuroprotective role for neuroglobin. *Int J Mol Sci.* 2010; 11(6): 2306–2321.
178. Sun Y, Jin K, Mao XO et al. Effect of aging on neuroglobin expression in rodent brain. *Neurobiol Aging.* Feb 2005; 26(2): 275–278.
179. Greenberg DA, Jin K, Khan AA. Neuroglobin: An endogenous neuroprotectant. *Curr Opin Pharmacol.* Feb 2008; 8(1): 20–24.
180. dos Santos VV, Santos DB, Lach G et al. Neuropeptide Y (NPY) prevents depressive-like behavior, spatial memory deficits and oxidative stress following amyloid-beta (Abeta(1–40)) administration in mice. *Behav Brain Res.* May 1 2013; 244: 107–115.
181. Algarzae N, Hebron M, Miessau M, Moussa CE. Parkin prevents cortical atrophy and Abeta-induced alterations of brain metabolism: (1)(3)C NMR and magnetic resonance imaging studies in AD models. *Neuroscience.* Dec 6 2012; 225: 22–34.
182. Itoh K, Chiba T, Takahashi S et al. An Nrf2/small Maf heterodimer mediates the induction of phase II detoxifying enzyme genes through antioxidant response elements. *Biochem Biophys Res Commun.* Jul 18 1997; 236(2): 313–322.
183. Hayes JD, Chanas SA, Henderson CJ et al. The Nrf2 transcription factor contributes both to the basal expression of glutathione S-transferases in mouse liver and to their induction by the chemopreventive synthetic antioxidants, butylated hydroxyanisole and ethoxyquin. *Biochem Soc Trans.* Feb 2000; 28(2): 33–41.
184. Chan K, Han XD, Kan YW. An important function of Nrf2 in combating oxidative stress: Detoxification of acetaminophen. *Proc Natl Acad Sci U S A.* Apr 10 2001; 98(8): 4611–4616.
185. Williamson TP, Johnson DA, Johnson JA. Activation of the Nrf2-ARE pathway by siRNA knockdown of Keap1 reduces oxidative stress and provides partial protection from MPTP-mediated neurotoxicity. *Neurotoxicology.* Jun 2012; 33(3): 272–279.
186. Niture SK, Kaspar JW, Shen J, Jaiswal AK. Nrf2 signaling and cell survival. *Toxicol Appl Pharmacol.* Apr 1 2010; 244(1): 37–42.
187. Xi YD, Yu HL, Ding J et al. Flavonoids protect cerebrovascular endothelial cells through Nrf2 and PI3K from beta-amyloid peptide-induced oxidative damage. *Curr Neurovasc Res.* Feb 2012; 9(1): 32–41.
188. Li XH, Li CY, Lu JM, Tian RB, Wei J. Allicin ameliorates cognitive deficits ageing-induced learning and memory deficits through enhancing of Nrf2 antioxidant signaling pathways. *Neurosci Lett.* Apr 11 2012; 514(1): 46–50.
189. Bergstrom P, Andersson HC, Gao Y et al. Repeated transient sulforaphane stimulation in astrocytes leads to prolonged Nrf2-mediated gene expression and protection from superoxide-induced damage. *Neuropharmacology.* Feb–Mar 2011; 60(2–3): 343–353.
190. Wruck CJ, Gotz ME, Herdegen T, Varoga D, Brandenburg LO, Pufe T. Kavalactones protect neural cells against amyloid beta peptide-induced neurotoxicity via extracellular signal-regulated kinase 1/2-dependent nuclear factor erythroid 2-related factor 2 activation. *Mol Pharmacol.* Jun 2008; 73(6): 1785–1795.
191. Hine CM, Mitchell JR. NRF2 and the phase II response in acute stress resistance induced by dietary restriction. *J Clin Exp Pathol.* Jun 19 2012; S4(4).

192. Suh JH, Shenvi SV, Dixon BM et al. Decline in transcriptional activity of Nrf2 causes age-related loss of glutathione synthesis, which is reversible with lipoic acid. *Proc Natl Acad Sci U S A*. Mar 9 2004; 101(10): 3381–3386.

193. Ramsey CP, Glass CA, Montgomery MB et al. Expression of Nrf2 in neurodegenerative diseases. *J Neuropathol Exp Neurol*. Jan 2007; 66(1): 75–85.

194. Kanninen K, Malm TM, Jyrkkanen HK et al. Nuclear factor erythroid 2-related factor 2 protects against beta amyloid. *Mol Cell Neurosci*. Nov 2008; 39(3): 302–313.

195. Zou Y, Hong B, Fan L et al. Protective effect of puerarin against beta-amyloid-induced oxidative stress in neuronal cultures from rat hippocampus: Involvement of the GSK-3beta/Nrf2 signaling pathway. *Free Radic Res*. Jan 2013; 47(1): 55–63.

196. Choi HK, Pokharel YR, Lim SC et al. Inhibition of liver fibrosis by solubilized coenzyme Q_{10}: Role of Nrf2 activation in inhibiting transforming growth factor beta 1 expression. *Toxicol Appl Pharmacol*. Nov 1 2009; 240(3): 377–384.

197. Trujillo J, Chirino YI, Molina-Jijon E, Anderica-Romero AC, Tapia E, Pedraza-Chaverri J. Renoprotective effect of the antioxidant curcumin: Recent findings. *Redox Biol*. 2013; 1(1): 448–456.

198. Steele ML, Fuller S, Patel M, Kersaitis C, Ooi L, Munch G. Effect of Nrf2 activators on release of glutathione, cysteinylglycine, and homocysteine by human U373 astroglial cells. *Redox Biol*. 2013; 1(1): 441–445.

199. Kode A, Rajendrasozhan S, Caito S, Yang SR, Megson IL, Rahman I. Resveratrol induces glutathione synthesis by activation of Nrf2 and protects against cigarette smoke-mediated oxidative stress in human lung epithelial cells. *Am J Physiol. Lung Cell Mol Physiol*. Mar 2008; 294(3): L478–488.

200. Gao L, Wang J, Sekhar KR et al. Novel n-3 fatty acid oxidation products activate Nrf2 by destabilizing the association between Keap1 and Cullin3. *J Biol Chem*. Jan 26 2007; 282(4): 2529–2537.

201. Saw CL, Yang AY, Guo Y, Kong AN. Astaxanthin and omega-3 fatty acids individually and in combination protect against oxidative stress via the Nrf2/ARE pathway. *Food Chem Toxicol*. Dec 2013; 62: 869–875.

202. Ji L, Liu R, Zhang XD et al. N-acetylcysteine attenuates phosgene-induced acute lung injury via upregulation of Nrf2 expression. *Inhal Toxicol*. Jun 2010; 22(7): 535–542.

203. Zambrano S, Blanca AJ, Ruiz-Armenta MV et al. The renoprotective effect of L-carnitine in hypertensive rats is mediated by modulation of oxidative stress-related gene expression. *Eur J Nutr*. Sep 2013; 52(6): 1649–1659.

204. Messier EM, Day BJ, Bahmed K et al. N-acetylcysteine protects murine alveolar type II cells from cigarette smoke injury in a nuclear erythroid 2-related factor-2-independent manner. *Am J Resp Cell Mol Biol*. May 2013; 48(5): 559–567.

205. Romanque P, Cornejo P, Valdes S, Videla LA. Thyroid hormone administration induces rat liver Nrf2 activation: Suppression by N-acetylcysteine pretreatment. *Thyroid*. Jun 2011; 21(6): 655–662.

206. Carlson DA, Smith AR, Fischer SJ, Young KL, Packer L. The plasma pharmacokinetics of R-(+)-lipoic acid administered as sodium R-(+)-lipoate to healthy human subjects. *Altern Med Rev*. Dec 2007; 12(4): 343–351.

207. Chng HT, New LS, Neo AH, Goh CW, Browne ER, Chan EC. Distribution study of orally administered lipoic acid in rat brain tissues. *Brain Res*. Jan 28 2009; 1251: 80–86.

208. Hager K, Kenklies M, McAfoose J, Engel J, Munch G. Alpha-lipoic acid as a new treatment option for Alzheimer's disease—a 48 months follow-up analysis. *J Neural Transm Suppl*. 2007(72): 189–193.

209. Moreira PI, Harris PL, Zhu X et al. Lipoic acid and N-acetyl cysteine decrease mitochondrial-related oxidative stress in Alzheimer disease patient fibroblasts. *J Alzheimers Dis*. Sep 2007; 12(2): 195–206.

210. Zhang L, Xing GQ, Barker JL et al. Alpha-lipoic acid protects rat cortical neurons against cell death induced by amyloid and hydrogen peroxide through the Akt signalling pathway. *Neurosci Lett.* Oct 26 2001; 312(3): 125–128.

211. Siedlak SL, Casadesus G, Webber KM et al. Chronic antioxidant therapy reduces oxidative stress in a mouse model of Alzheimer's disease. *Free Radic Res.* Feb 2009; 43(2): 156–164.

212. Quinn JF, Bussiere JR, Hammond RS et al. Chronic dietary alpha-lipoic acid reduces deficits in hippocampal memory of aged Tg2576 mice. *Neurobiol Aging.* Feb 2007; 28(2): 213–225.

213. Farr SA, Price TO, Banks WA, Ercal N, Morley JE. Effect of alpha-lipoic acid on memory, oxidation, and lifespan in SAMP8 mice. *J Alzheimers Dis.* 2012; 32(2): 447–455.

214. Suchy J, Chan A, Shea TB. Dietary supplementation with a combination of alpha-lipoic acid, acetyl-L-carnitine, glycerophosphocoline, docosahexaenoic acid, and phosphatidylserine reduces oxidative damage to murine brain and improves cognitive performance. *Nutr Res.* Jan 2009; 29(1): 70–74.

215. Zara S, De Colli M, Rapino M et al. Ibuprofen and lipoic acid conjugate neuroprotective activity is mediated by Ngb/Akt intracellular signaling pathway in Alzheimer's disease rat model. *Gerontology.* 2013; 59(3): 250–260.

216. Holmquist L, Stuchbury G, Berbaum K et al. Lipoic acid as a novel treatment for Alzheimer's disease and related dementias. *Pharmacol Ther.* Jan 2007; 113(1): 154–164.

217. Maczurek A, Hager K, Kenklies M et al. Lipoic acid as an anti-inflammatory and neuroprotective treatment for Alzheimer's disease. *Adv Drug Deliv Rev.* Oct–Nov 2008; 60(13–14): 1463–1470.

218. Yang X, Yang Y, Li G, Wang J, Yang ES. Coenzyme Q_{10} attenuates beta-amyloid pathology in the aged transgenic mice with Alzheimer presenilin 1 mutation. *J Mol Neurosci.* Feb 2008; 34(2): 165–171.

219. Ono K, Hasegawa K, Naiki H, Yamada M. Preformed beta-amyloid fibrils are destabilized by coenzyme Q_{10} *in vitro. Biochem Biophys Res Commun.* Apr 29 2005; 330(1): 111–116.

220. Moreira PI, Santos MS, Sena C, Nunes E, Seica R, Oliveira CR. Co Q_{10} therapy attenuates amyloid beta-peptide toxicity in brain mitochondria isolated from aged diabetic rats. *Exp Neurol.* Nov 2005; 196(1): 112–119.

221. de Bustos F, Molina JA, Jimenez-Jimenez FJ et al. Serum levels of coenzyme Q_{10} in patients with Alzheimer's disease. *J Neural Transm.* 2000; 107(2): 233–239.

222. McDonald SR, Sohal RS, Forster MJ. Concurrent administration of coenzyme Q_{10} and alpha-tocopherol improves learning in aged mice. *Free Radic Biol Med.* Mar 15 2005; 38(6): 729–736.

223. Feng Z, Qin C, Chang Y, Zhang JT. Early melatonin supplementation alleviates oxidative stress in a transgenic mouse model of Alzheimer's disease. *Free Radic Biol Med.* Jan 1 2006; 40(1): 101–109.

224. Olcese JM, Cao C, Mori T et al. Protection against cognitive deficits and markers of neurodegeneration by long-term oral administration of melatonin in a transgenic model of Alzheimer disease. *J Pineal Res.* Aug 2009; 47(1): 82–96.

225. Gehrman PR, Connor DJ, Martin JL, Shochat T, Corey-Bloom J, Ancoli-Israel S. Melatonin fails to improve sleep or agitation in double-blind randomized placebo-controlled trial of institutionalized patients with Alzheimer disease. *Am J Geriatr Psychiatry.* Feb 2009; 17(2): 166–169.

226. Furio AM, Brusco LI, Cardinali DP. Possible therapeutic value of melatonin in mild cognitive impairment: A retrospective study. *J Pineal Res.* Nov 2007; 43(4): 404–409.

227. Green KN, Steffan JS, Martinez-Coria H et al. Nicotinamide restores cognition in Alzheimer's disease transgenic mice via a mechanism involving sirtuin inhibition and selective reduction of Thr231-phosphotau. *J Neurosci.* Nov 5 2008; 28(45): 11500–11510.

228. Liu D, Pitta M, Mattson MP. Preventing NAD(+) depletion protects neurons against excitotoxicity: Bioenergetic effects of mild mitochondrial uncoupling and caloric restriction. *Ann NY Acad Sci.* Dec 2008; 1147: 275–282.

229. Liu D, Pitta M, Jiang H et al. Nicotinamide forestalls pathology and cognitive decline in Alzheimer mice: Evidence for improved neuronal bioenergetics and autophagy procession. *Neurobiol Aging.* Jun 2013; 34(6): 1564–1580.

230. Birkmayer JG. Coenzyme nicotinamide adenine dinucleotide: new therapeutic approach for improving dementia of the Alzheimer type. *Ann Clin Lab Sci.* Jan–Feb 1996; 26(1): 1–9.

231. Rex A, Spychalla M, Fink H. Treatment with reduced nicotinamide adenine dinucleotide (NADH) improves water maze performance in old Wistar rats. *Behav Brain Res.* Sep 23 2004; 154(1): 149–153.

232. Demarin V, Podobnik SS, Storga-Tomic D, Kay G. Treatment of Alzheimer's disease with stabilized oral nicotinamide adenine dinucleotide: A randomized, double-blind study. *Drugs Exp Clin Res.* 2004; 30(1): 27–33.

233. Rainer M, Kraxberger E, Haushofer M, Mucke HA, Jellinger KA. No evidence for cognitive improvement from oral nicotinamide adenine dinucleotide (NADH) in dementia. *J Neural Transm.* 2000; 107(12): 1475–1481.

234. Ono K, Yoshiike Y, Takashima A, Hasegawa K, Naiki H, Yamada M. Vitamin A exhibits potent antiamyloidogenic and fibril-destabilizing effects *in vitro*. *Exp Neurol.* Oct 2004; 189(2): 380–392.

235. Ding Y, Qiao A, Wang Z et al. Retinoic acid attenuates beta-amyloid deposition and rescues memory deficits in an Alzheimer's disease transgenic mouse model. *J Neurosci.* Nov 5 2008; 28(45): 11622–11634.

236. Peng QL, Buz'Zard AR, Lau BH. Pycnogenol protects neurons from amyloid-beta peptide-induced apoptosis. *Brain Res Mol Brain Res.* Jul 15 2002; 104(1): 55–65.

237. Sung S, Yao Y, Uryu K et al. Early vitamin E supplementation in young but not aged mice reduces Abeta levels and amyloid deposition in a transgenic model of Alzheimer's disease. *FASEB J.* Feb 2004; 18(2): 323–325.

238. Desrumaux C, Pisoni A, Meunier J et al. Increased amyloid-beta peptide-induced memory deficits in phospholipid transfer protein (PLTP) gene knockout mice. *Neuropsychopharmacology.* Apr 2013; 38(5): 817–825.

239. Isaac MG, Quinn R, Tabet N. Vitamin E for Alzheimer's disease and mild cognitive impairment. *Cochrane Database Syst Rev.* 2008(3): CD002854.

240. Farina N, Isaac MG, Clark AR, Rusted J, Tabet N. Vitamin E for Alzheimer's dementia and mild cognitive impairment. *Cochrane Database Syst Rev.* 2012; 11: CD002854.

241. Sano M, Ernesto C, Thomas RG et al. A controlled trial of selegiline, alpha-tocopherol, or both as treatment for Alzheimer's disease. The Alzheimer's Disease Cooperative Study. *N Engl J Med.* Apr 24 1997; 336(17): 1216–1222.

242. Fillenbaum GG, Kuchibhatla MN, Hanlon JT et al. Dementia and Alzheimer's disease in community-dwelling elders taking vitamin C and/or vitamin E. *Ann Pharmacother.* Dec 2005; 39(12): 2009–2014.

243. Gray SL, Anderson ML, Crane PK et al. Antioxidant vitamin supplement use and risk of dementia or Alzheimer's disease in older adults. *J Am Geriatr Soc.* Feb 2008; 56(2): 291–295.

244. Zandi PP, Anthony JC, Khachaturian AS et al. Reduced risk of Alzheimer disease in users of antioxidant vitamin supplements: The Cache County Study. *Arch Neurol.* Jan 2004; 61(1): 82–88.

245. Chen P, Wang RR, Ma XJ, Liu Q, Ni JZ. Different forms of selenoprotein M differentially affect Abeta aggregation and ROS generation. *Int J Mol Sci.* 2013; 14(3): 4385–4399.

246. Du X, Li H, Wang Z, Qiu S, Liu Q, Ni J. Selenoprotein P and selenoprotein M block Zn-mediated Abeta aggregation and toxicity. *Metallomics: Integrated Biometal Science.* May 8 2013.

247. Zhang GL, Zhang WG, Du Y et al. Edaravone ameliorates oxidative damage associated with Aβ25–35 treatment in PC12 cells. *J Mol Neurosci.* Jul 2013; 50(3): 494–503.
248. Jimenez-Jimenez FJ, Molina JA, de Bustos F et al. Serum levels of beta-carotene, alpha-carotene and vitamin A in patients with Alzheimer's disease. *Eur J Neurol.* Jul 1999; 6(4): 495–497.
249. Jimenez-Jimenez FJ, de Bustos F, Molina JA et al. Cerebrospinal fluid levels of alpha-tocopherol (vitamin E) in Alzheimer's disease. *J Neural Transm.* 1997; 104(6–7): 703–710.
250. Rinaldi P, Polidori MC, Metastasio A et al. Plasma antioxidants are similarly depleted in mild cognitive impairment and in Alzheimer's disease. *Neurobiol Aging.* Nov 2003; 24(7): 915–919.
251. Charlton KE, Rabinowitz TL, Geffen LN, Dhansay MA. Lowered plasma vitamin C, but not vitamin E, concentrations in dementia patients. *J Nutr Health Aging.* 2004; 8(2): 99–107.
252. Cole MG, Prchal JF. Low serum vitamin B_{12} in Alzheimer-type dementia. *Age Ageing.* Mar 1984; 13(2): 101–105.
253. Regland B, Gottfries CG, Oreland L. Vitamin B_{12}-induced reduction of platelet monoamine oxidase activity in patients with dementia and pernicious anaemia. *Eur Arch Psychiatry Clin Neurosci.* 1991; 240(4–5): 288–291.
254. Nadeau A, Roberge AG. Effects of vitamin B_{12} supplementation on choline acetyltransferase activity in cat brain. *Int J Vitam Nutr Res.* 1988; 58(4): 402–406.
255. Ikeda T, Yamamoto K, Takahashi K et al. Treatment of Alzheimer-type dementia with intravenous mecobalamin. *Clin Ther.* May–Jun 1992; 14(3): 426–437.
256. Malouf R, Grimley Evans J. Folic acid with or without vitamin B_{12} for the prevention and treatment of healthy elderly and demented people. *Cochrane Database Syst Rev.* 2008(4): CD004514.
257. Aisen PS, Schneider LS, Sano M et al. High-dose B vitamin supplementation and cognitive decline in Alzheimer disease: A randomized controlled trial. *JAMA.* Oct 15 2008; 300(15): 1774–1783.
258. van Dyck CH, Lyness JM, Rohrbaugh RM, Siegal AP. Cognitive and psychiatric effects of vitamin B_{12} replacement in dementia with low serum B12 levels: A nursing home study. *Int Psychogeriatr.* Feb 2009; 21(1): 138–147.
259. Vingtdeux V, Dreses-Werringloer U, Zhao H, Davies P, Marambaud P. Therapeutic potential of resveratrol in Alzheimer's disease. *BMC Neurosci.* 2008; 9 Suppl 2: S6.
260. Wang J, Ho L, Zhao Z et al. Moderate consumption of Cabernet Sauvignon attenuates Abeta neuropathology in a mouse model of Alzheimer's disease. *FASEB J.* Nov 2006; 20(13): 2313–2320.
261. Luchsinger JA, Tang MX, Siddiqui M, Shea S, Mayeux R. Alcohol intake and risk of dementia. *J Am Geriatr Soc.* Apr 2004; 52(4): 540–546.
262. Savaskan E, Olivieri G, Meier F, Seifritz E, Wirz-Justice A, Muller-Spahn F. Red wine ingredient resveratrol protects from beta-amyloid neurotoxicity. *Gerontology.* Nov–Dec 2003; 49(6): 380–383.
263. Marambaud P, Zhao H, Davies P. Resveratrol promotes clearance of Alzheimer's disease amyloid-beta peptides. *J Biol Chem.* Nov 11 2005; 280(45): 37377–37382.
264. Anekonda TS. Resveratrol—a boon for treating Alzheimer's disease? *Brain Res Rev.* Sep 2006; 52(2): 316–326.
265. Tang BL, Chua CE. SIRT1 and neuronal diseases. *Mol Aspects Med.* Jun 2008; 29(3): 187–200.
266. Wight RD, Tull CA, Deel MW et al. Resveratrol effects on astrocyte function: Relevance to neurodegenerative diseases. *Biochem Biophys Res Commun.* Sep 14 2012; 426(1): 112–115.

267. Jiang T, Zhi XL, Zhang YH, Pan LF, Zhou P. Inhibitory effect of curcumin on the Al(III)-induced Abeta(4)(2) aggregation and neurotoxicity in vitro. *Biochim Biophys Acta.* Aug 2012; 1822(8): 1207–1215.

268. Taylor M, Moore S, Mourtas S et al. Effect of curcumin-associated and lipid ligand-functionalized nanoliposomes on aggregation of the Alzheimer's Abeta peptide. *Nanomedicine.* Oct 2011; 7(5): 541–550.

269. Hamaguchi T, Ono K, Yamada M. REVIEW: Curcumin and Alzheimer's disease. *CNS Neurosci Ther.* Oct 2010; 16(5): 285–297.

270. DeKosky ST, Williamson JD, Fitzpatrick AL et al. Ginkgo biloba for prevention of dementia: a randomized controlled trial. *JAMA.* Nov 19 2008; 300(19): 2253–2262.

271. Augustin S, Rimbach G, Augustin K, Schliebs R, Wolffram S, Cermak R. Effect of a short- and long-term treatment with Ginkgo biloba extract on amyloid precursor protein levels in a transgenic mouse model relevant to Alzheimer's disease. *Arch Biochem Biophys.* Jan 15 2009; 481(2): 177–182.

272. Freund-Levi Y, Eriksdotter-Jonhagen M, Cederholm T et al. Omega-3 fatty acid treatment in 174 patients with mild to moderate Alzheimer disease: OmegAD study: A randomized double-blind trial. *Arch Neurol.* Oct 2006; 63(10): 1402–1408.

273. Fotuhi M, Mohassel P, Yaffe K. Fish consumption, long-chain omega-3 fatty acids and risk of cognitive decline or Alzheimer disease: A complex association. *Nat Clin Pract Neurol.* Mar 2009; 5(3): 140–152.

274. Kroger E, Verreault R, Carmichael PH et al. Omega-3 fatty acids and risk of dementia: The Canadian study of health and aging. *Am J Clin Nutr.* Jul 2009; 90(1): 184–192.

275. Chiu CC, Su KP, Cheng TC et al. The effects of omega-3 fatty acids monotherapy in Alzheimer's disease and mild cognitive impairment: A preliminary randomized double-blind placebo-controlled study. *Prog Neuropsychopharmacol Biol Psychiatry.* Aug 1 2008; 32(6): 1538–1544.

276. Rezai-Zadeh K, Arendash GW, Hou H et al. Green tea epigallocatechin-3-gallate (EGCG) reduces beta-amyloid mediated cognitive impairment and modulates tau pathology in Alzheimer transgenic mice. *Brain Res.* Jun 12 2008; 1214: 177–187.

277. Lim HJ, Shim SB, Jee SW et al. Green tea catechin leads to global improvement among Alzheimer's disease-related phenotypes in NSE/hAPP-C105 Tg mice. *J Nutr Biochem.* Jan 17 2013.

278. Arendash GW, Schleif W, Rezai-Zadeh K et al. Caffeine protects Alzheimer's mice against cognitive impairment and reduces brain beta-amyloid production. *Neuroscience.* Nov 3 2006; 142(4): 941–952.

279. Ma WW, Hou CC, Zhou X et al. Genistein alleviates the mitochondria-targeted DNA damage induced by beta-amyloid peptides 25–35 in C6 glioma cells. *Neurochem Res.* Jul 2013; 38(7): 1315–1323.

280. Xi YD, Yu HL, Ma WW et al. Genistein inhibits mitochondrial-targeted oxidative damage induced by beta-amyloid peptide 25–35 in PC12 cells. *J Bioenerg Biomembr.* Aug 2011; 43(4): 399–407.

281. Shoulson I. DATATOP: A decade of neuroprotective inquiry. Parkinson Study Group. Deprenyl and tocopherol antioxidative therapy of Parkinsonism. *Ann Neurol.* Sep 1998; 44(3 Suppl 1): S160–166.

282. Albanes D, Heinonen OP, Huttunen JK et al. Effects of alpha-tocopherol and beta-carotene supplements on cancer incidence in the alpha-tocopherol beta-carotene cancer prevention study. *Am J Clin Nutr.* Dec 1995; 62(6 Suppl): 1427S–1430S.

283. Chen RS, Huang CC, Chu NS. Coenzyme Q_{10} treatment in mitochondrial encephalomyopathies. Short-term double-blind, crossover study. *Eur Neurol.* 1997; 37(4): 212–218.

284. Gaziano JM, Sesso HD, Christen WG et al. Multivitamins in the prevention of cancer in men: The Physicians' Health Study II randomized controlled trial. *JAMA*. Nov 14 2012; 308(18): 1871–1880.

285. Baum MK, Campa A, Lai S et al. Effect of micronutrient supplementation on disease progression in asymptomatic, antiretroviral-naive, HIV-infected adults in Botswana: A randomized clinical trial. *JAMA*. Nov 27 2013; 310(20): 2154–2163.

286. Sharif SF, Hariri RJ, Chang VA, Barie PS, Wang RS, Ghajar JB. Human astrocyte production of tumour necrosis factor-alpha, interleukin-1 beta, and interleukin-6 following exposure to lipopolysaccharide endotoxin. *Neurol Res*. Apr 1993; 15(2): 109–112.

287. Rozemuller JM, Eikelenboom P, Pals ST, Stam FC. Microglial cells around amyloid plaques in Alzheimer's disease express leucocyte adhesion molecules of the LFA-1 family. *Neurosci Lett*. Jul 3 1989; 101(3): 288–292.

288. Breitner JC, Gau BA, Welsh KA et al. Inverse association of anti-inflammatory treatments and Alzheimer's disease: Initial results of a cotwin control study. *Neurology*. Feb 1994; 44(2): 227–232.

289. Andersen K, Launer LJ, Ott A, Hoes AW, Breteler MM, Hofman A. Do nonsteroidal anti-inflammatory drugs decrease the risk for Alzheimer's disease? The Rotterdam Study. *Neurology*. Aug 1995; 45(8): 1441–1445.

290. Aisen PS, Davis KL, Berg JD et al. A randomized controlled trial of prednisone in Alzheimer's disease. Alzheimer's disease cooperative study. *Neurology*. Feb 8 2000; 54(3): 588–593.

291. Cote S, Carmichael PH, Verreault R, Lindsay J, Lefebvre J, Laurin D. Nonsteroidal anti-inflammatory drug use and the risk of cognitive impairment and Alzheimer's disease. *Alzheimers Dement*. May 2012; 8(3): 219–226.

292. Scharf S, Mander A, Ugoni A, Vajda F, Christophidis N. A double-blind, placebo-controlled trial of diclofenac/misoprostol in Alzheimer's disease. *Neurology*. Jul 13 1999; 53(1): 197–201.

293. Sainati S, Ingram D, Talwalker S. Results of a double-blind, placebo-controlled study of Celecoxib in the treatment of progression of Alzheimer's disease. Paper presented at: *Sixth International Stockholm Springfield Symposium of Advances in Alzheimer's Therapy 2000*; Stockholm.

294. McGeer PL. Cyclo-oxygenase-2 inhibitors: Rationale and therapeutic potential for Alzheimer's disease. *Drugs Aging*. Jul 2000; 17(1): 1–11.

295. Choi SH, Aid S, Caracciolo L et al. Cyclooxygenase-1 inhibition reduces amyloid pathology and improves memory deficits in a mouse model of Alzheimer's disease. *J Neurochem*. Jan 2013; 124(1): 59–68.

296. Bernardi A, Frozza RL, Meneghetti A et al. Indomethacin-loaded lipid-core nanocapsules reduce the damage triggered by $A\beta 1$–42 in Alzheimer's disease models. *Intl J Nanomed*. 2012; 7: 4927–4942.

297. Candelario-Jalil E, Akundi RS, Bhatia HS et al. Ascorbic acid enhances the inhibitory effect of aspirin on neuronal cyclooxygenase-2-mediated prostaglandin E2 production. *J Neuroimmunol*. May 2006; 174(1–2): 39–51.

298. Mackenzie IR, Munoz DG. Nonsteroidal anti-inflammatory drug use and Alzheimer-type pathology in aging. *Neurology*. Apr 1998; 50(4): 986–990.

299. Lim GP, Yang F, Chu T et al. Ibuprofen suppresses plaque pathology and inflammation in a mouse model for Alzheimer's disease. *J Neurosci*. Aug 1 2000; 20(15): 5709–5714.

300. Abate A, Yang G, Dennery PA, Oberle S, Schroder H. Synergistic inhibition of cyclooxygenase-2 expression by vitamin E and aspirin. *Free Radic Biol Med*. Dec 2000; 29(11): 1135–1142.

301. Fotuhi M, Zandi PP, Hayden KM et al. Better cognitive performance in elderly taking antioxidant vitamins E and C supplements in combination with nonsteroidal anti-inflammatory drugs: The Cache County Study. *Alzheimers Dement*. May 2008; 4(3): 223–227.

302. Lopez-Pousa S, Turon-Estrada A, Garre-Olmo J et al. Differential efficacy of treatment with acetylcholinesterase inhibitors in patients with mild and moderate Alzheimer's disease over a 6-month period. *Dement Geriatr Cogn Disord.* 2005; 19(4): 189–195.

303. Birks J, Flicker L. Donepezil for mild cognitive impairment. *Cochrane Database Syst Rev.* 2006; 3: CD006104.

304. Lopez OL, Mackell JA, Sun Y et al. Effectiveness and safety of donepezil in Hispanic patients with Alzheimer's disease: A 12-week open-label study. *J Natl Med Assoc.* Nov 2008; 100(11): 1350–1358.

305. Mucha L, Shaohung S, Cuffel B, McRae T, Mark TL, Del Valle M. Comparison of cholinesterase inhibitor utilization patterns and associated health care costs in Alzheimer's disease. *J Manag Care Pharm.* Jun 2008; 14(5): 451–461.

306. Kurata T, Miyazaki K, Morimoto N et al. Atorvastatin and pitavastatin reduce oxidative stress and improve IR/LDL-R signals in Alzheimer's disease. *Neurol Res.* Mar 2013; 35(2): 193–205.

307. Prior M, Dargusch R, Ehren JL, Chiruta C, Schubert D. The neurotrophic compound J147 reverses cognitive impairment in aged Alzheimer's disease mice. *Alzheimers Res Ther.* May 14 2013; 5(3): 25.

4 Etiology of Parkinson's Disease

Prevention and Improved Management by Micronutrients

INTRODUCTION

Parkinson's disease (PD) is considered a slow progressive neurological disorder associated with defects in the function of the extrapyramidal system in the brain which controls voluntary movements. This disease is also associated with nonmotor deficits and neurological symptoms, including impaired olfaction, autonomic failure, cognitive impairment, and psychiatric symptoms. PD is the commonest form of neurodegenerative diseases after Alzheimer's disease. It is estimated that in normal individuals about 3–5% of dopaminergic (DA) neurons are lost every decade; however, in PD patients, the rate of loss is greater than that found in normal individuals.[1] The analysis of autopsied samples of PD brain revealed that about 70–75 of DA neurons are lost at the time the disease becomes detectable. This suggests that DA neurons possess a high degree of functional plasticity.

Some environmental-, dietary- or lifestyle-related factors that influence the incidence of PD have been identified. Research of the last several decades has identified major biochemical defects which participate in the initiation and progression of PD. These defects include increased oxidative stress, mitochondrial dysfunction, chronic inflammation, and proteasome inhibition. The genetic defects include overexpression of alpha-synuclein or mutation in alpha-synuclein. It is not certain which of the biochemical or genetic defects is the earliest event that initiates damage to DA neurons. Based on the above biochemical defects, it is possible to develop nontoxic agents that can be used for the prevention, and in combination with standard therapy, for the improved management of PD. Antioxidants which reduce oxidative stress and chronic inflammation may be one of the rational choices for the prevention and improved management of PD. Unfortunately, clinical trial with a single antioxidant has produced inconsistent results, varying from no effect to some transient beneficial effects in reducing the symptoms of the disease.

At present, there is no effective strategy for reducing the incidence or progression of PD in high-risk populations (familial cases, early stage PD, and individuals over the age of 65 years). The current drug and surgical treatments are very effective in improving the major symptoms of PD; but the efficacy of these treatments is only transient. In addition, the beneficial effects of the commonly used drug, levodopa, persists for about 5 years after which the symptoms of PD become aggravated. These side effects of levodopa are due to progressive damage to DA neurons. It is known that auto-oxidation of L-dopa and dopamine generates excessive amounts of free radicals that could damage not only DA neurons but neurons in other regions of the brain. The toxic side effects become a limiting factor for the continuation of levodopa therapy. None of the current treatments with drugs or surgical procedures affects the levels of oxidative stress and chronic inflammation. Therefore, DA neurons continue to die despite drug treatment.

The prevalence of PD is likely to increase in the future because of growth of the older population. Therefore, novel strategies based on the causes of the disease should be developed for the prevention and improved management of PD.

This chapter briefly describes incidence, cost, causes, neuropathology of PD, and proposes that increased oxidative stress is the earliest biochemical defect which initiates degeneration in the DA neurons. Other biochemical defects occur subsequent to increased oxidative stress. In addition, this chapter describes scientific rational and evidence for using a micronutrient formulation containing dietary and endogenous antioxidants, as well as certain polyphenolic compounds for reducing the incidence and progression of PD, and in combination with standard therapy, for the improved management of PD.

PREVALENCE AND INCIDENCE

USA

About 1 million people suffer from Parkinson's disease and about 60,000 new cases are diagnosed annually in the USA (Parkinson's Disease Foundation, 2013). About 3–4 million people remain undiagnosed. Average age of individuals for developing PD is around 60 years. Incidence rate of PD increases with age. Approximately 4% of people with PD are diagnosed before the age of 50 years. Men are one and a half times more likely to develop PD than women.

The age- and gender-adjusted annual incidence rates in ethnic groups were highest among Hispanics, followed by non-Hispanic Whites, Asians, and Blacks.[2] The data are summarized below.

Ethnic Group	Incidence (Cases/100,000 People)
Non-hispanic white	13.6
Hispanic	16.6
Asian	11.3
Black	10.2

WORLDWIDE

About 6.3 million people have PD. The World Health Organization (WHO) estimates that the prevalence of PD is about 160 cases per 100,000 people, and the annual incidence of this disease is about 16–19 cases per 100,000 (International Group Researchers and Development for Complimentary Medicine, 2013).

COST

The direct and indirect cost of PD is estimated to be about $25 billion per year in the USA. Average medical cost per person is about $2500.00 per year, and the therapeutic surgery may cost as high as $100,000.00 per patient (Parkinson's Disease Foundation, 2013).

NEUROPATHOLOGY AND SYMPTOMS

In 1917, Dr. James Parkinson, a British physician, published an article on "The Shaky Palsy" describing the major symptoms of the disease that would later bear his name. Since then, pathologists and neurologists have repeatedly reported the loss of dopamine (DA)-producing nerve cells (DA neurons) from the substantia nigra (SN) region of the brain of PD patients. Major symptoms of PD include tremor (trembling in hands, arms, legs, jaw, and face); rigidity, (stiffness of the limbs and trunk); bradykinesia (slowness of movement); and postural instability (impaired balance and coordination). This disease is characterized by the presence of Lewy bodies in the cytoplasm of the neuron and its neurites. In addition to the SN, other areas of the brain, such as locus coeruleus, reticular nuclei of the brainstem, dorsal motor nucleus of the vagus, and the amygdala and the CA2 of the hippocampus are also affected. Lewy bodies are also found in these locations of the brain. Lewy bodies contain predominantly neurofilaments that are important components of the neuronal cytoskeleton and ubiquitin that degrades abnormal proteins. Lewy bodies also contain high levels of alpha-synuclein. More recently, the presence of another protein FOXO3 (a transcriptional activator which can trigger neuronal death upon oxidative stress) was demonstrated in Lewy bodies in the autopsied brain samples of PD as well as in the Lewy body dementia.[3] Lewy bodies are considered consequences of neuronal damage. They can be transferred from one neuron to another by endocytosis. This was demonstrated by the fact that Lewy bodies were present in the neurons grafted in patients with PD and in a transgenic animal model of PD.[4] *In vitro* studies showed that extracellular alpha-synuclein oligomers can induce intracellular alpha-synuclein aggregation in neurons.

The major symptoms of PD include tremor, muscle rigidity, postural problems, gait disorders, speaking difficulties, cognitive dysfunction, and immobility that ultimately lead to total disability and death. Increased oxidative stress, mitochondrial dysfunction, and chronic inflammation play a central role in the pathogenesis of PD.

The nonmotor symptoms include sleep disorders due to a dysfunctional circadian system. This could be due to a defect in the signaling output from the suprachiasmatic nuclei caused by increased oxidative stress and mitochondrial dysfunction.[5]

CAUSES OF PD

The identification of agents which can increase or decrease the risk of developing PD may include environmental-, diet-, and lifestyle-related factors, and internal factors (increased oxidative stress, mitochondrial dysfunction, chronic inflammation, and genetic defects) are important in order to develop rational strategies for prevention and improved management of PD.

EXTERNAL FACTORS THAT INFLUENCE RISK OF DEVELOPING PD

ENVIRONMENTAL AGENTS THAT INCREASE RISK OF PD

Age is a risk factor for most idiopathic (sporadic) neurological diseases including PD. Exposure to excess of manganese (Mn) produces cognitive dysfunction, motor deficits, and psychiatric problems. Exposure to Mn occurs primarily among workers of the steel industry and welding. It is interesting to note that no degeneration of DA neurons occur in Mn-induced neurological disorders in nonhuman primates; however, welders who were exposed to high levels of Mn from the welding fumes exhibited dysfunction of DA neurons. In addition, smelter workers who were exposed to Mn showed defects in the function of the thalamus and frontal cortex.[6] An epidemiologic study on manganese miners showed increased incidence of the PD-like disease.[7] This is because increased brain levels of free manganese can enhance the production of free radicals, which then gradually cause damage to DA neurons.

A meta-analysis of 104 studies with 3087 references revealed that the risk of PD increased among individuals who were exposed to pesticide, herbicides, and solvents.[8] Exposure to fungicides did not increase the risk of PD.[9] Trichloroethylene (TCE) is the most common organic contaminant in the ground water, whereas perchloroethylene (PERC) and carbon tetrachloride (CCl) are ubiquitous in the environment. Among these solvents, TCE was most effective in increasing the risk of PD.[10] Paraquat, one of the herbicides, and neonatal iron exposure increased the risk of PD; however, a combination of the two increased neurodegeneration via increased oxidative stress in a synergistic manner.[11]

LIFESTYLE-RELATED FACTORS THAT INCREASE RISK OF PD

In 1980, increased incidence of PD-like disease was seen among users of the designer drug, meperidene, which contains 1-methyl-4-phenyl 1,2,3,6 tetrahydropyridine (MPTP), a neurotoxic byproduct formed during the synthesis of this drug.[12] At least one of the mechanisms of action of MPTP-induced degeneration of DA neurons is mediated by free radicals.

LIFESTYLE-RELATED FACTORS THAT REDUCE RISK OF PD

An epidemiologic study suggested that cigarette smoking may reduce the risk of PD. In order to clarify the role of smoking, a clinical study was performed on 113 twin pairs in which at least one twin had PD. The results showed that cigarette smoking reduced the risk of PD. The reduction in the incidence was most pronounced in genetically identical twin pairs.[13] An epidemiologic study showed that ibuprofen users, but not aspirin (acetylsalicylic acid) users, had reduced risk of PD.[14] Increased consumption of caffeine decreases the risk of PD.[15] A combination of cigarette smoking, coffee drinking, and nonsteroidal anti-inflammatory drug (NSAID) was associated with 87% reduction in the incidence of PD.[16]

DIET-RELATED FACTORS THAT REDUCE RISK OF PD

Although no particular dietary risk factors for PD were identified, the consumption of nuts and salad oil (pressed from seeds) appeared to be of protective value.[17] Vitamin E consumption was found to be lower among patients with PD than among normal control.[18] The role of dietary antioxidants in PD are discussed later in this chapter.

INTERNAL FACTORS INFLUENCING DEVELOPMENT AND PROGRESSION OF PD

Internal factors in the development and progression of PD include increased oxidative stress, mitochondrial dysfunction, chronic inflammation, and defects in certain genes. The role of these internal factors are discussed here.

INCREASED OXIDATIVE STRESS IN PD

STUDIES ON AUTOPSIED HUMAN BRAIN TISSUE

Several studies have demonstrated the presence of high levels of oxidative stress in the autopsied brain samples of PD patients. The normal brain has the highest concentration of unsaturated fatty acids of all organs, and these fatty acids are very susceptible to lipid peroxidation. Indeed, high levels of oxidative damage have been observed in the autopsied samples of substantia nigra of PD brains.[19–22] Autopsied samples of substantia nigra of PD brain contained reduced levels of antioxidant enzymes[23,24] and antioxidants.[25–27] Reduced glutathione levels were observed in the substantia nigra of the autopsied brain samples of PD patients indicating the presence of high oxidative stress.[28–30] Reduced glutathione can impair mitochondrial function. The antioxidant capacity in the autopsied substantia nigra of PD brain was lower than control subjects.[31]

Isofurans are products of lipid peroxidation, and their formation is favored in the presence of high oxygen tension. The levels of isofurans but not F2-isoprostane are elevated in the autopsied samples of the substantia nigra of PD patients.[32] Heme oxygenase-1 (HO-1) is a cellular stress protein expressed in brain and other tissues and becomes elevated in response to increased oxidative stress. The expression of HO-1 is upregulated in the autopsied samples of the substantia nigra of PD brain.[33]

Several studies have confirmed that PD is associated with a significant increase in free iron in the degenerating substantia nigra.[34–36] The effects of iron on degeneration of DA neurons are via increased oxidative stress. The mechanisms of accumulation of iron in the substantia nigra are unknown; however, an isoform of the divalent metal transporter-1 (DMT1) is elevated in the substantia nigra of PD brain.[37]

Glutamate is a major excitatory transmitter in the mammalian central nervous system and is neurotoxic when present in excess at the synapses. With the depletion of nigrostriatal DA neurons, the glutamatergic projections from subthalamic nucleus to the basal ganglia output nuclei become overactive.[38] The glutamatergic activity also increased in the striatal region of the PD brain.

It has been reported that the neuromelanin granules accumulate in the substantia nigra of PD patients. Neuromelanin is formed from auto-oxidation of catecholamines in the substantia nigra of PD brain and contains significant amounts of iron.[39,40] Neuromelanin can cause degeneration in DA neurons by generating H_2O_2 when it is intact, or by releasing redox active metals such as iron, if it is impaired. In addition, dying DA neurons can release melanin that can initiate chronic inflammatory responses by activating microglia cells.

Uric acid is a product of purine metabolism and exhibits antioxidant activity. The serum uric acid levels were lower in PD patients than in control subjects in the Chinese population. The levels of uric acid correlated with the progression of the disease.[41] Similar association between the uric acid levels and disease progression is found in both men and women.

STUDIES ON BRAIN OF ANIMAL MODEL OF PD

Using a MPTP model of rat PD, it was demonstrated that the expression of DMT1 and the levels of iron increased in treated animals. These two biological events were associated with increased oxidative stress and neuronal death.[37] The mutation in DMT1 protected rats against toxicity produced by MPTP or 6-hydroxydopamine. Manganese enhanced DA-induced apoptosis in mesencephalic neurons.[42] The effect of manganese is mediated by induction of NF-kappaB and activation of nitric oxide synthase that generates increased amounts of free radicals. Excessive production of NO by the treatment with MPTP plays a significant role in degeneration of DA neurons, because nitric oxide can be oxidized to form peroxynitrite, a form of nitrogen-derived free radicals that is highly neurotoxic. Therefore, the involvement of NO in the pathophysiology of PD has been proposed.[43]

The NADOH oxidases (NOXs) are the major source of reactive oxygen species (ROS). Therefore, the levels of these enzymes should be elevated in PD. Indeed, the levels of NOX-1 in the rat dopaminergic cells (N27 neuron) were increased after treatment with 6-hydroxydopamine. Injection of 6-hydroxydopamine directly into the striatum increased the levels of NOX-1 in dopaminergic neurons of the rat substantia nigra. Elevated levels of NOX-1 were also found in the dopaminergic neurons of the substantia nigra in the autopsied brain tissues.[44]

STUDIES ON HUMAN PERIPHERAL TISSUES

The levels of markers of oxidative damage and vitamin E were measured in 211 patients with PD and 135 healthy controls. The results showed that leukocyte 8-hydroxy-guanosine and plasma malondialdehyde (MDA) were elevated, whereas erythrocyte glutathione peroxidase and plasma vitamin E levels were reduced in PD patients compared to the control subjects.[45,46] The urine levels of 8-hydroxy-2'deoxyguanosine (8-OHdG) and the ratio of OHdG/2-dG were higher in patients with PD than in healthy control subjects; however, only the plasma levels of OHdG/2-dG increased in patients with PD compared to that in healthy control subjects.[47] It has been reported that the NADH (reduced form of nicotinamide adenine dehydrogenase) activity in the platelets of PD patients were lowered compared to healthy age- and gender-matched controls, whereas the activity of succinate dehydrogenase was similar in both groups.[48] Plasma levels of vitamin C and vitamin E were decreased in patients with vascular PD.[49] In contrast to above studies, the serum levels of vitamin A, vitamin E, or vitamin C in PD patients did not differ from controls.[49–52] These studies suggest that serum or plasma levels of vitamin A, vitamin C, or vitamin E should not be used as a marker of oxidative stress in the brain; therefore, they do not play any significant role in the pathogenesis of PD because they did not reflect the brain levels of antioxidants. Thus, brain tissue levels of antioxidants rather than the blood levels of antioxidants may play a significant role in the initiation and progression of both sporadic and familial PD.

EFFECT OF GLUTAMATE ON ANIMAL PD MODELS

In the animal model of PD, inhibitors of glutamate receptors ameliorated abnormality in motor movements.[53,54] Increased glutamate signaling in the substantia nigra played an important role in the mechanisms of neuronal death induced by chronic treatment of mice with MPTP.[55] Thus, increased glutamatergic activity may play an important role in the pathogenesis and symptoms of PD. Thus, antioxidants that can block the toxic effects of glutamate[56,57] should be useful in improving some of the symptoms of PD and in protecting neuron from glutamate-induced toxicity.

MITOCHONDRIAL DYSFUNCTION IN PD

Mitochondria are the major site for producing free radicals, and they are most sensitive to free radical damage. Mitochondrial dysfunction plays a central role in most neurodegenerative diseases including PD[58,59]; however, it occurs subsequent to increased oxidative stress and participates in the progression of PD. Mitochondrial dysfunction can be induced by diverse groups of external and internal agents. External agents include MPTP, insecticides, and pesticides, whereas internal agents include increased oxidative stress and chronic inflammation and mutated or aggregated alpha-synuclein, mutated PTEN-induced kinase 1 (PINK1), DJ-1, and PARKIN genes.[60–62] The mitochondrial dysfunctions include impaired electron transport chain, mutations in mitochondrial DNA, impaired calcium buffering, reduced ATP synthesis, and anomalies of morphology and dynamics of mitochondria.[63,64] The consequences of mitochondrial dysfunction include increased oxidative stress, release of cytochrome c, activation of caspase, chronic inflammation, release of calcium, upregulation of Bax expression and its translocation to mitochondria, and proteasome inhibition all of which contribute to degeneration of DA neurons and eventually to their death.[58,65,66] Importance of mitochondrial dysfunction in the pathogenesis of PD is further suggested by the fact that rotenone, an inhibitor of mitochondrial complex-1, induces clinical and biochemical features of human PD. Thus, reducing oxidative stress by antioxidants should protect mitochondria, and thereby, reduce the risk of PD.

In addition to antioxidant enzymes, mitochondrial uncoupling proteins (UCP1–5, UCP4, and UCP5 primarily expressed in the neurons) also provide protection against oxidative stress. The neuroprotective effect of UCP4 was demonstrated in neuronal cells treated with 1-methy-4-phenylpyridine (MPP+), a toxic metabolite of MPTP by preserving ATP levels and mitochondrial membrane potential, and reducing oxidative stress.[67] Activators of NF-kB can increase the expression of UCP4; therefore, protective effect of UCP4 is mediated by the NF-kB pathway.

INCREASED CHRONIC INFLAMMATION IN PD

STUDIES ON CHRONIC INFLAMMATION IN HUMAN PD

Microglia-initiated chronic inflammation responses also play an important role in the mechanism of degeneration of DA neurons in PD.[68,69] Aggregated or nitrated alpha-synuclein activates microglia that contributes to the degeneration of DA neurons by releasing proinflammatory cytokines and other neurotoxic factors.[70–72] It has been reported that nitric oxide and superoxide released by activated microglia may promote inflammation as well as abnormal alpha-synuclein (excessive amount or mutated form) to cause degeneration of DA neurons in transgenic mice model of PD.[73] In autopsied brain samples of PD brains, the number of activated microglia cells increased in the substantia nigra during the progression of PD. The levels of proinflammatory cytokines IL-6 and TNF-alpha increased in both PD and Lewy body disease.[74] The analysis of neuronal loss in autopsied samples of substantia nigra suggests that neurons containing melanin are primarily lost.[75] Indeed, pathologists have consistently observed depigmentation of the substantia nigra in the autopsied samples of PD brains. The addition of human neuromelanin to microglia cell cultures induced chemotactic effects and activated the proinflammatory transcription factor NF-kappaB.[75] This treatment of microglia cells also upregulated TNF-alpha, IL-6, and nitric oxide. These results suggest that the presence of extracellular neuromelanin serves as a source of chronic inflammation that aggravates the rate of degeneration of DA neurons. Although inflammatory response is considered a protective response, but chronic activation of microglia cells may produce excessive amounts of proinflammatory cytokines, complement proteins, adhesion molecules, and ROS all of which are neurotoxic. It has been reported that cyclooxygenase (COX) is the rate-limiting enzyme in the synthesis of prostaglandins that are neurotoxic in excessive amounts.[76] The inducible isoforms COX-2 is upregulated in the DA neurons of the autopsied brain samples of PD patients. The levels of COX-2 are also increased in chemical-induced animal PD models. The overexpression of COX-2 in human neuroblastoma cells facilitated oxidation of DA and proteins including alpha-synuclein.[77] The studies presented in this section clearly show that chronic inflammation plays an important role in degeneration and apoptosis of DA neurons in PD. Therefore, agents such as high-dose antioxidants and a low-dose NSAID, such as aspirin, may reduce the incidence of PD in high-risk populations. The same micronutrient preparation, when used as an adjunctive therapy, may improve the management of PD more than that produced by individual agents.

MUTATIONS OR OVEREXPRESSION IN PD-RELATED GENES

Mutations in six genes have been identified in familial PD, and their actions in degeneration of DA neurons have been elucidated. Mutations in alpha-synuclein (SNCA), PARKIN, PINK1, DJ-1, and leucin-rich repeat kinase 2 (LRRK2) are associated with familial PD,[60,78–80] and account for about 2–3% of all cases of PD. In addition, the levels of ATP13A2 gene that encodes a lysosomal ATPase increased in the brains of patients with sporadic or idiopathic PD.[81] The transgenic animal models confirm the role of these mutations in the pathology of PD.[82,83] Among familial PD, mutations in the PARKIN gene account for about 50%, PINK1 about 8–15%, and DJ-1 about 1% of cases.[84] The mutation in the LRRK2 gene is involved not only in familial PD but also in some sporadic PD. Several variants in LRRK2 and SNCA have been associated with an increased risk of sporadic PD.[85] There appears to be interaction between PARKIN, PINK1, and DJ-1 genes. It was demonstrated that these genes formed a complex referred to as PARKIN/PINK1/DJ-1 (PPD) complex to promote ubiquitination and degradation of PARKIN substrates, including PARKIN itself in neuroblastoma cells in culture and human brain lysates.[86] Genetic ablation of either PINK1 or DJ-1reduced ubiquitination of endogenous PARKIN and decreased degradation of aberrantly expressed PRKIN substrates. Expression of PINK1 increased PARKIN-mediated degradation of heat shock-induced misfolded protein. However, mutations in PARKIN and PINK1 reduced degradation of PARKIN substrates by impairing ubiquitin E3 ligase activity.[86]

DJ-1 GENE

DJ-1 originally identified as an oncogene is a ubiquitous redox-responsive protein with diverse biological functions, including protecting against oxidative stress. It acts as a transcriptional regulator of antioxidant-mediated gene expression.[87] DJ-1 is very sensitive to oxidative stress, and oxidized form of DJ-1 is considered as a biomarker for neurodegenerative diseases including sporadic PD.[88] The oxidized form of DJ-1 has been found in the autopsied brain tissues of sporadic as well as in familial PD.[89] Overexpression of wild-type DJ-1 made cells more resistant to oxidative stress induced by H_2O_2,[90] protected neurons against DA- and 6-hydroxydopamine-induced toxicity and reduced intracellular levels of ROS.[91,92] The levels of wild-type DJ-1 can be upregulated by antioxidant treatment in rats.[93] Mutations in DJ-1 and PARKIN genes make animals more sensitive to oxidative stress and mitochondrial toxins implicated in sporadic PD. Mutated DJ-1 make DA neurons more vulnerable to oxidative stress-induced apoptosis.[94] An inactivated form of DJ-1 may also promote aggregation of alpha-synuclein that impairs mitochondrial function causing DA neurons to degenerate slowly.[95] Human DJ-1 binds with copper and mercury and thereby prevents metal-induced toxicity in DA neurons.[96]

A novel compound, comp-23, binds to DJ-1. Treatment with comp-23 prevented oxidative stress-induced neuronal death, but it failed to do so in neurons lacking DJ-1, suggesting that neuroprotective action of comp-23 requires the presence of DJ-1.[89] Comp-23 also prevented death of DA neurons in the substantia nigra and restored movement disorders in 6-hydroxydopamine-injected and rotenone-treated PD model rats and mice. DJ-1 acts as a stress sensor, and its levels increase in response to increased oxidative stress.[97]

Loss of DJ-1 leads to mitochondrial dysfunction and fragmentation in human DA neurons via increased oxidative stress.[98] This is supported by the fact that treatment with n-acetylcysteine reversed the above effects of DJ-1. Like PINK1 and PARKIN, DJ-1 also protects mitochondrial damage produced by rotenone, a mitochondrial toxin. Overexpression of PARKIN protected against loss of DJ-1. DJ-1 continues to act as a mitochondrial protective agent in the absence of PINK1. Thus, the neuro-protective effect of DJ-1 against oxidative stress-induced mitochondrial dysfunction occurs in parallel to the PINK1/PARKIN pathways.[98]

The vesicular monoamine transporter-2 (VMAT-2) transfers dopamine into syn-aptic vesicles for exocytotic release and prevents its cytoplasmic oxidation. It has been reported that overexpression of DJ-1 protected DA neurons and vesicular sequestration of dopamine by upregulating VMAT-2.[99] Thus, DJ-1 acts as a transcrip-tional factor for VMAT-2. Dopamine vesicular sequestration and its release upon depolarization were dependent upon the levels of DJ-1. It has been reported that the nuclear pool of DJ-1 increased in DA neurons after treatment with 6-hydroxydopa-mine, whereas its level decreased in the cytoplasm. Treatment with n-acetylcysteine blocked the 6-hydroxydopamine-induced translocation of DJ-1 from the cytoplasm to the nucleus.[100] This suggests that increased oxidative stress may be involved in translocation of DJ-1 to the nucleus. The 6-hydroxydopamine treatment of DA neu-rons failed to translocate mutant DJ-1 to the nucleus. This suggests that only an active form of DJ-1 responds to increased oxidative stress, and that nuclear transloca-tion of DJ-1 is necessary for neuroprotection.

ALPHA-SYNUCLEIN GENE

A family of homologous proteins, alpha- and beta-synuclein, is located primarily in the presynaptic regions of brain neurons, whereas gamma-synuclein is present in the peripheral nervous system and retina.[101] Lewy bodies that are the hallmark of PD contain predominantly alpha-synuclein in aggregated form which has been impli-cated in the pathogenesis of PD.

The overexpression of wild-type alpha-synuclein caused degenerative changes in human DA neurons in culture[102] and in transgenic rat DA neurons.[103,104] The overex-pression of human wild-type alpha-synuclein in differentiated neuroblastoma cells decreased their viability and increased their sensitivity to oxidative stress and neu-rotoxins such as H_2O_2, nitric oxide, and prostaglandin E2.[105] Increased oxidative stress, proteasome inhibition, and endoplasmic reticulum stress upregulated wild-type alpha-synuclein expression in fibroblasts obtained from patients with PD com-pared to those obtained from normal subjects.[106]

Increased oxidative stress also causes aggregation of alpha-synuclein that is toxic to DA neurons. It has been shown that not only insoluble aggregated alpha-synuclein but also soluble oligomer aggregates alpha-synuclein is toxic to DA neurons.[107]

The mechanisms of action of alpha-synuclein are not well understood; however, it has been suggested that alpha-synuclein-induced neurotoxicity is related to increased oxidative stress[108,109] that is caused by impaired mitochondria. Alpha-synuclein enters mitochondria through import receptors located in both outer and inner mitochondrial membranes,[110] and excessive accumulation of alpha-synuclein cause mitochondrial dysfunction. This is due to the fact that overexpression of alpha-synuclein caused nitration of mitochondrial proteins and the release of cytochrome c from the mitochondria.[111] These biological events that are related to increased oxidative stress may initiate degeneration of DA neurons. The overexpression of human wild-type or mutant (A53T or A30P) alpha-synuclein in human neuroblastoma cells in culture enhanced aggregation of alpha-synuclein.[112] Mutant alpha-synuclein (A53T) transfected mice developed intraneuronal Lewy body-like inclusions, mitochondrial dysfunction, and apoptotic death in neocortical, brain stem, and motor neurons.[113]

Dopamine metabolite, 3,4-dihydroxyphenylacetaldehyde, interacts with alpha-synuclein proteins causing them to aggregate.[104] The aggregated form of alpha-synuclein plays an important role in the pathogenesis of PD.[114] Mitochondrial dysfunction can also induce alpha-synuclein oligomerization through increased protein oxidation and microtubule depolymerization.[115] Alpha-synuclein-knockout mice developed without gross abnormality, but are resistant to MPTP-induced degeneration of DA neurons. In addition, genetic ablation of alpha-synuclein protected neuronal cells in culture against oxidative stress[114] and increased the resistance of human DA neuron-like cells to MPP+.[116,117] Conversely, overexpression of wild-type alpha-synuclein or mutant alpha-synuclein (A53T) increased the sensitivity of neurons to MPP+ which induced mitochondrial dysfunction, and 6-hydroxydopamine increased oxidative stress in human neuroblastoma cells in culture.[118] Antioxidants such as Edaravone protected only against MPP+-induced toxicity, and epigallocatechin-3-o-gallate protected only against 6-hydroxydopamine-induced neurodegeneration.[118] This study suggests that one type of antioxidant is not sufficient to affect neurodegeneration induced by diverse groups of toxins. Mutant alpha-synuclein (A53T), but not other variants such as A30P, induced adult onset of PD in transgenic mice, and this effect was associated with abnormal accumulation of detergent insoluble alpha-synuclein protein.[119]

Overexpression of wild-type alpha-synuclein or mutated alpha-synuclein had no effect on proteasome activity in neuronal cells in culture or in transgenic mice,[120,121] although alpha-synuclein directly inhibited the activity of purified 20S subunits of proteasome reversibly *in vitro*.[121] The inhibition of proteasome in human neuroblastoma cells in culture failed to induce alpha-synuclein aggregation.[121] These results suggest that proteasome inhibition and overexpression of alpha-synuclein that are associated with PD are not related. It is likely that increased oxidative stress that upregulates alpha-synuclein and inhibits proteasome activity is a primary event in the pathogenesis of PD.

Since alpha-synuclein is degraded by proteasome and by autophagic pathways,[122,123] any defects in one or both pathways can lead to an accumulation of alpha synuclein in neurons. Whether or not a protein forms aggregation depends upon the cellular concentration of the protein and thermodynamic properties inherent to each protein. Therefore, an increase in cellular concentration of alpha-synuclein can lead to aggregation. In addition, oxidation of alpha-synuclein can also cause aggregation. Tyrosinase, a rate-limiting enzyme in the synthesis of melanin, in combination with

alpha-synuclein, allows aggregation of alpha-synuclein.[124] The abnormal aggregation of alpha-synuclein plays a central role in the degeneration of DA neurons.[122]

It has been demonstrated that alpha-synuclein and Nrf2 deficiency cooperate in
the formation of aggregation, neuroinflammation, and neuronal death in mice.[125] It
has been shown that oxidative stress-induced nuclear translocated alpha-synuclein
binds to the promoter for the master mitochondrial transcription activator PGC1
alpha. This binding reduced the promoter activity of PGC1 alpha, which may account
for inducing mitochondrial dysfunction in PD.[126]

It has been reported that expression of full length alpha-synuclein caused activation of microglia and induction of major histocompatability complex class II
(MHCII) and neurodegeneration in mice, whereas in MHCII knockout mice, alpha-
synuclein did not activate microglia and prevented degeneration of DA neurons.[127]
This suggested that MCHII is necessary for the neurotoxicity of alpha-synuclein.

PTEN-INDUCED PUTATIVE KINASE 1 GENE

PINK1, a mitochondrial Ser/Thr kinase, is a ubiquitous protein expressed throughout the human brain and is primarily located at the mitochondrial membrane and
the cytosol. One of the functions of wild-type PINK1 is to protect the mitochondria against a variety of stress signaling pathways. Genetic ablation of wild-type
PINK1 caused loss of mitochondrial membrane potential, decrease in ATP synthesis, complex IV activity, and mitochondrial electron transport chain function.[128]
Impairment of mitochondrial electron transport chain and an increased frequency
of deletions of mitochondrial DNA which codes some of the subunits of mitochondrial electron transport chain have been found in the autopsied samples of
the substantia nigra of PD brains. PINK1 is also present in the Lewy bodies.[129]
Like mutated alpha-synuclein, mutated PINK1 also impairs mitochondrial function. Mutant PINK1 (W437X) enhanced the levels of mutant synuclein (A53T)-
induced mitochondrial dysfunction. This effect was associated with increased
intracellular calcium levels.[130] Coexpression of mutated PINK1 and alpha-synuclein
altered mitochondrial structure and neurite growth that were totally blocked by
the inhibitor of mitochondrial calcium flux.[130] Mutant PINK1 or PINK1 reduced
mitochondrial respiration, and ATP synthesis inhibited proteasome activity and
increased alpha-synuclein aggregation in neuronal cells in culture.[131] Mutated
PINK1 increased oxidative damage in the fibroblasts obtained from PD patients as
well as upregulated wild-type alpha-synuclein expression in fibroblasts obtained
from normal subjects.[106]

PARKIN GENE

PARKIN is E3-ubiquitin-protein ligase that ubiquitinates itself and promotes its own
degradation. Mutation in the PARKIN gene impairs this function which eventually
can lead to the death of DA neurons. It is interesting to note that Lewy bodies are
absent in the brain of patients with mutated PARKIN, suggesting that the wild-type
PARKIN is needed to form Lewy bodies.[132] The interaction between PARKIN and
alpha-synuclein protein and synphilin-1 participates in the formation of Lewy bodies.

Nitric oxide and oxidative stress inhibit PARKIN function that may be involved in the pathogenesis of sporadic PD.

The wild-type PARKIN is considered one of the most important factors that improve mitochondrial dysfunction.[133] PINK1 and PARKIN play a central role in the regulation of mitochondrial dynamic and function (fission, fusion, and migration and energy generation); therefore, mutations in these genes can impair mitochondrial function and dynamics.[86] Mitochondrial dysfunction interferes with the generation of energy and produces more free radicals that initiate degeneration of DA neurons and eventually causes neuronal death.

To define the role of the PARKIN gene further, pluripotent stem cells from normal subjects and PD patients with the mutated PARKIN gene have been studied. The results showed that loss of the PARKIN gene in human midbrain DA neurons increases transcription of monoamine oxidases and oxidative stress, reduces DA uptake, and enhances spontaneous release of DA. Insertion of a wild-type PARKIN gene into these DA neurons prevents the above changes. These results suggest that the PARKIN gene controls dopamine utilization in human midbrain DA neurons by increasing the precision of DA neurotransmission and suppressing DA oxidation.[134]

The transcriptional factor ATF4 (activating transcriptional factor 4) can be upregulated by increased oxidative damage or by endoplasmic reticulum stress. The levels of ATF4 were increased in neuromelanin-positive neurons in the substantia nigra of a subset of PD patients compared to control subjects.[135] ATF levels were also elevated in neuronal cells (PC12 rat neuroblastoma cells) after treatment with 6-hydroxydopamine (6-OHDA) or MPP+ which selectively causes degeneration in DA neurons. It was demonstrated that silencing the ATF4 enhanced cell death produced by the treatment with 6-OHDA or MPP+, whereas overexpression of ATF4 reduced cell death caused by OHDA or MPP+ treatments. In addition, treatment of neuronal cells with OHDA or MPP+ decreased the levels of PARKIN, despite an increase in mRNA levels. Silencing ATF4 enhanced toxin-induced reduction of PARKIN, whereas overexpression of ATF4 partially preserved PARKIN levels. Furthermore, silencing the PARKIN gene prevented the protective effect of ATF4. These results suggest that ATF4 exerts its neuroprotective effect through the regulation of PARKIN.

MUTATION IN LYSOSOMAL GENE SMPD1

The PD patients with Ashkenazi Jewish ancestry exhibited a strong association between mutation in sphingomyelin phosphodiesterase 1 (SMPD1) (p.L302P), a lysosomal enzyme gene, and increased risk of PD. This study suggests that the defects in the activities of lysosomal enzymes may participate in the pathogenesis of PD.[136]

PROTEOMIC PROFILING OF SUBSTANTIA NIGRA IN PD

The analysis of proteins in the autopsied samples of the substantia nigra from PD patients revealed that the levels of the cytosolic nonspecific dipeptidase 2 (CNDP2), a relatively unknown protein, were increased. Immunohistochemical analysis of the substantia nigra tissue demonstrated the presence of CNDP2 in the cytoplasm of DA neurons. This study suggests a possible role of CNDP2 in PD neurodegeneration. It was suggested that CNDP2-induced neurodegeneration could involve increased oxidaitive stress, protein aggregation, or inflammation.[137]

The studies discussed above strongly suggest that increased oxidative stress play a central role in the initiation and progression of damage; therefore, inhibiting oxidative stress may reduce the risk of developing of PD. Because of complexity of regulation of oxidative stress in humans, it is not possible to reduce oxidative stress optimally by the use of a single antioxidant for the prevention of PD.

HOW TO REDUCE OXIDATIVE STRESS OPTIMALLY

Oxidative stress in the body occurs when the antioxidant system fails to provide adequate protection against damage produced by free radicals (reactive oxygen species and reactive nitrogen species). Increased oxidative stress in the body is reduced by upregulating antioxidant enzymes as well as by existing levels of dietary and endogenous antioxidant chemicals because they work by different mechanisms. For example, antioxidant enzymes reduce free radicals by catalysis, whereas dietary and endogenous antioxidant chemicals reduce free radicals by directly scavenging them. In response to ROS, a nuclear transcriptional factor, Nrf2 (nuclear factor-erythroid 2-related factor 2) is translocated from the cytoplasm to the nucleus where it binds with ARE (antioxidant response element) which increases the levels of antioxidant enzymes (gamma-glutamylcysteine ligase, glutathione peroxidase, glutathione reductase, and heme oxygenase-1) and phase 2 detoxifying enzymes (NAD(P)H): quinine oxidoreductase 1 and glutathione-S-transferase in order to reduce oxidative damage.[138–140] In response to increased oxidative stress, existing levels of dietary and endogenous antioxidant chemicals levels cannot be elevated without supplementation.

FACTORS REGULATING RESPONSE OF NRF2

Antioxidant enzymes are elevated by activation of Nrf2 which depends upon ROS-dependent and ROS-independent mechanisms. In addition, elevated levels of antioxidant enzymes are also dependent upon the binding ability of Nrf2 with ARE in the nucleus. These studies are described here.

ROS-Dependent Regulation of Nrf2

Normally, Nrf2 is associated with Kelch-like ECH associated protein 1 (Keap1) protein which acts as an inhibitor of Nrf2 (INrf2).[141] INrf2 protein serves as an adaptor to link Nrf2 to the ubiquitin ligase CuI-Rbx1 complex for degradation by proteasomes and maintains the steady levels of Nrf2 in the cytoplasm. INrf2 acts as a sensor for ROS/electrophilic stress. In response to increased ROS, Nrf2 dissociates itself from INrf2-CuI-Rbx1 complex and translocates into the nucleus where it binds with ARE that increases antioxidant genes. It has been demonstrated that Nrf2 regulates INrf2 levels by controlling its transcription, whereas INrf2 regulates Nrf2 levels by controlling its degradation by proteasome.[142]

ROS-Independent Regulation of Nrf2

Antioxidants such as vitamin E, genistein (a flavonoid),[143] allicin, a major organo-sulfur compound found in garlic,[144] sulforaphane, an organosulfur compound, found in cruciferous vegetables,[145] kavalactones (methysticin, kavain, and yangonin)[146] and dietary restriction[147] activate Nrf2 without stimulation by ROS.

Reduced Binding of Nrf2 with ARE

Age-related decline in antioxidant enzymes in the liver of older rats compared to that in younger rats was due to reduction in the binding ability of Nrf2 with ARE; however, treatment with alpha-lipoic acid restored this defect, increased the levels of antioxidant enzymes, and restored the loss of glutathione from the liver of old rats.[148]

DIFFERENTIAL RESPONSE OF Nrf2 TO ROS STIMULATION DURING ACUTE AND CHRONIC OXIDATIVE STRESS

It appears that Nrf2 responds to ROS generated during acute and chronic oxidative stress differently. For example, acute oxidative stress during strenuous exercise translocates Nrf2 from the cytoplasm to the nucleus where it binds with ARE to upregulate antioxidant genes. However, during chronic oxidative stress commonly observed in older individuals and in neurodegenerative diseases, such as Parkinson's disease and Alzheimer's disease, the Nrf2/ARE pathway becomes unresponsive to ROS. A reduction in the binding ability of Nrf2 with ARE was demonstrated in older rats.[148] The reasons for the Nrf2/ARE pathway to become unresponsive to ROS during chronic oxidative stress are unknown.

Nrf2 IN PARKINSON'S DISEASE

6-hydroxydopamine (6-OHDA) is considered one of the PD-related neurotoxins which cause death of neurons *in vitro* and *in vivo* by increasing production of free radicals. 3,4-Dihydroxybenzalacetone (DBL), a small catechol-containing compound isolated from Inonotus obliquus, exhibits antioxidant, anti-inflammation activities. Pretreatment of human neuroblastoma cells (SH-SYPY cell) with DBL improved the survival of 6-OHDA-treated cells by activating Nrf2/ARE pathway through PI3K/AKT, although it did not reduce 6-OHDA-induced ROS.[149] Pretreatment of human neuroblastoma cells in culture and mice with naringenin, a natural flavonoid, protected neurons against 6-OHDA-induced toxicity. The protective effect of naringenin was dependent upon the presence of Nrf2, because deletion of Nrf2 blocked its protective effect.[150] Puerarin treatment reduced neurodegeneration in the substantia nigra of rats following injection with 6-OHDA by activation Nrf2/ARE pathway and elevating the levels of brain-derived neurotrophic factor (BDNF).[151] Resveratrol reduced paraquat-induced ROS and inflammation by activating Nrf2/ARE pathway.[152]

Aggregation of alpha-synuclein plays an important role in the pathogenesis of PD. Iron (ferrous form)-induced aggregation of alpha-synuclein appears to be due to the downregulation of the Nrf2 pathway which causes increased neurotoxicity. This creates a vicious cycle of iron accumulation, increased alpha-synuclein aggregation, and increased neurotoxicity.[153] It has been demonstrated that deficiency of alpha-synuclein and Nrf2 enhance alpha-synuclein aggregation and chronic inflammation that contribute to the DA neurons in PD.[125]

Nrf2 deficiency increased the sensitivity of mice to MPTP. Overexpression of Nrf2 in astrocytes was sufficient to provide neuroprotection in the MPTP mouse model of PD.[154] Licochalcone E (Lico-E), a Glycyrrhiza inflate-derived chaocone, reduced inflammation in microglia cells and protected human neuroblastoma cells against 6-OHDA- and MPTP-induced neurotoxicity by activating the Nrf2/ARE pathway.[155]

It has been demonstrated that the neuroprotective effect of DJ-1 against oxidative damage is mediated through activating the Nrf2/ARE pathway which enhances the expression of thioredoxin.[156]

Bromocriptine, a dopamine agonist, is used clinically for the treatment of PD. In addition to activating DA D2 receptor, this drug is also neuroprotective and exhibits antioxidant activity. Treatment of dopaminergic cells (PC12) with Bromocriptine reduced oxidative damage by activating, the Nrf2/ARE pathway through PI3K/AKT.[157]

Therefore, the following groups of selected nontoxic agents in combination may be useful in reducing oxidative stress optimally:

1. *Agents that can reduce oxidative stress by directly scavenging free radicals*: Some examples are dietary antioxidants, such as vitamin A, beta-carotene (BC), vitamin C, and vitamin E, and endogenous antioxidants, such as glutathione, alpha-lipoic acid, and coenzyme Q_{10}.
2. *Agents that can reduce oxidative stress by activating Nrf2-regulated antioxidant genes without ROS stimulation*: Some examples are organosulfur compound sulforaphane found in cruciferous vegetables, kavalactones, found in Kava shrubs, and Puerarin, a major flavonoid from the root of *Pueraria lobata*,[145,146,158] genistein and vitamin E[143] and coenzyme Q_{10}[159] activate Nrf2 without ROS stimulation.
3. *Agents that can reduce oxidative stress directly by scavenging free radicals as well as indirectly by activating the Nrf2/ARE pathway*: Some examples are vitamin E,[143] alpha-lipoic acid,[148] curcumin,[160] resveratrol,[161,162] omega-3-fatty acids,[163,164] and NAC.[165]
4. *Agents reducing oxidative stress by ROS-dependent mechanism*: They include L-carnitine which generates transient ROS.[166]

Treatment of primary culture of hippocampal neurons with Puerarin, a major flavonoid from the root of *Pueraria lobata,* significantly reduced beta-amyloid-induced oxidative stress by activating the Nrf2/ARE pathway.[158] Genistein, a flavonoid, and vitamin E reduced oxidative damage produced by beta-amyloids (Aβ25–35) in transformed cerebrovascular mouse endothelial cells in culture by activating Nrf2-regulated antioxidant genes.[143]

A study on the aged mouse hippocampus revealed that supplementation with allicin, a major organosulfur compound found in garlic, which has an electrophilic center (electron deficient) prevented age-related decline in cognitive function. This effect of allicin was due to enhancement of antioxidant enzymes via the Nrf2/ARE pathway.[144] This study suggests that the INrf2/Nrf2 complex and binding of Nrf2 with ARE remain responsive to allicin. Repeated administration of another organo-sulfur compound, sulforaphane, found in cruciferous vegetables, simulated Nrf2-dependent increase of Nqo1 gene which codes for NAD(P)H: quinone oxidoreductase and Hmox1 gene which codes for HO-1 enzyme in astrocytes in culture and reduced oxidative damage.[145] It is also possible that sulforaphane-induced activation of Nrf2 does not require ROS stimulation. Indeed, kavalactones (methysticin, kavain, and yangonin)-induced activation of Nrf2 is not dependent upon ROS stimulation in neuronal cells and astroglia cells in culture.[146]

In a study on murine alveolar cells in culture, NAC, which directly scavenges free radicals via increasing intracellular glutathione levels, requires the presence of Nrf2 for an optimal reduction in oxidative stress.[167] For example, cigarette smoking produces greater damage in alveolar cells obtained from Nrf2-deleted mice (Nrf2-/-) than in cells obtained from wild-type mice.[167] Pretreatment of alveolar cells with NAC reduced cigarette smoke-induce damage more in cells obtained from the wild-type mice than in cells from Nrf2-deleted mice. In another study on rat liver, pretreatment with NAC prevents the ROS-induced activation of Nrf2.[168] If NAC scavenge all ROS, then ROS was not available for activating the Nrf2/ARE pathway.

The studies discussed above strongly suggest that increased oxidative stress play a central role in the initiation and progression of damage; therefore, inhibiting oxidative stress may reduce the risk of developing PD. Because of complexity of regulation of oxidative stress in humans, it is not possible to reduce oxidative stress optimally by the use of a single antioxidant for prevention of PD.

LABORATORY AND HUMAN STUDIES IN PD AFTER TREATMENT WITH ANTIOXIDANTS AND POLYPHENOLIC COMPOUNDS

Several *in vitro* and animal studies suggest that supplementation with individual antioxidants may be useful in reducing the risk and progression of PD; however, the efficacy of individual antioxidants on risk factors for developing PD varied, depending upon the type of antioxidants, cell type, and biochemical risk factor. The clinical studies with individual antioxidants have produced inconsistent results varying from no effect to minimal beneficial effects. These studies are briefly described here.

STUDIES OF IN VITRO PD MODELS

VITAMIN A, BETA-CAROTENE, VITAMIN C, OR COENZYME Q_{10} ON ALPHA-SYNUCLEIN

Alpha-synuclein fibrils are considered toxic to DA neurons. It has been reported that certain antioxidants such as vitamin A, BC, and coenzyme Q_{10} inhibited formation of alpha-synuclein fibrils in a dose-dependent manner, whereas vitamin B_2, vitamin B_6, vitamin C, and vitamin E were ineffective *in vitro*.[169] In addition, vitamin A, BC, and coenzyme Q_{10} destabilized preformed alpha-synuclein fibrils in a dose-dependent manner. The results of these studies cannot be extrapolated to human PD, but they would suggest that supplementation with these antioxidants may help reduce the risk of PD by preventing the aggregation of alpha-synuclein and by destabilizing the preformed alpha-synuclein fibrils.

NAC, Vitamin C, Vitamin E, Trolox, or Quercetin

Dopamine is known to induce apoptosis in several lines of neuronal cells in culture by increasing oxidative stress. The viability of DA-treated human melanocytes significantly decreased in a dose-dependent manner, whereas keratinocytes exhibited less sensitivity to DA treatment. NAC or glutathione protected against DA-induced toxicity in normal human melanocytes, whereas other antioxidants such as vitamin C, vitamin E, trolox, and quercetin were ineffective.[170]

Melatonin, Deprenyl, Vitamin E, or Vitamin C

Melatonin, deprenyl, and vitamin E inhibited auto-oxidation of DA in a dose-dependent manner, whereas vitamin C was ineffective.[171] These studies further confirmed that only certain antioxidants could protect DA neuron against free radicals generated by auto-oxidation of DA.

Vitamin E, NAC, or Coenzyme Q_{10} on Glutamate-Induced Toxicity

Glutamate, an excitatory neurotransmitter, in excessive amounts is toxic to DA neurons by increasing oxidative stress. This effect of glutamate can be blocked by an analog of NAC,[172] vitamin E,[56] and coenzyme Q_{10}.[57]

B Vitamins

In a cellular model of PD, pretreatment with B vitamins for a period of 4 weeks prevented rotenone-induced mitochondrial dysfunction, increased oxidative stress, accumulation of alpha-synuclein, and polyubiquitin in neurons.[173] Treatment of human neuroblastoma cells in culture with a relatively high dose of nicotinamide protected from MPP+-induced cellular toxicity and decrease in complex I and alpha-ketoglutarate dehydrogenase activities, increase in ROS, and oxidation of DNA and protein.[174] These studies also revealed that the presence of B vitamins in a micronutrient preparation is essential for producing an optimal beneficial effect in experimental models of PD.

STUDIES ON ANIMAL MODELS OF PD

Vitamin E

6-OHDA or MPTP induced some neurological and biochemical abnormalities in rodents similar to those observed in human PD. Therefore, they have been used in evaluating the efficacy of antioxidants in reducing neurological and behavior abnormalities. Pretreatment of rats with D-alpha tocopherol or DL-alpha-tocopherol significantly reduced 6-OHDA-induced behavior and biochemical abnormalities.[175,176] Intramuscular administration of D-alpha-tocopheryl succinate, the most effective form of vitamin E,[177] protected 6-OHDA-induced death of locus coeruleus neurons as well as behavioral and biochemical changes in rats.[178,179]

MELATONIN AND DEPRENYL

Melatonin, a neurohormone secreted by the pineal gland, exhibits antioxidant activity. Melatonin and deprenyl prevent auto-oxidation of DA in a synergistic manner. Melatonin, but not deprenyl, prevented MPTP-induced inhibition of mitochondrial complex I activity and oxidative damage in nigrostriatal neuron.[180] Deprenyl significantly restored MPTP-induced decrease in DA levels and tyrosine hydroxylase activity; however, the combination of melatonin and deprenyl was more effective than the individual agents.[180]

L-CARNITINE

Quinolinic acid, an excitotoxin and free radical generator, and 3-nitropropionic acid, a mitochondrial toxin, induced oxidative damage and behavioral alterations in animals similar to those observed in PD patients. Administration of L-carnitine at micromolar concentrations reduced neurotoxin-induced oxidative damage and behavior abnormalities.[181]

L-CARNITINE, COENZYME Q_{10}, ALPHA-LIPOIC ACID, VITAMIN E, OR RESVERATROL

Analysis of laboratory studies revealed that L-carnitine, coenzyme Q_{10}, alpha-lipoic acid, vitamin E, and resveratrol reduced damage to neurons induced by diverse groups of neurotoxins such as MPTP, rotenone, and 3-nitropropionic acid.[182]

NICOTINAMIDE (VITAMIN B_3)

Nicotinamide, a precursor of nicotinamide adenine dinucleotide (NAD+) also attenuated glutamate-induced toxicity and preserved cellular levels of NAD+ to support the activity of silent information regulator-1 (SIRT1), a regulator of mitochondrial biogenesis.[183] This vitamin inhibits oxidative damage and improves mitochondrial function and thus can protect neurodegeneration and improve motor functions. In addition, in *Drosophila melanogaster* model of PD (an alpha-synuclein transgenic fly), nicotinamide treatment significantly improved the motor function (climbing ability).[174] These studies also revealed that the presence of B vitamins in any preparation of multiple antioxidants is essential for producing consistent beneficial effects in experimental models of PD.

RESVERATROL

Resveratrol, an activator of SIRT1 (silent information regulator-2), stimulated mitochondrial biogenesis in mice and reduced production of reactive oxygen species.[184] In contrast to SIRT1, SIRT2 promotes formation of alpha-synuclein fibrils that are toxic to nerve cells. Potent inhibitors of SIRT2 prevented formation of alpha-synuclein fibrils. Thus, inhibitors of SIRT2 could be useful in the treatment of PD.[185] It also protected DA neurons from chemical-induced cell death and improved symptoms of PD in a Drosophila model of PD.[186] This suggests that SIRT2 promotes formation of alpha-synuclein fibrils.

FISH OIL, MELATONIN, AND VITAMIN E

It has been demonstrated that treatment of mice with MPTP increased the activity of the COX-2 enzyme and lipid peroxides in the homogenates of midbrain; however, pretreatment with fish oil, melatonin, or vitamin E decreased the levels of the above biochemical changes. Treatment with fish oil was more effective in reducing MPTP-induced rise in COX-2 activity than vitamin E or melatonin, whereas melatonin was more effective in reducing MPTP-induced rise in lipid peroxides than fish oil or vitamin E.[187] These results suggest that different antioxidants affect markers of increased oxidative stress and chronic inflammation differently.

GINKGO BILOBA EXTRACT 761

This leaf extract is a patented product containing 24% flavonoids and 6% terpenoids. It has been demonstrated that administration of *Ginkgo biloba* extract 761 in an animal model of PD protected DA neurons in the midbrain against oxidative damage.[188]

CURCUMIN AND A MIXTURE OF DIETARY AND ENDOGENOUS ANTIOXIDANT

In collaboration with Dr. Clive Charlton of Meharry Medical College, Nashville, TN, we have found that both curcumin and a mixture of dietary and endogenous antioxidants (a gift from Premier Micronutrient Corporation, Nashville, TN) reduced the incidence of death and hypokinesia induced by MPTP treatment in mice. Although both curcumin and an antioxidant mixture markedly blocked MPTP-induced depletion of tyrosine hydroxylase (TH) activity, only the antioxidant mixture enhanced the TH activity. This suggested that an antioxidant mixture treatment was more effective than the curcumin treatment in reducing the adverse effects of MPTP in mice.

BLACK AND GREEN TEA EXTRACT

Black tea extract exhibited antioxidant activity, reduced 6-OHDA-induced degeneration of the nigrostriatal dopaminergic system, and improved motor and neurochemical deficits.[189] Green tea phenolic compound, epigallocatechin-3-gallate, exhibited antioxidant properties and reduced MPTP-induced PD in mice through inhibition of nitric oxide synthase activity.[190]

FIBROBLASTIC GROWTH FACTOR

The fibroblastic growth factor (FGF) family consists of 22 members with diverse biological functions in development and metabolism. Administration of FGF20 protected DA neurons in rat PD model. Treatment of neuronal and embryonic stem cells with FGF20 caused preferential differentiation of these cells into DA neurons, which attenuated the symptom of PD in an animal model of PD.[191]

SODIUM PHENYLBUTYRATE

Sodium phenylbutyrate (NaPB), an FDA-approved drug for other health conditions, can suppress the levels of ROS and pro-inflammatory cytokines. Oral administration of NaPB-protected DA neurons, normalized striatal neurotransmitters, and improved motor functions in MPTP mouse PD model.[192] These effects of NaPB are mediated via decreased oxidative damage and chronic inflammation.

STUDIES ON HUMAN PD

VITAMIN E AND DEPRENYL

Most clinical trials utilized a single antioxidant, primarily vitamin E, that may have contributed to the inconsistent results. Deprenyl and Tocopherol Antioxidative Therapy of Parkinsonism (DATATOP), a randomized, double-blind, placebo-controlled, multicenter clinical trial, was initiated in 1989 in order to evaluate the efficacy of deprenyl (10 mg per day) and DL-tocopherol (2000 IU per day) individually and in combination in patients with early stage of PD when no therapy was required. The primary outcome was prolongation of the time needed for levodopa therapy. After a follow-up period of 8.2 years, deprenyl significantly delayed the time when levodopa therapy was needed, but alpha tocopherol was ineffective.[193,194] The use of a single dietary antioxidant, vitamin E, was a major flaw in this study design in view of the fact that glutathione deficiency in the brain is a consistent finding in most neurodegenerative diseases including PD; therefore, addition of glutathione-elevating agents such as alpha-lipoic acid and n-acetylcysteine would have been useful. In addition, mitochondrial dysfunction is also commonly observed in PD and other neurodegenerative diseases; therefore, addition of coenzyme Q_{10} and L-carnitine that improve the function of mitochondria would have been useful. There was another flaw in the DATATOP study design with respect to the selection of antioxidants for control and treatment groups. A multiple vitamin preparation (One-a-Day™) was allowed for all individuals who wished to take it. It was argued that the effect of 30 IU of vitamin E, which was present in the multiple vitamin preparation, would not significantly contribute to the effect of 2000 IU of vitamin E that was given to the treatment group. This argument may not be valid, since it has been shown that antioxidants when used individually had no effect of growth of mammalian cancer cells in culture, but when they are combined at the same doses produced pronounced effect on growth inhibition, suggesting that they may interact with each other in a synergistic manner,[195,196] Therefore, the impact of 30 IU of vitamin E in a multiple vitamin preparation would be more pronounced than that produced by 30 IU of vitamin E alone. Hence, the consumption of a multiple vitamin preparation containing a low dose of vitamin E by control subjects is likely to create an unacceptable variable while evaluating the efficacy of high dose of vitamin E alone in early PD patients, especially when both experimental and placebo group were allowed to have a multiple vitamin preparation in an uncontrolled fashion. The patients with PD have a high-oxidative environment in the brain. It is known that individual antioxidants when oxidized act as pro-oxidants. Therefore, the conclusion of the DATATOP study that antioxidants are not useful in reducing the progression of PD is not valid.

Several epidemiologic studies suggested that diet rich in vitamin E may reduce the risk of PD.[18,197,198] These epidemiologic studies with vitamin E conflict with the results obtained from those obtained from the intervention trials. It is possible that the diet contains antioxidants other than vitamin E, and therefore, its interaction with other antioxidants may have contributed to the beneficial effect on reducing the risk of PD. Thus, epidemiologic studies would favor the use of multiple antioxidants in any clinical study on PD.

VITAMIN E AND VITAMIN C IN COMBINATION WITH ANTICHOLINERGIC DRUGS

In an open-labeled clinical trial, the efficacy of high doses of alpha-tocopherol and ascorbate was tested in early PD patients. Patients were allowed to receive amantadine (increases dopamine release and prevents reuptake of dopamine) and anticholinergic, but not levodopa or a DA agonist. The primary outcome was delay of the time when levodopa therapy is needed. The results showed that these antioxidants delayed the time when levodopa therapy was needed by 2.5 years.[199] This study shows that a mixture of antioxidants may be a better approach for delaying the time when levodopa therapy is needed than a single antioxidant in patients with an early-stage PD.

COENZYME Q_{10}

In a multicenter, randomized, double-blind, placebo-controlled trial on 80 early-stage PD patients who did not require any therapy, the efficacy of coenzyme Q_{10} at doses of 300, 600, or 1200 mg per day was evaluated. The primary outcome was Unified Parkinson's disease Rating Score (UPDRS), and the patients were followed up for 16 months or until disability requiring levodopa therapy is needed. The results showed that coenzyme Q_{10} at the highest dose of 1200 mg per day was safe and well tolerated by patients. The results also revealed that less disability developed in patients receiving coenzyme Q_{10} compared to placebo controls; the benefit was greater in patients receiving the highest dosage.[200] Reviews of several open and controlled clinical studies revealed that daily supplementation with coenzyme Q_{10} either has no effect or has minimal benefit in early stage PD patients.[201,202]

NAD/NADH

No studies have been performed with NAD or nicotinamide (vitamin B_3), a precursor of NAD. A review on the clinical efficacy of reduced NAD (NADH) has concluded that it is premature to recommend NADH alone for the treatment of PD.[203] Thus, NADH alone is not sufficient to produce any beneficial effects on prevention or improved treatment of PD; however, the use of nicotinamide in a micronutrient preparation may be useful in enhancing the effectiveness of this therapy.

PREVENTION OF PD

Before discussing the strategies for PD prevention, it is essential to define primary and secondary prevention. The purpose of primary prevention is to protect healthy individuals, such as individuals 50 years or older and individuals with a family history of PD who have no symptoms of PD. The purpose of secondary prevention is to stop or slow the progression of PD. Individuals who exhibit early signs of PD, but are not taking any medication, may be included in secondary prevention.

PRIMARY PREVENTION

In order to develop primary prevention strategies, it is essential to identify external risk factors that increase the risk of developing PD. Some human epidemiologic studies have identified environment- and lifestyle-related agents that increase the risk of developing PD. These agents include exposure to Mn, pesticides, herbicides, and certain solvents, such as trichloroethylene (TCE), perchloroethylene (PERC), and carbon tetrachloride (CCl), and the designer drug meperidene. I would suggest that exposure to the above agents should be avoided for primary prevention of PD. Although epidemiologic studies suggest that cigarette smoking reduced the risk of PD, I would not recommend it because of serious adverse health consequences of smoking. In addition, a preparation of multiple dietary and endogenous antioxidants, certain phenolic compounds (curcumin and resveratrol), vitamin D, selenium, L-carnitine, B vitamin including high-dose vitamin B_3 is recommended. These agents would reduce oxidative stress indirectly by increasing the levels of antioxidant enzymes through activation of the Nrf2/ARE pathway, and directly by scavenging free radicals.

SECONDARY PREVENTION

In order to develop secondary prevention strategies, it is essential to identify external risk factors that increase the risk of developing PD and internal risk factors that participate in the progression of PD. In addition to external risk factors mentioned in the above paragraph, internal risk factors include increased oxidative stress, mitochondrial dysfunction, and chronic inflammation. Therefore, attenuation of oxidative stress and chronic inflammation may be one of the rational choices for secondary prevention of PD. The same micronutrient preparation recommended for primary prevention can also be used for secondary prevention. Aspirin, a nonsteroidal anti-inflammatory agent, in combination with antioxidants would reduce chronic inflammation maximally.

PROBLEMS OF USING A SINGLE ANTIOXIDANT IN PD PATIENTS

Laboratory studies consistently showed that supplementation with individual antioxidants may reduce the symptoms and improve neurochemical changes in animal models of PD. Although epidemiologic studies revealed that diet rich in vitamin E may reduce the risk of PD, the clinical trials with an individual antioxidant has been inconsistent producing minimal benefit at best. In PD patients, the levels of oxidative stress are high in the brain. Administration of a single antioxidant in such patients may not be effective, because this antioxidant may be oxidized in the presence of a high internal oxidative environment and then acts as a pro-oxidant.

Previous studies in other chronic diseases, such as BC in male heavy smokers for reducing the risk of lung cancer, vitamin E in Alzheimer's disease (AD) for improving cognitive function and vitamin E in PD for improving the symptoms and as expected, produced inconsistent results varying from no effect as in PD,[193] to modest beneficial[204] or no effect effects as in AD,[205] and harmful effects as in heavy male smokers.[206] Because of the failure to obtain consistent beneficial effects with individual agents, a preparation of multiple micronutrients containing dietary and endogenous antioxidants, vitamin D, B vitamins, certain minerals and herbs (resveratrol and curcumin), and omega-3-fatty acids for reducing the risk of PD and for improving the efficacy of standard therapy in the management of PD is proposed.

RATIONALE FOR USING MULTIPLE MICRONUTRIENTS IN PD

The references for this section are described in a review.[207] The mechanisms of action of various antioxidants and polyphenolic compounds are in part different; and their distribution in various organs and cells, their affinity to various types of free radicals, and their biological half-lives are also different. BC is more effective in quenching oxygen radicals than most other antioxidants. BC can perform certain biological functions that cannot be produced by its metabolite vitamin A, and vice versa. It has been reported that BC treatment enhances the expression of the connexin gene which codes for a gap junction protein in mammalian fibroblasts in culture, whereas vitamin A treatment does not produce such an effect. Vitamin A can induce differentiation in certain normal and cancer cells, whereas BC and other carotenoids do not. Thus, BC and vitamin A have, in part, different biological functions in the body. The gradient of oxygen pressure varies within cells. Some antioxidants, such as vitamin E, are more effective as quenchers of free radicals in reduced oxygen pressure, whereas BC and vitamin A are more effective in higher atmospheric pressures. Vitamin C is necessary to protect cellular components in aqueous environments, whereas carotenoids and vitamins A and E protect cellular components in lipid environments. Vitamin C also plays an important role in maintaining cellular levels of vitamin E by recycling vitamin E radical (oxidized) to the reduced (antioxidant) form.

The form of vitamin E used in a preparation of micronutrients is also important. It has been established that d-alpha-tocopheryl succinate (vitamin E succinate) is the most effective form of vitamin both *in vitro* and *in vivo*. This form of vitamin E is more soluble than alpha-tocopherol and enters cells more readily, and therefore, it is expected that vitamin E succinate would cross the blood–brain barrier in greater amounts than alpha-tocopherol. However, this idea has not yet been tested in animals or humans. We have reported that an oral ingestion of vitamin E succinate (800 IU/day) in humans increased plasma levels of not only alpha-tocopherol but also of vitamin E succinate, suggesting that a portion of this form of vitamin E can be absorbed from the intestinal tract before hydrolysis to alpha-tocopherol, provided that the plasma pool of alpha-tocopherol is saturated. This observation is important because the conventional assumption based on the studies in rodents has been that esterified forms of vitamin E such as alpha-tocopheryl succinate, alpha-tocopheryl nicotinate, and alpha-tocopheryl acetate can be absorbed from the intestinal tract only after they are hydrolyzed to alpha-tocopherol. Our preliminary data showed that this assumption may not be true for the absorption of vitamin E succinate in humans provided that the plasma pool of alpha-tocopherol is saturated.

An endogenous antioxidant, glutathione, is effective in catabolizing H_2O_2 and anions. However, oral supplementation with glutathione failed to significantly increase plasma levels of glutathione in human subjects, suggesting that this tripeptide is completely hydrolyzed in the GI tract. Therefore, I propose to utilize N-acetylcysteine and alpha-lipoic acid that increase the cellular levels of glutathione by different mechanisms in a multiple micronutrient preparation.

Another endogenous antioxidant, coenzyme Q_{10}, may have some potential value in prevention and improved treatment of PD. Since mitochondrial dysfunction is associated with PD and since coenzyme Q_{10} is needed for the generation of ATP by mitochondria, it is essential to add this antioxidant in multiple micronutrient preparation. A study has shown that coenzyme Q_{10} scavenges peroxy radicals faster than alpha-tocopherol, and like vitamin C, can regenerate vitamin E in a redox cycle. However, it is a weaker antioxidant than alpha-tocopherol. Coenzyme Q_{10} administration has been shown to improve clinical symptoms in patients with mitochondrial encephalomyopathies.[208]

Nicotinamide (vitamin B_3), a precursor of NAD+ also attenuated glutamate-induced toxicity and preserved cellular levels of NAD+ to support the activity of SIRT1, a regulatory mitochondrial biogenesis. This vitamin B_3 inhibits oxidative damage and improves mitochondrial functions and thus can protect DA neurons and can improve motor function. Thus, oral supplementation with nicotinamide may be safe and useful in the prevention and improved treatment of PD.

Selenium is a cofactor of glutathione peroxidase, and Se-glutathione peroxidase acts as an antioxidant by increasing the intracellular level of glutathione. Therefore, selenium should be added to a multiple micronutrient preparation for prevention and in combination with standard care, for improved management of PD.

In addition to dietary and endogenous antioxidants, B vitamins, especially high doses of vitamin B_3 (nicotinamide), should be added to a multiple micronutrient preparation. B vitamins are also essential for normal health.

Two recent studies showed that supplementation with multiple vitamin preparations reduced cancer incidence by 10% in men[209] and improved clinical outcomes in patients with HIV/AIDS who were not taking medication.[210]

RATIONALE FOR USING A NSAID IN PD PREVENTION

Since inflammatory reactions represent one of the major factors that initiate and promote degeneration of DA neurons in PD brain, the use of an NSAID in prevention and treatment of PD appears rational. Laboratory data have shown that products of inflammatory reactions such as prostaglandins,[76,211] cytokines,[212,213] complement proteins,[214-218] adhesion molecules,[219-221] and free radicals[222-224] are neurotoxic.

Thus, the use of low-dose NSAIDs for the prevention and for reducing the progression of PD remains one of the viable options. These drugs do not improve the function of surviving neurons but protect them from further damage caused by increased chronic inflammatory reactions.

CAN THE FAMILIAL PD BE PREVENTED OR DELAYED?

It is often believed that the familial PD cannot be prevented or delayed by any pharmacological and/or physiological means. Laboratory experiments on the genetic basis of another disease model (cancer) in *Drosophila melanogaster* (fruit fly) show that it may be possible to prevent or at least delay the onset of the familial basis of human diseases.

The gene HOP (TUM-1) is essential for the development of fruit flies. A mutation in this gene markedly increases the risk of developing a leukemia-like tumor in female flies (unpublished observation in collaboration with Dr. Bhattacharya et al. of NASA, Moffat Field, CA). Proton radiation is a powerful cancer-causing agent. Whole-body irradiation of these flies with proton radiation dramatically increased the incidence of cancer compared to that in unirradiated flies. The question arose as to whether or not a preparation of multiple antioxidants can reduce the incidence of cancer which is due to a specific gene defect. To test this possibility, a mixture of multiple dietary and endogenous antioxidants were fed to these flies through diet 7 days before proton irradiation and continued after irradiation throughout the experimental period of 7 days. The results showed that antioxidant treatment before and after irradiation totally blocked the proton radiation-induced cancer in fruit flies. This finding on fruit flies is of particular interest, because to my knowledge, this is a first demonstration in which genetic basis of a disease can be prevented by antioxidant treatment. This observation made on fruit flies cannot readily be extrapolated to humans. It is unknown whether daily supplementation with antioxidants in children of parents who had heritable mutations that increases the risk of PD can prevent or delay the onset of the disease. A clinical study is needed to evaluate the effectiveness of multiple antioxidants in prevention of or delayed onset of PD in children of parents carrying heritable mutations in alpha-synuclein, DJ-1, PARKIN, or PINK1 gene that increases the risk of developing PD.

RECOMMENDED MICRONUTRIENT SUPPLEMENT IN COMBINATION WITH LOW DOSES OF NSAID FOR PRIMARY PREVENTION OF PD

The high-risk populations include individuals with a family history of PD and those aged 50 years or older who have no symptoms of PD. These populations are very suitable to investigate the effectiveness of proposed micronutrients in combination with a low-dose aspirin in prevention of PD. The selected combination of nontoxic agents include vitamin A (retinyl palmitate), vitamin E (both D-alpha-tocopherol and D-alpha-tocopheryl succinate), natural mixed carotenoids, vitamin C (calcium ascorbate), vitamin D, B vitamins with higher levels of vitamin-B_3 (nicotinamide), selenium, coenzyme Q_{10}, alpha-lipoic acid, NAC, L-carnitine omega-3-fatty acids, resveratrol, and curcumin. The combination of the above agents were selected because they would reduce oxidative stress and chronic inflammation optimally by activating the Nrf2/ARE pathway without ROS stimulation and by directly scavenging free radicals. No iron, copper, manganese, or heavy metals (vanadium, zirconium, and molybdenum) would be added in the above preparation. The daily doses can be divided into two (half in the morning and half in the evening preferably with meal). No iron, copper, or manganese should be included because these trace minerals are known to interact with vitamin C to produce free radicals. These trace minerals are absorbed from the intestinal tract more in the presence of antioxidants than in their absence that could result in increased body stores of these minerals. Increased iron stores have been linked to increased risk of several chronic diseases including PD.[225]

A low-dose aspirin (81 mg/day) is recommended because of its anti-inflammatory effect, and because in combination with vitamin E, it produced a synergetic effect on inhibition of cyclooxygenase activity[226]; therefore, the combination of multiple micronutrients and aspirin may be more effective in reducing the levels of chronic inflammation than the individual agents. The efficacy of proposed micronutrient formulation in combination with aspirin remains to be tested in high-risk populations or in patients with an early-stage PD, but they have been used in humans for several decades without reported significant toxicity. In the meantime, the proposed micronutrient and aspirin recommendations may be adopted by the individuals among high-risk populations and those with an early-stage PD in consultation with their physicians or health professionals. It is expected that the proposed recommendations would reduce the risk of developing PD in high-risk populations.

The recommended micronutrient supplements should be taken orally and divided into two doses, half in the morning and the other half in the evening with meal. This is because the biological half-lives of micronutrients are highly variable which can create high levels of fluctuations in the tissue levels of micronutrients. A two-fold difference in the levels of certain micronutrients such as alpha-tocopheryl succinate can cause a marked difference in the expression of gene profiles (our unpublished data). In order to maintain relatively consistent levels of micronutrients in the brain, the proposed micronutrients should be taken twice a day. A clinical study should be initiated to test the efficacy of proposed recommendations for primary prevention.

RECOMMENDED MICRONUTRIENTS IN COMBINATION WITH LOW DOSES OF NSAID FOR SECONDARY PREVENTION

Individuals with early symptoms of PD who are not taking levodopa therapy can be included in secondary prevention. The strategies proposed for the primary prevention may also be used in combination with standard care for secondary prevention in patients with early-phase PD. A clinical study should be initiated to test the efficacy of the proposed strategies in reducing the progression of PD. A clinical study should be initiated to test the efficacy of proposed recommendations for secondary prevention.

TREATMENTS OF PD

The purpose of treatment is to slow down the progression of disease and improve the symptoms of the disease. At present, there is no cure for PD, but a variety of medications provide dramatic relief from the symptoms. Usually, patients are given levodopa combined with carbidopa. Carbidopa delays the conversion of levodopa into dopamine until it reaches the brain. Nerve cells can use levodopa to make dopamine and replenish the brain's dwindling supply. Although levodopa helps at least three-quarters of PD patients, not all symptoms respond equally to the drug. Bradykinesia and rigidity respond best, while tremor may be only marginally reduced. Problems with balance and other symptoms may not be alleviated at all. Anticholinergics may help to control tremor and rigidity. Other drugs, such as bromocriptine, pramipex-ole, and ropinirole, mimic the role of dopamine in the brain, causing the neurons to react as they would to dopamine. An antiviral drug, amantadine, also appears to reduce symptoms. In May 2006, the FDA approved rasagiline to be used along with levodopa for patients with advanced PD or as a single-drug treatment for early PD.

In some cases, surgery may be appropriate if the disease doesn't respond to drugs. A therapy called deep brain stimulation (DBS) has now been approved by the U.S. Food and Drug Administration. In DBS, electrodes are implanted into the brain and connected to a small electrical device called a pulse generator that can be externally programmed. DBS can reduce the need for levodopa and related drugs, which in turn decreases the involuntary movements called dyskinesia that are a common side effect of levodopa. It also helps to alleviate fluctuations of symptoms and to reduce tremors, slowness of movements, and gait problems. DBS requires careful program-ming of the stimulator device in order to work correctly.

The current treatment strategies involve increasing the function of surviving DA neurons by maintaining adequate levels of DA. To accomplish this, L-dopa, a pre-cursor of DA and DA receptor agonists, are used. Deprenyl and catechol-o-methyl transferase (COMT) inhibitor are used to prevent degradation of DA. In addition, in some cases, acetylcholinesterase inhibitor is utilized in order to balance between two neurotransmitters, DA and acetylcholine, by reducing the levels of acetylcholine. In cases where drug therapy becomes ineffective, highly effective surgical methods to relieve some of the symptoms of PD such as tremor are available. None of these treatments prevents the DA neuron from dying due to increased oxidative stress and chronic inflammation.

RATIONALE FOR USING MICRONUTRIENT SUPPLEMENT AND NSAID IN COMBINATION WITH STANDARD THERAPY IN PD PATIENTS

Increased oxidative stress, chronic inflammation, and mitochondrial dysfunction play an important role in the progression of PD. Levodopa therapy is considered a gold standard for the treatment of PD, but its toxicity becomes a limiting fac-tor, and the treatment is discontinued after about 5 years. The reasons for this effect of levodopa are unknown. *In vitro* studies have suggested that treatment of neuronal cells in culture with L-dopa is very toxic. This is due to the fact that

L-dopa generates excessive amounts of free radicals during auto-oxidation as well as during oxidative metabolism of its product, DA; however, from animal studies, it appears that there is no evidence of similar effects of L-dopa *in vivo*.[227] In a randomized, double-blind, placebo-controlled trial involving 361 patients with an early-stage PD, the effects of various doses of levodopa for a period of 40 weeks were investigated.[228] The results showed that the patients receiving the highest dose of levodopa had significantly more dyskinesia, hypertonia, infection, headache, and nausea than those receiving placebo. The clinical data showed that levodopa treatment either slowed the progression of PD or has improved the symptoms of the disease. However, neuroimaging data suggested that levodopa treatment increased the rate of loss of nigrostriatal DA nerve terminals or it reduced the levels of DA transporter more than that produced by placebo treatment. A further investigation on this issue revealed that dose of levodopa is a factor in producing motor complications of dyskinesia and wearing-off, and these can develop as early as 5 to 6 months at high levodopa doses.[229] Since L-dopa has a potential to cause increased oxidative damage peripherally and/or centrally, it appears rational to propose that supplementation with multiple antioxidants in combination with levodopa therapy may improve the efficacy of this therapy by reducing the side effects of levodopa. This would then allow levodopa treatment to be effective for a period longer than that currently expected. Furthermore, if the oxidation of L-dopa is reduced by antioxidants, it would then be possible to reduce the dosage of levodopa without sacrificing its efficacy.

In a rat PD model (induced by rotenone), the efficacy of oral L-dopa therapy with or without various doses of coenzyme Q_{10} was evaluated.[230] The results showed that L-dopa therapy improved the symptoms and restored striatal DA levels, but it did not show any significant effect on striatal mitochondrial complex I activity, ATP levels, or the expression of Bcl2. Administration of coenzyme Q_{10} at a high dose with L-dopa increased striatal complex I activity, ATP levels, DA levels, and Bcl2 expression compared to coenzyme Q_{10} treatment at low doses with L-dopa.

RECOMMENDED MICRONUTRIENT SUPPLEMENT AND LOW DOSES OF NSAID IN COMBINATION WITH STANDARD THERAPY IN PD PATIENTS

The proposed strategies recommended for secondary prevention can also be used in combination with standard medications in the management of PD. It is expected that adoption of these recommendations may reduce the progression of the disease and prolong the efficacy of medications.

DIET AND LIFESTYLE RECOMMENDATIONS FOR PD

Even though there is no direct link between the diet- and lifestyle-related factors and the initiation or progression of PD, it is always useful to include a balanced diet that contains low fat and plenty of fruits and vegetables. Among fruits, blueberries and raspberries are particularly important because of their protective role against oxidative injuries in the brain. Lifestyle recommendations include daily moderate exercise, reduced stress, and no tobacco smoking or drug use.

CONCLUSIONS

The results of many studies presented in this review suggest that increased oxidative stress, mitochondrial dysfunction, and chronic inflammation play a dominant role in the initiation and progression of sporadic PD. Even in familial PD, these biological events play a crucial role in the pathogenesis of PD. Mitochondria are very sensitive to increased oxidative stress which induce mitochondrial dysfunction. Damaged mitochondria produce more free radicals.

At present, there are no effective strategies to reduce the incidence of PD. It is proposed that a combination of agents which can increase the levels of antioxidant enzymes by activating the Nrf2/ARE pathway without ROS stimulation, and which can directly scavenge free radicals, may be necessary to reduce oxidative stress and chronic inflammation optimally in PD. Dietary and endogenous antioxidants, curcumin, resveratrol, and omega-3-fatty acids can fulfill the above requirements for reducing oxidative stress and chronic inflammation optimally. Thus, a preparation of the above antioxidants in combination with a low-dose of NSAIDs, such as aspirin, may be useful in reducing chronic inflammation optimally. The same multiple antioxidants and phenolic compounds would also protect against glutamate-induced damage to the nerve cells. All the agents described here are of low toxicity, which would allow their prolonged safe usage among high-risk populations not expressing any symptoms of PD. The same preparation of micronutrient can also be used for secondary prevention as well as in combination with medications for the treatment of PD. Separate clinical studies using the proposed micronutrient recommendations for primary prevention, secondary prevention, and treatment should be initiated. In the meantime, those individuals interested in micronutrient approach in reducing risk and the rate of progression of PD or improving the efficacy of standard therapy in the treatment of PD may like to adopt these recommendations in consultation with their physicians or health professionals.

REFERENCES

1. Mandel S, Grunblatt E, Riederer P, Gerlach M, Levites Y, Youdim MB. Neuroprotective strategies in Parkinson's disease: An update on progress. *CNS Drugs*. 2003; 17(10): 729–762.
2. Van Den Eeden SK, Tanner CM, Bernstein AL et al. Incidence of Parkinson's disease: Variation by age, gender, and race/ethnicity. *Am J Epidemiol*. Jun 1 2003; 157(11): 1015–1022.
3. Su B, Liu H, Wang X et al. Ectopic localization of FOXO3a protein in Lewy bodies in Lewy body dementia and Parkinson's disease. *Mol Neurodegener*. 2009; 4: 32.
4. Desplats P, Lee HJ, Bae EJ et al. Inclusion formation and neuronal cell death through neuron-to-neuron transmission of alpha-synuclein. *Proc Natl Acad Sci U S A*. Aug 4 2009; 106(31): 13010–13015.
5. Willison LD, Kudo T, Loh DH, Kuljis D, Colwell CS. Circadian dysfunction may be a key component of the non-motor symptoms of Parkinson's disease: Insights from a transgenic mouse model. *Exp Neurol*. May 2013; 243: 57–66.

6. Racette BA, Aschner M, Guilarte TR, Dydak U, Criswell SR, Zheng W. Pathophysiology of manganese-associated neurotoxicity. *Neurotoxicology.* Aug 2012; 33(4): 881–886.
7. Mena I, Horiuchi K, Burke K, Cotzias GC. Chronic manganese poisoning. Individual susceptibility and absorption of iron. *Neurology.* Oct 1969; 19(10): 1000–1006.
8. Pezzoli G, Cereda E. Exposure to pesticides or solvents and risk of Parkinson disease. *Neurology.* May 28 2013; 80(22): 2035–2041.
9. van der Mark M, Brouwer M, Kromhout H, Nijssen P, Huss A, Vermeulen R. Is pesticide use related to Parkinson disease? Some clues to heterogeneity in study results. *Environ Health Perspect.* Mar 2012; 120(3): 340–347.
10. Goldman SM, Quinlan PJ, Ross GW et al. Solvent exposures and Parkinson disease risk in twins. *Ann Neurol.* Jun 2012; 71(6): 776–784.
11. Peng J, Stevenson FF, Oo ML, Andersen JK. Iron-enhanced paraquat-mediated dopaminergic cell death due to increased oxidative stress as a consequence of microglial activation. *Free Radic Biol Med.* Jan 15 2009; 46(2): 312–320.
12. Ballard PA, Tetrud JW, Langston JW. Permanent human parkinsonism due to 1-methyl-4-phenyl-1,2,3,6-tetrahydropyridine (MPTP): Seven cases. *Neurology.* Jul 1985; 35(7): 949–956.
13. Tanner CM, Goldman SM, Aston DA et al. Smoking and Parkinson's disease in twins. *Neurology.* Feb 26 2002; 58(4): 581–588.
14. Samii A, Etminan M, Wiens MO, Jafari S. NSAID use and the risk of Parkinson's disease: Systematic review and meta-analysis of observational studies. *Drug Aging.* 2009; 26(9): 769–779.
15. Hancock DB, Martin ER, Stajich JM et al. Smoking, caffeine, and nonsteroidal anti-inflammatory drugs in families with Parkinson disease. *Arch Neurol.* Apr 2007; 64(4): 576–580.
16. Powers KM, Kay DM, Factor SA et al. Combined effects of smoking, coffee, and NSAIDs on Parkinson's disease risk. *Mov Disord.* Jan 2008; 23(1): 88–95.
17. Golbe LI, Farrell TM, Davis PH. Case-control study of early life dietary factors in Parkinson's disease. *Arch Neurol.* Dec 1988; 45(12): 1350–1353.
18. de Rijk MC, Breteler MM, den Breeijen JH et al. Dietary antioxidants and Parkinson disease. The Rotterdam Study. *Arch Neurol.* Jun 1997; 54(6): 762–765.
19. Dexter DT, Holley AE, Flitter WD et al. Increased levels of lipid hydroperoxides in the parkinsonian substantia nigra: An HPLC and ESR study. *Mov Disord.* Jan 1994; 9(1): 92–97.
20. Dexter DT, Carter CJ, Wells FR et al. Basal lipid peroxidation in substantia nigra is increased in Parkinson's disease. *J Neurochem.* Feb 1989; 52(2): 381–389.
21. Sanchez-Ramos J, Overvik E, Ames B. A marker of oxyradical-mediated DNA damage (8-hydroxy-2'-deoxyguanosine) is increased in nigro-striatum of Parkinson's disease brain. *Neurodegeneration.* 1994; 3: 197–204.
22. Ebadi M, Srinivasan SK, Baxi MD. Oxidative stress and antioxidant therapy in Parkinson's disease. *Prog Neurobiol.* Jan 1996; 48(1): 1–19.
23. Ambani LM, Van Woert MH, Murphy S. Brain peroxidase and catalase in Parkinson disease. *Arch Neurol.* Feb 1975; 32(2): 114–118.
24. Kish SJ, Morito C, Hornykiewicz O. Glutathione peroxidase activity in Parkinson's disease brain. *Neurosci Lett.* Aug 5 1985; 58(3): 343–346.
25. Riederer P, Sofic E, Rausch WD et al. Transition metals, ferritin, glutathione, and ascorbic acid in parkinsonian brains. *J Neurochem.* Feb 1989; 52(2): 515–520.
26. Perry TL, Godin DV, Hansen S. Parkinson's disease: A disorder due to nigral glutathione deficiency? *Neurosci Lett.* Dec 13 1982; 33(3): 305–310.
27. Sofic E, Lange KW, Jellinger K, Riederer P. Reduced and oxidized glutathione in the substantia nigra of patients with Parkinson's disease. *Neurosci Lett.* Aug 17 1992; 142(2): 128–130.

28. Sian J, Dexter DT, Lees AJ et al. Alterations in glutathione levels in Parkinson's disease and other neurodegenerative disorders affecting basal ganglia. *Ann Neurol.* Sep 1994; 36(3): 348–355.

29. Jenner P. Oxidative mechanisms in nigral cell death in Parkinson's disease. *Mov Disord.* 1998; 13 Suppl 1: 24–34.

30. Fitzmaurice PS, Ang L, Guttman M, Rajput AH, Furukawa Y, Kish SJ. Nigral glutathione deficiency is not specific for idiopathic Parkinson's disease. *Mov Disord.* Sep 2003; 18(9): 969–976.

31. Sofic E, Sapcanin A, Tahirovic I et al. Antioxidant capacity in postmortem brain tissues of Parkinson's and Alzheimer's diseases. *J Neural Transm Suppl.* 2006 (71): 39–43.

32. Fessel JP, Hulette C, Powell S, Roberts LJ, 2nd, Zhang J. Isofurans, but not F2-isoprostanes, are increased in the substantia nigra of patients with Parkinson's disease and with dementia with Lewy body disease. *J Neurochem.* May 2003; 85(3): 645–650.

33. Schipper HM, Liberman A, Stopa EG. Neural heme oxygenase-1 expression in idiopathic Parkinson's disease. *Exp Neurol.* Mar 1998; 150(1): 60–68.

34. Double KL, Gerlach M, Youdim MB, Riederer P. Impaired iron homeostasis in Parkinson's disease. *J Neural Transm Suppl.* 2000 (60): 37–58.

35. Graham JM, Paley MN, Grunewald RA, Hoggard N, Griffiths PD. Brain iron deposition in Parkinson's disease imaged using the PRIME magnetic resonance sequence. *Brain.* Dec 2000; 123 Pt 12: 2423–2431.

36. Andersen JK. Iron dysregulation and Parkinson's disease. *J Alzheimers Dis.* Dec 2004; 6(6 Suppl): S47–S52.

37. Salazar J, Mena N, Hunot S et al. Divalent metal transporter 1 (DMT1) contributes to neurodegeneration in animal models of Parkinson's disease. *Proc Natl Acad Sci U S A.* Nov 25 2008; 105(47): 18,578–18,583.

38. Blandini F, Porter RH, Greenamyre JT. Glutamate and Parkinson's disease. *Mol Neurobiol.* Feb 1996; 12(1): 73–94.

39. Enochs WS, Sarna T, Zecca L, Riley PA, Swartz HM. The roles of neuromelanin, binding of metal ions, and oxidative cytotoxicity in the pathogenesis of Parkinson's disease: A hypothesis. *J Neural Transm Park Dis Dement Sect.* 1994; 7(2): 83–100.

40. Good PF, Olanow CW, Perl DP. Neuromelanin-containing neurons of the substantia nigra accumulate iron and aluminum in Parkinson's disease: A LAMMA study. *Brain Res.* Oct 16 1992; 593(2): 343–346.

41. Zhang HN, Guo JF, He D et al. Lower serum UA levels in Parkinson's disease patients in the Chinese population. *Neurosci Lett.* Apr 18 2012; 514(2): 152–155.

42. Prabhakaran K, Ghosh D, Chapman GD, Gunasekar PG. Molecular mechanism of manganese exposure-induced dopaminergic toxicity. *Brain Res Bull.* Jul 1 2008; 76(4): 361–367.

43. Ebadi M, Sharma SK. Peroxynitrite and mitochondrial dysfunction in the pathogenesis of Parkinson's disease. *Antioxid Redox Signal.* Jun 2003; 5(3): 319–335.

44. Choi DH, Cristovao AC, Guhathakurta S et al. NADPH oxidase 1-mediated oxidative stress leads to dopamine neuron death in Parkinson's disease. *Antioxid Redox Signal.* May 15 2012; 16(10): 1033–1045.

45. Chen CM, Liu JL, Wu YR et al. Increased oxidative damage in peripheral blood correlates with severity of Parkinson's disease. *Neurobiol Dis.* Mar 2009; 33(3): 429–435.

46. Sanyal J, Bandyopadhyay SK, Banerjee TK et al. Plasma levels of lipid peroxides in patients with Parkinson's disease. *Eur Rev Med Pharmacol Sci.* Mar-Apr 2009; 13(2): 129–132.

47. Bolner A, Pilleri M, De Riva V, Nordera GP. Plasma and urinary HPLC-ED determination of the ratio of 8-OHdG/2-dG in Parkinson's disease. *Clinical laboratory.* 2011; 57(11–12): 859–866.

48. Varghese M, Pandey M, Samanta A, Gangopadhyay PK, Mohanakumar KP. Reduced NADH coenzyme Q dehydrogenase activity in platelets of Parkinson's disease, but not Parkinson plus patients, from an Indian population. *J Neurol Sci.* Apr 15 2009; 279(1–2): 39–42.
49. Paraskevas GP, Kapaki E, Petropoulou O, Anagnostouli M, Vagenas V, Papageorgiou C. Plasma levels of antioxidant vitamins C and E are decreased in vascular parkinsonism. *J Neurol Sci.* Nov 15 2003; 215(1–2): 51–55.
50. Fernandez-Calle P, Jimenez-Jimenez FJ, Molina JA et al. Serum levels of ascorbic acid (vitamin C) in patients with Parkinson's disease. *J Neurol Sci.* Aug 1993; 118(1): 25–28.
51. Fernandez-Calle P, Molina JA, Jimenez-Jimenez FJ et al. Serum levels of alpha-tocopherol (vitamin E) in Parkinson's disease. *Neurology.* May 1992; 42(5): 1064–1066.
52. King D, Playfer JR, Roberts NB. Concentrations of vitamins A, C and E in elderly patients with Parkinson's disease. *Postgrad Med J.* Aug 1992; 68(802): 634–637.
53. Bonsi P, Cuomo D, Picconi B et al. Striatal metabotropic glutamate receptors as a target for pharmacotherapy in Parkinson's disease. *Amino Acids.* Feb 2007; 32(2): 189–195.
54. Ossowska K, Konieczny J, Wardas J et al. An influence of ligands of metabotropic glutamate receptor subtypes on parkinsonian-like symptoms and the striatopallidal pathway in rats. *Amino Acids.* Feb 2007; 32(2): 179–188.
55. Meredith GE, Totterdell S, Beales M, Meshul CK. Impaired glutamate homeostasis and programmed cell death in a chronic MPTP mouse model of Parkinson's disease. *Exp Neurol.* Sep 2009; 219(1): 334–340.
56. Schubert D, Kimura H, Maher P. Growth factors and vitamin E modify neuronal glutamate toxicity. *Proc Natl Acad Sci U S A.* Sep 1 1992; 89(17): 8264–8267.
57. Sandhu JK, Pandey S, Ribecco-Lutkiewicz M et al. Molecular mechanisms of glutamate neurotoxicity in mixed cultures of NT2-derived neurons and astrocytes: Protective effects of coenzyme Q_{10}. *J Neurosci Res.* Jun 15 2003; 72(6): 691–703.
58. Arduino DM, Esteves AR, Cardoso SM, Oliveira CR. Endoplasmic reticulum and mitochondria interplay mediates apoptotic cell death: Relevance to Parkinson's disease. *Neurochem Int.* Sep 2009; 55(5): 341–348.
59. Gubellini P, Picconi B, Di Filippo M, Calabresi P. Downstream mechanisms triggered by mitochondrial dysfunction in the basal ganglia: From experimental models to neurodegenerative diseases. *Biochim Biophys Acta.* Aug 14 2009.
60. Dodson MW, Guo M. Pink1, Parkin, DJ-1 and mitochondrial dysfunction in Parkinson's disease. *Curr Opin Neurobiol.* Jun 2007; 17(3): 331–337.
61. Gautier CA, Kitada T, Shen J. Loss of PINK1 causes mitochondrial functional defects and increased sensitivity to oxidative stress. *Proc Natl Acad Sci U S A.* Aug 12 2008; 105(32): 11364–11369.
62. Lee SJ. alpha-synuclein aggregation: A link between mitochondrial defects and Parkinson's disease? *Antioxid Redox Signal.* Jun 2003; 5(3): 337–348.
63. Banerjee R, Starkov AA, Beal MF, Thomas B. Mitochondrial dysfunction in the limelight of Parkinson's disease pathogenesis. *Biochim Biophys Acta.* Jul 2009; 1792(7): 651–663.
64. Yang JL, Weissman L, Bohr VA, Mattson MP. Mitochondrial DNA damage and repair in neurodegenerative disorders. *DNA Repair (Amst).* Jul 1 2008; 7(7): 1110–1120.
65. Perier C, Bove J, Wu DC et al. Two molecular pathways initiate mitochondria-dependent dopaminergic neurodegeneration in experimental Parkinson's disease. *Proc Natl Acad Sci U S A.* May 8 2007; 104(19): 8161–8166.
66. Domingues AF, Arduino DM, Esteves AR, Swerdlow RH, Oliveira CR, Cardoso SM. Mitochondria and ubiquitin-proteasomal system interplay: Relevance to Parkinson's disease. *Free Radic Biol Med.* Sep 15 2008; 45(6): 820–825.

67. Ho PW, Ho JW, Liu HF et al. Mitochondrial neuronal uncoupling proteins: A target for potential disease-modification in Parkinson's disease. *Translat Neurodegener.* 2012; 1(1): 3.

68. Whitton PS. Inflammation as a causative factor in the aetiology of Parkinson's disease. *Br J Pharmacol.* Apr 2007; 150(8): 963–976.

69. McGeer PL, McGeer EG. Glial reactions in Parkinson's disease. *Mov Disord.* Mar 15 2008; 23(4): 474–483.

70. Reynolds AD, Glanzer JG, Kadiu I et al. Nitrated alpha-synuclein-activated microglial profiling for Parkinson's disease. *J Neurochem.* Mar 2008; 104(6): 1504–1525.

71. Zhang W, Wang T, Pei Z et al. Aggregated alpha-synuclein activates microglia: A process leading to disease progression in Parkinson's disease. *FASEB J.* Apr 2005; 19(6): 533–542.

72. Roodveldt C, Christodoulou J, Dobson CM. Immunological features of alpha-synuclein in Parkinson's disease. *J Cell Mol Med.* Oct 2008; 12(5B): 1820–1829.

73. Gao HM, Kotzbauer PT, Uryu K, Leight S, Trojanowski JQ, Lee VM. Neuroinflammation and oxidation/nitration of alpha-synuclein linked to dopaminergic neurodegeneration. *J Neurosci.* Jul 23 2008; 28(30): 7687–7698.

74. Sawada M, Imamura K, Nagatsu T. Role of cytokines in inflammatory process in Parkinson's disease. *J Neural Transm Suppl.* 2006(70): 373–381.

75. Wilms H, Zecca L, Rosenstiel P, Sievers J, Deuschl G, Lucius R. Inflammation in Parkinson's diseases and other neurodegenerative diseases: Cause and therapeutic implications. *Curr Pharm Des.* 2007; 13(18): 1925–1928.

76. Prasad KN, Hovland AR, La Rosa FG, Hovland PG. Prostaglandins as putative neurotoxins in Alzheimer's disease. *Proc Soc Exp Biol Med.* Nov 1998; 219(2): 120–125.

77. Chae SW, Kang BY, Hwang O, Choi HJ. Cyclooxygenase-2 is involved in oxidative damage and alpha-synuclein accumulation in dopaminergic cells. *Neurosci Lett.* May 9 2008; 436(2): 205–209.

78. Gandhi PN, Chen SG, Wilson-Delfosse AL. Leucine-rich repeat kinase 2 (LRRK2): A key player in the pathogenesis of Parkinson's disease. *J Neurosci Res.* May 1 2009; 87(6): 1283–1295.

79. Giaime E, Sunyach C, Druon C et al. Loss of function of DJ-1 triggered by Parkinson's disease-associated mutation is due to proteolytic resistance to caspase-6. *Cell Death Differ.* Aug 14 2009.

80. Fitzgerald JC, Plun-Favreau H. Emerging pathways in genetic Parkinson's disease: Autosomal-recessive genes in Parkinson's disease—a common pathway? *FEBS J.* Dec 2008; 275(23): 5758–5766.

81. Klein C, Lohmann-Hedrich K. Impact of recent genetic findings in Parkinson's disease. *Curr Opin Neurol.* Aug 2007; 20(4): 453–464.

82. Li Y, Liu W, Oo TF et al. Mutant LRRK2(R1441G) BAC transgenic mice recapitulate cardinal features of Parkinson's disease. *Nat Neurosci.* Jul 2009; 12(7): 826–828.

83. Giasson BI, Van Deerlin VM. Mutations in LRRK2 as a cause of Parkinson's disease. *Neurosignals.* 2008; 16(1): 99–105.

84. da Costa CA. DJ-1: A newcomer in Parkinson's disease pathology. *Curr Mol Med.* Nov 2007; 7(7): 650–657.

85. Wider C, Wszolek ZK. Clinical genetics of Parkinson's disease and related disorders. *Parkinsonism Relat Disord.* 2007; 13 Suppl 3: S229–S232.

86. Bueler H. Impaired mitochondrial dynamics and function in the pathogenesis of Parkinson's disease. *Exp Neurol.* Aug 2009; 218(2): 235–246.

87. Kahle PJ, Waak J, Gasser T. DJ-1 and prevention of oxidative stress in Parkinson's disease and other age-related disorders. *Free Radic Biol Med.* Aug 14 2009.

88. Bandopadhyay R, Kingsbury AE, Cookson MR et al. The expression of DJ-1 (PARK7) in normal human CNS and idiopathic Parkinson's disease. *Brain.* Feb 2004; 127(Pt 2): 420–430.

89. Kitamura Y, Watanabe S, Taguchi M et al. Neuroprotective effect of a new DJ-1-binding compound against neurodegeneration in Parkinson's disease and stroke model rats. *Mol Neurodegener.* 2011; 6(1): 48.

90. Gu L, Cui T, Fan C et al. Involvement of ERK1/2 signaling pathway in DJ-1-induced neuroprotection against oxidative stress. *Biochem Biophys Res Commun.* Jun 12 2009; 383(4): 469–474.

91. Lev N, Ickowicz D, Barhum Y, Lev S, Melamed E, Offen D. DJ-1 protects against dopamine toxicity. *J Neural Transm.* Feb 2009; 116(2): 151–160.

92. Lev N, Ickowicz D, Melamed E, Offen D. Oxidative insults induce DJ-1 upregulation and redistribution: Implications for neuroprotection. *Neurotoxicology.* May 2008; 29(3): 397–405.

93. Nunome K, Miyazaki S, Nakano M, Iguchi-Ariga S, Ariga H. Pyrroloquinoline quinone prevents oxidative stress-induced neuronal death probably through changes in oxidative status of DJ-1. *Biol Pharm Bull.* Jul 2008; 31(7): 1321–1326.

94. Xu J, Zhong N, Wang H et al. The Parkinson's disease-associated DJ-1 protein is a transcriptional co-activator that protects against neuronal apoptosis. *Hum Mol Genet.* May 1 2005; 14(9): 1231–1241.

95. Batelli S, Albani D, Rametta R et al. DJ-1 modulates alpha-synuclein aggregation state in a cellular model of oxidative stress: Relevance for Parkinson's disease and involvement of HSP70. *PLoS One.* 2008; 3(4): e1884.

96. Bjorkblom B, Adilbayeva A, Maple-Grodem J et al. Parkinson disease protein DJ-1 binds metals and protects against metal-induced cytotoxicity. *J Biol Chem.* Aug 2 2013; 288(31): 22,809–22,820.

97. Ariga H, Takahashi-Niki K, Kato I, Maita H, Niki T, Iguchi-Ariga SM. Neuroprotective function of DJ-1 in Parkinson's disease. *Oxid Med Cell Longev.* 2013; 2013: 683920.

98. Thomas KJ, McCoy MK, Blackinton J et al. DJ-1 acts in parallel to the PINK1/parkin pathway to control mitochondrial function and autophagy. *Hum Mol Genet.* Jan 1 2011; 20(1): 40–50.

99. Lev N, Barhum Y, Pilosof NS et al. DJ-1 protects against dopamine toxicity: Implications for Parkinson's disease and aging. *J Gerontol A Biol Sci Med Sci.* Mar 2013; 68(3): 215–225.

100. Kim SJ, Park YJ, Hwang IY, Youdim MB, Park KS, Oh YJ. Nuclear translocation of DJ-1 during oxidative stress-induced neuronal cell death. *Free Radic Biol Med.* Aug 15 2012; 53(4): 936–950.

101. Duda JE, Shah U, Arnold SE, Lee VM, Trojanowski JQ. The expression of alpha-, beta-, and gamma-synucleins in olfactory mucosa from patients with and without neurodegenerative diseases. *Exp Neurol.* Dec 1999; 160(2): 515–522.

102. Zhou W, Schaack J, Zawada WM, Freed CR. Overexpression of human alpha-synuclein causes dopamine neuron death in primary human mesencephalic culture. *Brain Res.* Feb 1 2002; 926(1–2): 42–50.

103. Lo Bianco C, Ridet JL, Schneider BL, Deglon N, Aebischer P. Alpha-synucleinopathy and selective dopaminergic neuron loss in a rat lentiviral-based model of Parkinson's disease. *Proc Natl Acad Sci U S A.* Aug 6 2002; 99(16): 10,813–10,818.

104. Galvin JE. Interaction of alpha-synuclein and dopamine metabolites in the pathogenesis of Parkinson's disease: A case for the selective vulnerability of the substantia nigra. *Acta Neuropathol.* Aug 2006; 112(2): 115–126.

105. Prasad JE, Kumar B, Andreatta C et al. Overexpression of alpha-synuclein decreased viability and enhanced sensitivity to prostaglandin E(2), hydrogen peroxide, and a nitric oxide donor in differentiated neuroblastoma cells. *J Neurosci Res.* May 1 2004; 76(3): 415–422.

106. Hoepken HH, Gispert S, Azizov M et al. Parkinson patient fibroblasts show increased alpha-synuclein expression. *Exp Neurol.* Aug 2008; 212(2): 307–313.

107. Kalia LV, Kalia SK, McLean PJ, Lozano AM, Lang AE. Alpha-synuclein oligomers and clinical implications for Parkinson disease. *Ann Neurol.* Feb 2013; 73(2): 155–169.

108. Lucking CB, Brice A. Alpha-synuclein and Parkinson's disease. *Cell Mol Life Sci.* Dec 2000; 57(13–14): 1894–1908.

109. el-Agnaf OM, Irvine GB. Aggregation and neurotoxicity of alpha-synuclein and related peptides. *Biochem Soc Trans.* Aug 2002; 30(4): 559–565.

110. Devi L, Anandatheerthavarada HK. Mitochondrial trafficking of APP and alpha synuclein: Relevance to mitochondrial dysfunction in Alzheimer's and Parkinson's diseases. *Biochim Biophys Acta.* Jul 18 2009.

111. Parihar MS, Parihar A, Fujita M, Hashimoto M, Ghafourifar P. Mitochondrial association of alpha-synuclein causes oxidative stress. *Cell Mol Life Sci.* Apr 2008; 65(7–8): 1272–1284.

112. Parihar MS, Parihar A, Fujita M, Hashimoto M, Ghafourifar P. Alpha-synuclein over-expression and aggregation exacerbates impairment of mitochondrial functions by augmenting oxidative stress in human neuroblastoma cells. *Int J Biochem Cell Biol.* May 19 2009.

113. Martin LJ, Pan Y, Price AC et al. Parkinson's disease alpha-synuclein transgenic mice develop neuronal mitochondrial degeneration and cell death. *J Neurosci.* Jan 4 2006; 26(1): 41–50.

114. Junn E, Lee KW, Jeong BS, Chan TW, Im JY, Mouradian MM. Repression of alpha-synuclein expression and toxicity by microRNA-7. *Proc Natl Acad Sci U S A.* Aug 4 2009; 106(31): 13,052–13,057.

115. Esteves AR, Arduino DM, Swerdlow RH, Oliveira CR, Cardoso SM. Oxidative Stress involvement in alpha-synuclein oligomerization in Parkinsons disease cybrids. *Antioxid Redox Signal.* Aug 21 2008.

116. Fountaine TM, Venda LL, Warrick N et al. The effect of alpha-synuclein knockdown on MPP+ toxicity in models of human neurons. *Eur J Neurosci.* Dec 2008; 28(12): 2459–2473.

117. Wu F, Poon WS, Lu G et al. alpha-Synuclein knockdown attenuates MPP(+) induced mitochondrial dysfunction of SH-SY5Y cells. *Brain Res.* Jul 29 2009.

118. Ma L, Cao TT, Kandpal G et al. Genome-wide microarray analysis of the differential neuroprotective effects of antioxidants in neuroblastoma cells overexpressing the familial Parkinson's disease alpha-synuclein A53T mutation. *Neurochem Res.* Aug 2 2009.

119. Lee MK, Stirling W, Xu Y et al. Human alpha-synuclein-harboring familial Parkinson's disease-linked Ala-53→Thr mutation causes neurodegenerative disease with alpha-synuclein aggregation in transgenic mice. *Proc Natl Acad Sci U S A.* Jun 25 2002; 99(13): 8968–8973.

120. Martin-Clemente B, Alvarez-Castelao B, Mayo I et al. alpha-Synuclein expression levels do not significantly affect proteasome function and expression in mice and stably transfected PC12 cell lines. *J Biol Chem.* Dec 17 2004; 279(51): 52,984–52,990.

121. Dyllick-Brenzinger M, D'Souza CA, Dahlmann B, Kloetzel PM, Tandon A. Reciprocal effects of alpha-synuclein overexpression and proteasome inhibition in neuronal cells and tissue. *Neurotox Res.* Aug 4 2009.

122. Kim C, Lee SJ. Controlling the mass action of alpha-synuclein in Parkinson's disease. *J Neurochem.* Oct 2008; 107(2): 303–316.

123. Xilouri M, Vogiatzi T, Vekrellis K, Stefanis L. alpha-Synuclein degradation by autophagic pathways: A potential key to Parkinson's disease pathogenesis. *Autophagy.* Oct 1 2008; 4(7): 917–919.

124. Tessari I, Bisaglia M, Valle F et al. The reaction of alpha-synuclein with tyrosinase: Possible implications for Parkinson disease. *J Biol Chem.* Jun 13 2008; 283(24): 16,808–16,817.

125. Lastres-Becker I, Ulusoy A, Innamorato NG et al. alpha-Synuclein expression and Nrf2 deficiency cooperate to aggravate protein aggregation, neuronal death and inflammation in early-stage Parkinson's disease. *Hum Mol Genet.* Jul 15 2012; 21(14): 3173–3192.
126. Siddiqui A, Chinta SJ, Mallajosyula JK et al. Selective binding of nuclear alpha-synuclein to the PGC1alpha promoter under conditions of oxidative stress may contribute to losses in mitochondrial function: Implications for Parkinson's disease. *Free Radic Biol Med.* Aug 15 2012; 53(4): 993–1003.
127. Harms AS, Cao S, Rowse AL et al. MHCII is required for alpha-synuclein-induced activation of microglia, CD4 T cell proliferation, and dopaminergic neurodegeneration. *J Neurosci.* Jun 5 2013; 33(23): 9592–9600.
128. Gegg ME, Cooper JM, Schapira AH, Taanman JW. Silencing of PINK1 expression affects mitochondrial DNA and oxidative phosphorylation in dopaminergic cells. *PLoS One.* 2009; 4(3): e4756.
129. Gandhi S, Muqit MM, Stanyer L et al. PINK1 protein in normal human brain and Parkinson's disease. *Brain.* Jul 2006; 129(Pt 7): 1720–1731.
130. Marongiu R, Spencer B, Crews L et al. Mutant Pink1 induces mitochondrial dysfunction in a neuronal cell model of Parkinson's disease by disturbing calcium flux. *J Neurochem.* Mar 2009; 108(6): 1561–1574.
131. Liu W, Vives-Bauza C, Acin-Perez R et al. PINK1 defect causes mitochondrial dysfunction, proteasomal deficit and alpha-synuclein aggregation in cell culture models of Parkinson's disease. *PLoS One.* 2009; 4(2): e4597.
132. Dawson TM. Parkin and defective ubiquitination in Parkinson's disease. *J Neural Transm Suppl.* 2006; (70): 209–213.
133. Mitsui T, Kuroda Y, Kaji R. [Parkin and mitochondria]. *Brain Nerve.* Aug 2008; 60(8): 923–929.
134. Jiang H, Ren Y, Yuen EY et al. Parkin controls dopamine utilization in human midbrain dopaminergic neurons derived from induced pluripotent stem cells. *Nat Commun.* 2012; 3: 668.
135. Sun X, Liu J, Crary JF et al. ATF4 protects against neuronal death in cellular Parkinson's disease models by maintaining levels of parkin. *J Neurosci.* Feb 6 2013; 33(6): 2398–2407.
136. Gan-Or Z, Ozelius LJ, Bar-Shira A et al. The p.L302P mutation in the lysosomal enzyme gene SMPD1 is a risk factor for Parkinson disease. *Neurology.* Apr 23 2013; 80(17): 1606–1610.
137. Licker V, Cote M, Lobrinus JA et al. Proteomic profiling of the substantia nigra demonstrates CNDP2 overexpression in Parkinson's disease. *J Proteomics.* Aug 3 2012; 75(15): 4656–4667.
138. Itoh K, Chiba T, Takahashi S et al. An Nrf2/small Maf heterodimer mediates the induction of phase II detoxifying enzyme genes through antioxidant response elements. *Biochem Biophys Res Commun.* Jul 18 1997; 236(2): 313–322.
139. Hayes JD, Chanas SA, Henderson CJ et al. The Nrf2 transcription factor contributes both to the basal expression of glutathione S-transferases in mouse liver and to their induction by the chemopreventive synthetic antioxidants, butylated hydroxyanisole and ethoxyquin. *Biochem Soc Trans.* Feb 2000; 28(2): 33–41.
140. Chan K, Han XD, Kan YW. An important function of Nrf2 in combating oxidative stress: Detoxification of acetaminophen. *Proc Natl Acad Sci USA.* Apr 10 2001; 98(8): 4611–4616.
141. Williamson TP, Johnson DA, Johnson JA. Activation of the Nrf2-ARE pathway by siRNA knockdown of Keap1 reduces oxidative stress and provides partial protection from MPTP-mediated neurotoxicity. *Neurotoxicology.* Jun 2012; 33(3): 272–279.
142. Niture SK, Kaspar JW, Shen J, Jaiswal AK. Nrf2 signaling and cell survival. *Toxicol aAppl Pharmacol.* Apr 1 2010; 244(1): 37–42.

143. Xi YD, Yu HL, Ding J et al. Flavonoids protect cerebrovascular endothelial cells through Nrf2 and PI3K from beta-amyloid peptide-induced oxidative damage. *Curr Neurovasc Res.* Feb 2012; 9(1): 32–41.

144. Li XH, Li CY, Lu JM, Tian RB, Wei J. Allicin ameliorates cognitive deficits ageing-induced learning and memory deficits through enhancing of Nrf2 antioxidant signaling pathways. *Neurosci Lett.* Apr 11 2012; 514(1): 46–50.

145. Bergstrom P, Andersson HC, Gao Y et al. Repeated transient sulforaphane stimulation in astrocytes leads to prolonged Nrf2-mediated gene expression and protection from superoxide-induced damage. *Neuropharmacology.* Feb–Mar 2011; 60(2–3): 343–353.

146. Wruck CJ, Gotz ME, Herdegen T, Varoga D, Brandenburg LO, Pufe T. Kavalactones protect neural cells against amyloid beta peptide-induced neurotoxicity via extracellular signal-regulated kinase 1/2-dependent nuclear factor erythroid 2-related factor 2 activation. *Mol Pharmacol.* Jun 2008; 73(6): 1785–1795.

147. Hine CM, Mitchell JR. NRF2 and the phase II response in acute stress resistance induced by dietary restriction. *J Clin Exp Pathol.* Jun 19 2012; S4(4).

148. Suh JH, Shenvi SV, Dixon BM et al. Decline in transcriptional activity of Nrf2 causes age-related loss of glutathione synthesis, which is reversible with lipoic acid. *Proc Natl Acad Sci USA.* Mar 9 2004; 101(10): 3381–3386.

149. Gunjima K, Tomiyama R, Takakura K et al. 3,4-Dihydroxybenzalacetone protects against Parkinson's disease-related neurotoxin 6-OHDA through Akt/Nrf2/glutathione pathway. *J Cell Biochem.* Jan 2014; 115(1): 151–160.

150. Lou H, Jing X, Wei X, Shi H, Ren D, Zhang X. Naringenin protects against 6-OHDA-induced neurotoxicity via activation of the Nrf2/ARE signaling pathway. *Neuropharmacology.* Dec 10 2013.

151. Li R, Liang T, Xu L, Zheng N, Zhang K, Duan X. Puerarin attenuates neuronal degeneration in the substantia nigra of 6-OHDA-lesioned rats through regulating BDNF expression and activating the Nrf2/ARE signaling pathway. *Brain Res.* Jul 26 2013; 1523: 1–9.

152. He X, Wang L, Szklarz G, Bi Y, Ma Q. Resveratrol inhibits paraquat-induced oxidative stress and fibrogenic response by activating the nuclear factor erythroid 2-related factor 2 pathway. *J Pharmacol Exp Ther.* Jul 2012; 342(1): 81–90.

153. He Q, Song N, Jia F et al. Role of alpha-synuclein aggregation and the nuclear factor E2-related factor 2/heme oxygenase-1 pathway in iron-induced neurotoxicity. *Int J Biochem Cell Biol.* Jun 2013; 45(6): 1019–1030.

154. Chen PC, Vargas MR, Pani AK et al. Nrf2-mediated neuroprotection in the MPTP mouse model of Parkinson's disease: Critical role for the astrocyte. *Proc Natl Acad Sci U S A.* Feb 24 2009; 106(8): 2933–2938.

155. Kim SS, Lim J, Bang Y et al. Licochalcone E activates Nrf2/antioxidant response element signaling pathway in both neuronal and microglial cells: Therapeutic relevance to neurodegenerative disease. *J Nutr Biochem.* Oct 2012; 23(10): 1314–1323.

156. Im JY, Lee KW, Woo JM, Junn E, Mouradian MM. DJ-1 induces thioredoxin 1 expression through the Nrf2 pathway. *Hum Mol Genet.* Jul 1 2012; 21(13): 3013–3024.

157. Lim JH, Kim KM, Kim SW, Hwang O, Choi HJ. Bromocriptine activates NQO1 via Nrf2-PI3K/Akt signaling: Novel cytoprotective mechanism against oxidative damage. *Pharmacol Res.* May 2008; 57(5): 325–331.

158. Zou Y, Hong B, Fan L et al. Protective effect of puerarin against beta-amyloid-induced oxidative stress in neuronal cultures from rat hippocampus: Involvement of the GSK-3beta/Nrf2 signaling pathway. *Free Radic Res.* Jan 2013; 47(1): 55–63.

159. Choi HK, Pokharel YR, Lim SC et al. Inhibition of liver fibrosis by solubilized coenzyme Q_{10}: Role of Nrf2 activation in inhibiting transforming growth factor-beta1 expression. *Toxicol Appl Pharmacol.* Nov 1 2009; 240(3): 377–384.

160. Trujillo J, Chirino YI, Molina-Jijon E, Anderica-Romero AC, Tapia E, Pedraza-Chaverri J. Renoprotective effect of the antioxidant curcumin: Recent findings. *Redox Biol.* 2013; 1(1): 448–456.

161. Steele ML, Fuller S, Patel M, Kersaitis C, Ooi L, Munch G. Effect of Nrf2 activators on release of glutathione, cysteinylglycine and homocysteine by human U373 astroglial cells. *Redox Biol.* 2013; 1(1): 441–445.

162. Kode A, Rajendrasozhan S, Caito S, Yang SR, Megson IL, Rahman I. Resveratrol induces glutathione synthesis by activation of Nrf2 and protects against cigarette smoke-mediated oxidative stress in human lung epithelial cells. *Am J Physiol Lung Cell Mol Physiol.* Mar 2008; 294(3): L478–L488.

163. Gao L, Wang J, Sekhar KR et al. Novel n-3 fatty acid oxidation products activate Nrf2 by destabilizing the association between Keap1 and Cullin3. *J Biol Chem.* Jan 26 2007; 282(4): 2529–2537.

164. Saw CL, Yang AY, Guo Y, Kong AN. Astaxanthin and omega-3 fatty acids individually and in combination protect against oxidative stress via the Nrf2-ARE pathway. *Food Chem Toxicol.* Dec 2013; 62: 869–875.

165. Ji L, Liu R, Zhang XD et al. N-acetylcysteine attenuates phosgene-induced acute lung injury via upregulation of Nrf2 expression. *Inhal Toxicol.* Jun 2010; 22(7): 535–542.

166. Zambrano S, Blanca AJ, Ruiz-Armenta MV et al. The renoprotective effect of L-carnitine in hypertensive rats is mediated by modulation of oxidative stress-related gene expression. *Eur J Nutr.* Sep 2013; 52(6): 1649–1659.

167. Messier EM, Day BJ, Bahmed K et al. N-acetylcysteine protects murine alveolar type II cells from cigarette smoke injury in a nuclear erythroid 2-related factor-2-independent manner. *Am J Respir Cell Mol Biol.* May 2013; 48(5): 559–567.

168. Romanque P, Cornejo P, Valdes S, Videla LA. Thyroid hormone administration induces rat liver Nrf2 activation: Suppression by N-acetylcysteine pretreatment. *Thyroid.* Jun 2011; 21(6): 655–662.

169. Ono K, Yamada M. Vitamin A potently destabilizes preformed alpha-synuclein fibrils in vitro: Implications for Lewy body diseases. *Neurobiol Dis.* Feb 2007; 25(2): 446–454.

170. Park ES, Kim SY, Na JI et al. Glutathione prevented dopamine-induced apoptosis of melanocytes and its signaling. *J Dermatol Sci.* Aug 2007; 47(2): 141–149.

171. Khaldy H, Escames G, Leon J, Vives F, Luna JD, Acuna-Castroviejo D. Comparative effects of melatonin, L-deprenyl, Trolox and ascorbate in the suppression of hydroxyl radical formation during dopamine autoxidation in vitro. *J Pineal Res.* Sep 2000; 29(2): 100–107.

172. Penugonda S, Mare S, Goldstein G, Banks WA, Ercal N. Effects of N-acetylcysteine amide (NACA), a novel thiol antioxidant against glutamate-induced cytotoxicity in neuronal cell line PC12. *Brain Res.* Sep 21 2005; 1056(2): 132–138.

173. Jia H, Liu Z, Li X et al. Synergistic anti-Parkinsonism activity of high doses of B vitamins in a chronic cellular model. *Neurobiol Aging.* Jul 16 2008.

174. Jia H, Li X, Gao H et al. High doses of nicotinamide prevent oxidative mitochondrial dysfunction in a cellular model and improve motor deficit in a Drosophila model of Parkinson's disease. *J Neurosci Res.* Jul 2008; 86(9): 2083–2090.

175. Cadet JL, Katz M, Jackson-Lewis V, Fahn S. Vitamin E attenuates the toxic effects of intrastriatal injection of 6-hydroxydopamine (6-OHDA) in rats: Behavioral and biochemical evidence. *Brain Res.* Jan 2 1989; 476(1): 10–15.

176. Heim C, Kolasiewicz W, Kurz T, Sontag KH. Behavioral alterations after unilateral 6-hydroxydopamine lesions of the striatum. Effect of alpha-tocopherol. *Pol J Pharmacol.* Sep–Oct 2001; 53(5): 435–448.

177. Prasad KN, Kumar B, Yan XD, Hanson AJ, Cole WC. Alpha-tocopheryl succinate, the most effective form of vitamin E for adjuvant cancer treatment: A review. *J Am Coll Nutr.* Apr 2003; 22(2): 108–117.

178. Pasbakhsh P, Omidi N, Mehrannia K et al. The protective effect of vitamin E on locus coeruleus in early model of Parkinson's disease in rat: Immunoreactivity evidence. *Iran Biomed J.* Oct 2008; 12(4): 217–222.

179. Roghani M, Behzadi G. Neuroprotective effect of vitamin E on the early model of Parkinson's disease in rat: Behavioral and histochemical evidence. *Brain Res.* Feb 16 2001; 892(1): 211–217.

180. Khaldy H, Escames G, Leon J, Bikjdaouene L, Acuna-Castroviejo D. Synergistic effects of melatonin and deprenyl against MPTP-induced mitochondrial damage and DA depletion. *Neurobiol Aging.* May–Jun 2003; 24(3): 491–500.

181. Silva-Adaya D, Perez-De La Cruz V, Herrera-Mundo MN et al. Excitotoxic damage, disrupted energy metabolism, and oxidative stress in the rat brain: Antioxidant and neuroprotective effects of L-carnitine. *J Neurochem.* May 2008; 105(3): 677–689.

182. Virmani A, Gaetani F, Binienda Z. Effects of metabolic modifiers such as carnitines, coenzyme Q_{10}, and PUFAs against different forms of neurotoxic insults: Metabolic inhibitors, MPTP, and methamphetamine. *Ann N Y Acad Sci.* Aug 2005; 1053: 183–191.

183. Liu D, Pitta M, Mattson MP. Preventing NAD(+) depletion protects neurons against excitotoxicity: Bioenergetic effects of mild mitochondrial uncoupling and caloric restriction. *Ann N Y Acad Sci.* Dec 2008; 1147: 275–282.

184. Guarente L. Sirtuins in aging and disease. *Cold Spring Harb Symp Quant Biol.* 2007; 72: 483–488.

185. Alcain FJ, Villalba JM. Sirtuin inhibitors. *Expert Opin Ther Pat.* Mar 2009; 19(3): 283–294.

186. Garske AL, Smith BC, Denu JM. Linking SIRT2 to Parkinson's disease. *ACS Chem Biol.* Aug 17 2007; 2(8): 529–532.

187. Ortiz GG, Pacheco-Moises FP, Gomez-Rodriguez VM, Gonzalez-Renovato ED, Torres-Sanchez ED, Ramirez-Anguiano AC. Fish oil, Melatonin and vitamin E attenuates midbrain cyclooxygenase-2 activity and oxidative stress after administration of 1-methyl-4-phenyl-1,2,3,6-tetrahydropyridine. *Matab Brain Dis.* 2013; May 24 (Epub ahead of publication).

188. Rojas P, Montes P, Rojas C, Serrano-Garcia N, Rojas-Castaneda JC. Effect of a phytopharmaceutical medicine, Ginko biloba extract 761, in an animal model of Parkinson's disease: Therapeutic perspectives. *Nutrition.* Nov–Dec 2012; 28(11–12): 1081–1088.

189. Chaturvedi RK, Shukla S, Seth K et al. Neuroprotective and neurorescue effect of black tea extract in 6-hydroxydopamine-lesioned rat model of Parkinson's disease. *Neurobiol Dis.* May 2006; 22(2): 421–434.

190. Choi JY, Park CS, Kim DJ et al. Prevention of nitric oxide-mediated 1-methyl-4-phenyl-1,2,3,6-tetrahydropyridine-induced Parkinson's disease in mice by tea phenolic epigallocatechin 3-gallate. *Neurotoxicology.* Sep 2002; 23(3): 367–374.

191. Itoh N, Ohta H. Roles of FGF20 in dopaminergic neurons and Parkinson's disease. *Front Mol Neurosci.* 2013; 6: 15.

192. Roy A, Ghosh A, Jana A et al. Sodium phenylbutyrate controls neuroinflammatory and antioxidant activities and protects dopaminergic neurons in mouse models of Parkinson's disease. *PLoS One.* 2012; 7(6): e38113.

193. Shoulson I. DATATOP: A decade of neuroprotective inquiry. Parkinson Study Group. Deprenyl and tocopherol antioxidative therapy of Parkinsonism. *Ann Neurol.* Sep 1998; 44(3 Suppl 1): S160–S166.

194. Group TPS. Effects of tocopherol and deprenyl on the progression of disability in early Parkinson's disease. *N Engl J Med.* 1993: 176–183.

195. Prasad KN, Hernandez C, Edwards-Prasad J, Nelson J, Borus T, Robinson WA. Modification of the effect of tamoxifen, cis-platin, DTIC, and interferon-alpha 2b on human melanoma cells in culture by a mixture of vitamins. *Nutr Cancer.* 1994; 22(3): 233–245.

196. Prasad KN, Kumar R. Effect of individual and multiple antioxidant vitamins on growth and morphology of human nontumorigenic and tumorigenic parotid acinar cells in culture. *Nutr Cancer.* 1996; 26(1): 11–19.

197. Zhang SM, Hernan MA, Chen H, Spiegelman D, Willett WC, Ascherio A. Intakes of vitamins E and C, carotenoids, vitamin supplements, and PD risk. *Neurology.* Oct 22 2002; 59(8): 1161–1169.

198. Etminan M, Gill SS, Samii A. Intake of vitamin E, vitamin C, and carotenoids and the risk of Parkinson's disease: A meta-analysis. *Lancet Neurol.* Jun 2005; 4(6): 362–365.

199. Fahn S. A pilot trial of high-dose alpha-tocopherol and ascorbate in early Parkinson's disease. *Ann Neurol.* 1992; 32 Suppl: S128–S132.

200. Shults CW, Oakes D, Kieburtz K et al. Effects of coenzyme Q_{10} in early Parkinson disease: Evidence of slowing of the functional decline. *Arch Neurol.* Oct 2002; 59(10): 1541–1550.

201. Weber CA, Ernst ME. Antioxidants, supplements, and Parkinson's disease. *Ann Pharmacother.* May 2006; 40(5): 935–938.

202. Storch A, Jost WH, Vieregge P et al. Randomized, double-blind, placebo-controlled trial on symptomatic effects of coenzyme Q(10) in Parkinson disease. *Arch Neurol.* Jul 2007; 64(7): 938–944.

203. Swerdlow RH. Is NADH effective in the treatment of Parkinson's disease? *Drugs Aging.* Oct 1998; 13(4): 263–268.

204. Sano M, Ernesto C, Thomas RG et al. A controlled trial of selegiline, alpha-tocopherol, or both as treatment for Alzheimer's disease. The Alzheimer's Disease Cooperative Study. *N Engl J Med.* Apr 24 1997; 336(17): 1216–1222.

205. Farina N, Isaac MG, Clark AR, Rusted J, Tabet N. Vitamin E for Alzheimer's dementia and mild cognitive impairment. *Cochrane Database Syst Rev.* 2012; 11: CD002854.

206. Albanes D, Heinonen OP, Huttunen JK et al. Effects of alpha-tocopherol and beta-carotene supplements on cancer incidence in the Alpha-Tocopherol Beta-Carotene Cancer Prevention Study. *Am J Clin Nutr.* Dec 1995; 62(6 Suppl): 1427S–1430S.

207. Prasad KN, Cole WC, Prasad KC. Risk factors for Alzheimer's disease: Role of multiple antioxidants, non-steroidal anti-inflammatory and cholinergic agents alone or in combination in prevention and treatment. *J Am Coll Nutr.* Dec 2002; 21(6): 506–522.

208. Chen RS, Huang CC, Chu NS. Coenzyme Q_{10} treatment in mitochondrial encephalomyopathies. Short-term double-blind, crossover study. *Eur Neurol.* 1997; 37(4): 212–218.

209. Gaziano JM, Sesso HD, Christen WG et al. Multivitamins in the prevention of cancer in men: The Physicians' Health Study II randomized controlled trial. *JAMA.* Nov 14 2012; 308(18): 1871–1880.

210. Baum MK, Campa A, Lai S et al. Effect of micronutrient supplementation on disease progression in asymptomatic, antiretroviral-naive, HIV-infected adults in Botswana: A randomized clinical trial. *JAMA.* Nov 27 2013; 310(20): 2154–2163.

211. Prasad KN, La Rosa FG, Prasad JE. Prostaglandins act as neurotoxin for differentiated neuroblastoma cells in culture and increase levels of ubiquitin and beta-amyloid. *In Vitro Cell Dev Biol Anim.* Mar 1998; 34(3): 265–274.

212. Shalit F, Sredni B, Stern L, Kott E, Huberman M. Elevated interleukin-6 secretion levels by mononuclear cells of Alzheimer's patients. *Neurosci Lett.* Jun 20 1994; 174(2): 130–132.

213. Sharif SF, Hariri RJ, Chang VA, Barie PS, Wang RS, Ghajar JB. Human astrocyte production of tumour necrosis factor-alpha, interleukin-1 beta, and interleukin-6 following exposure to lipopolysaccharide endotoxin. *Neurol Res.* Apr 1993; 15(2): 109–112.

214. Eikelenboom P, Rozemuller JM, Kraal G et al. Cerebral amyloid plaques in Alzheimer's disease but not in scrapie-affected mice are closely associated with a local inflammatory process. *Virchows Arch B Cell Pathol Incl Mol Pathol.* 1991; 60(5): 329–336.

215. Eikelenboom P, Stam FC. Immunoglobulins and complement factors in senile plaques. An immunoperoxidase study. *Acta Neuropathol (Berl).* 1982; 57(2–3): 239–242.
216. Rogers J, Cooper NR, Webster S et al. Complement activation by beta-amyloid in Alzheimer disease. *Proc Natl Acad Sci U S A.* Nov 1 1992; 89(21): 10,016–10,020.
217. Rogers J, Lue L-F, Brachova L, Webster S, Schultz J. Inflammation as a response and a cause of Alzheimer's pathophysiology. *Dementia.* 1995; 9: 133–138.
218. Webster S, O'Barr S, Rogers J. Enhanced aggregation and beta structure of amyloid beta peptide after coincubation with C1q. *J Neurosci Res.* Nov 1 1994; 39(4): 448–456.
219. Frohman EM, Frohman TC, Gupta S, de Fougerolles A, van den Noort S. Expression of intercellular adhesion molecule 1 (ICAM-1) in Alzheimer's disease. *J Neurol Sci.* Nov 1991; 106(1): 105–111.
220. Rozemuller JM, Eikelenboom P, Pals ST, Stam FC. Microglial cells around amyloid plaques in Alzheimer's disease express leucocyte adhesion molecules of the LFA-1 family. *Neurosci Lett.* Jul 3 1989; 101(3): 288–292.
221. Verbeek MM, Otte-Holler I, Westphal JR, Wesseling P, Ruiter DJ, de Waal RM. Accumulation of intercellular adhesion molecule-1 in senile plaques in brain tissue of patients with Alzheimer's disease. *Am J Pathol.* Jan 1994; 144(1): 104–116.
222. Anderton B. Free radicals on the mind. Hydrogen peroxide mediates amyloid beta protein toxicity. *Hum Exp Toxicol.* Oct 1994; 13(10): 719.
223. Harman D. Free radical theory of aging. *Mutat Res.* Sep 1992; 275(3–6): 257–266.
224. Smith MA, Sayre LM, Monnier VM, Perry G. Radical AGEing in Alzheimer's disease. *Trends Neurosci.* Apr 1995; 18(4): 172–176.
225. Olanow CW, Arendash GW. Metals and free radicals in neurodegeneration. *Curr Opin Neurol.* Dec 1994; 7(6): 548–558.
226. Abate A, Yang G, Dennery PA, Oberle S, Schroder H. Synergistic inhibition of cyclo-oxygenase-2 expression by vitamin E and aspirin. *Free Radic Biol Med.* Dec 2000; 29(11): 1135–1142.
227. Melamed E, Offen D, Shirvan A, Djaldetti R, Barzilai A, Ziv I. Levodopa toxicity and apoptosis. *Ann Neurol.* Sep 1998; 44(3 Suppl 1): S149–S154.
228. Fahn S, Oakes D, Shoulson I et al. Levodopa and the progression of Parkinson's disease. *N Engl J Med.* Dec 9 2004; 351(24): 2498–2508.
229. Fahn S. Does levodopa slow or hasten the rate of progression of Parkinson's disease? *J Neurol.* Oct 2005; 252 Suppl 4: IV37–IV42.
230. Abdin AA, Hamouda HE. Mechanism of the neuroprotective role of coenzyme Q_{10} with or without L-dopa in rotenone-induced parkinsonism. *Neuropharmacology.* Dec 2008; 55(8): 1340–1346.

5 Huntington's Disease
Prevention and Improved Management by Micronutrients

INTRODUCTION

The wild-type huntington protein plays an important role during embryogenesis, development, and survival of neurons in the brain, especially in those areas of brain most effected in Huntington's disease (HD). HD is a rare fatal hereditary neurodegenerative disease of the brain in which neurons (primarily in striatum and cortex) involved in movement, intellect, and emotions are gradually destroyed. This disease is characterized by jerking uncontrollable movements of the limbs, trunk, and face (chorea), progressive loss of cognitive functions, and the development of psychiatric problems. Each child of HD parent has a 50–50 chance of inheriting a mutated HD gene. The child with a HD gene will develop the disease at an early age that can vary from one individual to another, generally between 30 and 50 years. The disease progresses over 10–25 years, and patients ultimately become unable to take care of themselves. Juvenile HD generally appears before the age of 20 and progresses rapidly. Muscle rigidity progresses at a rapid rate leading to akinesia (loss of control of voluntary muscle movements). If a child has not inherited HD gene, his or her subsequent children will not develop the HD.

Despite overwhelming evidence for the role of increased oxidative stress in the initiation and progression of HD, very few studies with individual antioxidants primarily in animal HD models have been performed. The results of these studies revealed that supplement with individual antioxidants improved some symptoms of HD. No studies have been conducted on a preparation of micronutrients containing multiple dietary and endogenous antioxidants. At present, there are no effective strategies for prevention or delaying the onset of HD in humans. The current management of HD with standard care involving drugs, psychotherapy, physical therapy, and speech therapy is unsatisfactory, because the disease progresses despite these treatments.

This chapter describes briefly incidence, cost, and causes of HD and provides scientific data in support of a hypothesis that increased oxidative stress and chronic inflammation are one of the earliest events that play an important role in the initiation and progression of HD. This chapter also presents scientific rationale and published studies for the use of a preparation of micronutrients containing multiple dietary and endogenous antioxidants, certain polyphenolic compounds, and B vitamins for prevention and/or delaying the onset of HD. The same micronutrient preparation in combination with standard care may improve the management of HD by reducing the progression and improving the symptoms of disease.

INCIDENCE, PREVALENCE, AND COST

It is estimated that the incidence of HD in the USA is about 1550 per year. The prevalence of this disease in the USA, Europe, and Australia is 5–7 cases/100,000 individuals; in Asia, it is 0.4/100,000, and in the world, it is about 2.7/100,000.[1] It remains uncertain why the prevalence of HD is so low in Asia, compared to western countries. The annual cost of treating HD may vary. HD affects both male and female and all ethnic groups. Average annual medical cost per individual is about $10,500, but it could be $47,000, if the cost of care givers is included.

HUNTINGTON GENE

The wild-type Huntington protein plays an important role in embryogenesis, development, and survival of neurons in the brain, especially in those areas of brain most affected in HD. In the wild-type huntington gene, trinucleotide CAG (cytosine, adenine, and guanosine) codes for glutamine. However, in 1993, it was discovered that a mutation in the wild-type huntington gene causes repeated expansion of the trinucleotide CAG coding region. This causes translation of uninterrupted glutamine forming polyglutamine tract in the N-terminus of the huntington protein. The wild-type huntington gene contains 1–34 copies of trinucleotide CAG repeats; however, the number of triplet CAG repeats increases in HD gene. The number of trinucleotide CAG repeats in HD can be as high as 141. The larger the number of triplet CAG repeats, the earlier the onset of the symptoms of disease. Mutated huntington gene is referred to as HD gene and mutated huntington protein as HD protein. HD protein is sensitive to aggregation and aggregated form of HD protein causes selective degeneration and ultimately neuronal death in the striatum and cortex. The mechanisms of neurodegeneration involve increased oxidative stress, mitochondrial dysfunction, chronic inflammation, release of an excitatory neurotransmitter glutamate, impaired proteasome activity, altered expression of brain-derived trophic factors, and transcriptional deregulation. However, increased oxidative stress appears to be one of the earliest events in the development of HD, because it is also found in asymptomatic patients carrying HD gene. Other biochemical abnormalities, which together with increased oxidative stress participate in the progression of HD, occur later.

SYMPTOMS AND NEUROPATHOLOGY OF HD

SIGNS AND SYMPTOMS

In most cases of HD, symptoms appear in young adult life and become progressively worst. The major symptoms of HD include movement disorders, cognitive dysfunction, and psychiatric problems. The sequence of their appearance varies from one individual to another (http://www.healthcommunities.com/huntington-disease/symptoms.shtml). The movement disorders are characterized by uncontrolled movement or tics in the fingers, feet, face, or trunk which become more intense when the individuals are anxious or disturbed. As the disease progresses, other symptoms, such as clumsiness, jaw clenching (bruxism), loss of coordination and balance, slurred speech, swallowing/eating difficulty, uncontrolled continual muscular contractions (dystonia) and walking difficulty, stumbling, and falling, appear. Weight loss is commonly associated with HD.

The cognitive dysfunctions are characterized by the progressive loss of memory, and ability to concentrate, answering questions, and recognize familiar objects. These cognitive dysfunctions appear later in the course of the disease.

The major psychiatric problems include depression which appears early during progression of HD. The major signs of depression include hostility/irritability, lack of energy, and inability to enjoy pleasure in life. Some individuals may develop manic depression or bipolar disorder during the course of the disease. Some individuals may exhibit psychotic behavior, such as delusions, hallucinations, unprovoked aggression, and paranoia.

NEUROPATHOLOGY

It has been reported that HD protein is present in the form of N-terminal fragments, oligomers, and polymers primarily in the striatum and cortex. Oligomers are mostly soluble; however, N-terminal fragments, polymers, and other proteins attach with each other and form the insoluble aggregates that are toxic to neurons.[2] The aggregated form of HD protein fragments produced reactive oxygen species (ROS). Treatment with MW7 antibody to HD protein inhibited HD protein aggregation and prevented ROS production.[3]

Although HD protein is found throughout the body, it principally damages only the brain. The exact reasons for this are unknown. I propose that HD protein by itself may not be toxic; however, in the presence of increased oxidative stress, and availability of neurotransmitters, such as dopamine, glutamate, acetylcholine, and gamma-aminobutyric acid (GABA), this protein becomes toxic. Such conditions do not exist in non-nerve cells outside the brain; therefore, HD protein is not toxic for these cells. Damage to the striatum appears early and becomes severe at a later stage of the disease. Other regions of the brain, such as the cortex, thalamus, and subthalamus, also show degenerative changes at a later stage. Within the striatum, the medium spiny projection neurons are selectively degenerated in HD; however, interneurons are relatively spared.[4]

ANIMAL MODELS OF HD

Both chemical- and genetic-induced animal models of HD are commonly used to investigate the mechanisms of HD and to identify potential targets for the development of new drugs for the treatment of HD. Quinolinic acid, a NMDA (N-methyl-D-aspartate) receptor agonist and 3-nitropropionic acid (3-NP), an inhibitor of mitochondrial dehydrogenase, induced HD phenotype in the striatum similar to that observed in human HD. Administration of quinolinic acid directly into the striatum region of the rat brain produces some biochemical, morphological, and behavioral characteristics of HD. It has been reported that NAD(P)H oxidase activity, which catalyzes superoxide anion production, increased in the quinolinic acid treated striatal neurons. Treatment with apocynin, a specific inhibitor of NAD(P) oxidase, decreased quinolinic acid-induced NAD(P) oxidase activity, lipid peroxidation, circling behavior, and histological changes in the brain.[5] Increased oxidative and nitrosylative stress are involved in neurodegeneration caused by quinolinic acid[6] and 3-NP.[7]

Several genetic mouse models of HD have been developed to investigate the biochemical events and transcriptional regulations that are impaired in HD. These HD mice mimic the neuropathology and symptoms similar to those observed in human HD. Transgenic HD mouse models expressing short N-terminals fragments (R6/1 and R6/2) or full length HD gene (YAC128) exhibited rapid effects on gene expressions in the striatal neurons similar to those observed in human HD.[8]

INCREASED OXIDATIVE STRESS IN HD

HUMAN STUDIES

There is substantial evidence for the involvement of increased oxidative stress in the pathogenesis of HD.[9] Metabolic defects in the brain and muscle, and progressive weight loss have been observed in patients with HD. In addition, respiratory chain deficits have been found in the autopsied brain samples of HD patients. It has been suggested that HD protein accumulate in the mitochondria that may cause mitochondrial dysfunction which is associated with the progression of HD.[10] However, it is not adequately known how HD protein causes mitochondrial dysfunction. It is possible that HD protein binds with the respiratory chain complexes of mitochondria and inhibits their activities that reduce energy metabolism, one of the characteristic features of HD. Mitochondrial dysfunction can also increase the production of ROS. Thus, increased oxidative stress plays a significant role in the initiation and progression of HD symptoms.

Analysis of certain markers of oxidative stress in 19 patients with HD and 47 age- and sex-matched healthy subjects revealed that a 20% increase in plasma lipid peroxidation levels and 28% decrease in glutathione levels occurred in HD patients compared to in healthy controls. Similar changes in the levels of these markers of oxidative stress were observed in 11 asymptomatic HD gene carriers compared to in 22 age- and sex-matched healthy subjects. These results suggest that increased oxidative stress occurs prior to the onset of HD symptoms in asymptomatic individuals carrying the HD gene.[11]

Increased oxidative stress and mitochondrial dysfunction as evidenced by decreased activities of complexes II, III, and IV in the striatum of HD patients has been consistently observed. This observation was tested on the skin fibroblast cultures from 13 HD patients and 13 age- and sex-matched healthy subjects. The activities of respiratory chain complexes, total superoxide dismutase (SOD), glutathione peroxidase, and catalase, and the levels of coenzyme Q_{10} were measured. The results showed that only the activity of catalase decreased in fibroblasts obtained from HD patients compared to those obtained from healthy subjects.[12] These results suggest that HD fibroblasts in culture are not a good model to study the mechanisms of HD or to test the potential agents that could be useful in prevention and improved management of HD.

In a human study involving 16 HD patients and 36 age- and gender-matched healthy individuals, it was found that markers of oxidative stress, such as leukocyte 8-hydroxydeoxyguanosine (8-OHdG) and plasma malondialdehyde (MDA) were increased, whereas the activities of erythrocyte Cu/Znsuperoxide dismutase (Cu/Zn-SOD) and glutathione peroxidase were reduced in HD patients compared to those in healthy controls.[13] Plasma MDA levels were significantly correlated with the severity of the disease. Increased mitochondrial DNA defects possibly induced by HD protein were also observed in the autopsied brain samples of HD patients compared to those in healthy controls. These results again suggest that increased oxidative stress and mitochondrial dysfunction play an important role in the development and progression of HD.

In a clinical study involving the postmortem brain tissues from HD patients, it was found that activities of oxidative phosphorylation enzymes were impaired only in the basal ganglia.[14] In addition, the levels of markers of oxidative stress increased in the caudate of HD brain. These results suggest that increased oxidative stress and energy insufficiency contribute to the pathogenesis of HD.

CELL CULTURE STUDIES

It has been shown that increased oxidative stress caused aggregation of HD protein that contributes to neuronal cell death.[15] Increased oxidative stress also inhibited proteasome function in neurons expressing HD gene. Furthermore, overexpression of Cu/Zn-superoxide dismutase (SOD1), heat shock protein 70 (Hsp70) or Hsp40 reversed the oxidative stress-induced proteasome inhibition, HD protein aggregation and death of neuronal cells in culture.

AGGREGATION OF HD PROTEIN

Protein aggregation is one of the early events in the initiation of neurodegeneration in certain neurodegenerative diseases, including in HD. The mechanisms of protein aggregation-induced neurodegeneration in HD are not well understood. Using a transgenic HD mouse model, it was demonstrated that caspase-1 and caspase-3 were transcriptionally upregulated and activated in this disease.[16] This is consistent with the observation in which caspase-1 is activated in the autopsied brain samples of HD patients. Activation of caspases causes cleavage of key proteins including HD protein that eventually leads to neuronal death. The degree of activation of caspases correlated with the progression of this disease in HD mice. It has been demonstrated that activation of enzyme caspase-2 cleaves HD protein selectively at amino acid 552, and fragmented HD proteins become aggregated. Aggregated form of HD protein causes selective neuronal cell death in the striatum and cortex in HD. This has been demonstrated in the autopsied brain samples of human HD as well as in HD mouse model expressing full length HD gene (YAC72 mice).[17] Inhibitors of caspase delayed the onset of the symptoms of HD in transgenic HD mouse model. Treatment of animals with quinolinic acid and 3-NP induces HD phenotypes in the brain by increasing oxidative stress. However, an aggregated form of HD protein produces free radicals.[3] HD protein also activates microglia that release ROS, in addition to proinflammatory cytokines. Additionally, aggregated HD protein binds with mitochondria and induces mitochondrial dysfunction. The presence of these aggregates in the nucleus may induce transcriptional deregulation by binding to the histone. The studies presented in this section suggest that increased oxidative stress plays an important role in the initiation of HD symptoms.

Although trace metals like copper and iron are essential for survival, increased levels of these trace minerals may cause neurodegeneration in the striatum of certain neurodegenerative diseases, such as HD, Alzheimer's disease (AD), and Parkinson disease (PD). These trace metals cause neuronal death by protein aggregation and excessive generation of ROS.[18] It has been reported that copper-HD protein interaction caused increased oxidative stress that plays an important role in the progression of HD.[19] In addition, it appears that levels of lactate dehydrogenase (LDH) play a role in the progression of HD in animal model of HD. This is supported by the fact that oxamate, an inhibitor of LDH, when administered directly into the striatum of healthy mice, caused degeneration of neurons. These data suggest that increased oxidative stress and energy insufficiency due to mitochondrial dysfunction contribute to the progression of HD.

MITOCHONDRIAL DYSFUNCTION IN HD

Mitochondria are the major site of free radical production, and they are most sensitive to damage produced by free radicals. Mitochondrial dysfunction is associated with the neurodegenerative diseases, including with HD. In patients with HD, the number of mitochondria in spiny striatal neurons decreased. In addition, mitochondrial transcriptional factor A and peroxisome proliferator-activated receptor coactivator gamma-1 alpha (PGC-1 alpha), a key transcriptional regulator of energy metabolism and mitochondrial biogenesis, were reduced with increasing severity of disease. These results suggest that mitochondrial dysfunction plays an important role in the pathogenesis of HD.[20] Mitochondrial dysfunctions include reduction of Ca^{2+} buffering capacity, loss of membrane potential, and decreased expression of oxidative phosphorylation enzymes.[21] Mitochondrial dysfunction also increases the production of free radicals.

DOWNREGULATION OF PGC-1 ALPHA

It has been demonstrated that HD protein in humans and animal models downregulated the expression of PGC-1 alpha that regulates mitochondrial biogenesis and oxidative stress.[22] This suggested that overexpression of PGC-1 alpha may provide protection against neurodegeneration in HD. Indeed, overexpression of PGC-1 alpha partially reversed the toxic effect of HD protein in the striatal neuronal cells in culture. Administration of lentiviral-mediated delivery of PGC-1 alpha in the striatum protected neurons in the brain of transgenic HD mice.[23] Using mouse HD model, it was shown that induction of PGC-1 alpha eliminated HD protein aggregation and prevented neurodegeneration by reducing oxidative stress.[24] It was further demonstrated that PGC-1 alpha promoted turnover of HD protein and eliminated protein aggregates by activating transcriptional factor EB (TFEB). This transcriptional factor recognizes E-box sequence, a key regulator of the autophagy-lysosomal pathway that regulates protein degradation. Therefore, it was suggested that PGC-1 alpha and TFEB could be used as targets for developing new therapeutic agents for the treatment of HD.

It has been demonstrated that mitogen- and stress-activated kinase (MSK-1), a nuclear protein kinase involved in chromatin remodeling through histone H3 phosphorylation, was reduced in the striatum of patients with HD and animal models of HD.[25] Restoring MSK-1 expression in the striatal neurons in culture prevented HD protein-induced neuronal degeneration and death. Furthermore, deletion of MSK-1 in wild-type mice showed spontaneous striatal degeneration as they aged and increased sensitivity of striatal neuron to mitochondrial neurotoxin 3-NP. It was also shown that overexpression of MSK-1 upregulated PGC-1 alpha, suggesting that the neuroprotective effect of MSK-1 is mediated through increased expression of PGC-1 alpha.

INCREASED CHRONIC INFLAMMATION IN HD

Activation of microglia has been implicated in the pathogenesis of HD. Examination of the autopsied brain samples revealed that activated microglia is present in the area of neuronal loss. Activated microglia produces excessive amounts of neurotoxic factors, such as free radicals, proinflammatory cytokines, and prostaglandins. Measurement of [11]C(R)-PK11195, a radioactive marker of microglia activation, and ^{11}C raclopride, a radioactive marker of dopamine D2 receptor by PET (positron emission tomography) technique in HD patients at different stages of the disease, showed that an increase in microglia activation correlated with the severity of the disease. In addition, reduction in binding of dopamine D2 receptors and the Unified Huntington Disease Scale Score were observed.[26] Using the same PET technique as above in asymptomatic HD patients, it was shown that microglia activation was an early event in pathogenesis of HD and was associated with subclinical progression of disease.[27] In addition, atrophy in the sensorimotor striatum, substantia nigra, orbitofrontal, and anterior prefrontal cortex was found in asymptomatic HD patients. Also, the binding of dopamine D2/D3 receptors was reduced and activation of microglia increased in these patients. The above abnormalities in the striatum and cortex progressively increased in symptomatic HD patients. From these results, it was concluded that activated microglia occurs in the areas of brain responsible for cognitive function.[28] Using corticostriatal slices and primary neuronal cultures expressing HD protein, it was demonstrated that the number of activated microglia increased in the vicinity of neurons expressing HD protein. Activated microglia was found along the irregular neuritis. Increase in the levels of interleukin-6 (IL-6) and complement protein 1q occurred as neurodegeneration progressed.[29]

A clinical study reported that plasma levels of IL-6 were elevated in asymptomatic individuals carrying HD gene 16 years before the onset of symptoms of the disease.[30] In addition, monocytes from the subjects expressing HD gene were hyperactive in response to stimulation. Furthermore, cerebrospinal fluid from the striatum of HD patients exhibited increased immune activation. These results suggest that immune activation mediated by microglia plays a role in pathogenesis of HD.

It appears that abnormal concentration of oxidized tryptophan metabolites contribute to progressive degeneration of neuron in HD. Blood levels of proinflammatory cytokines IL-23 and the soluble human leukocyte antigen- G (sHLA-G) were increased in most severe cases of HD, and a significant correlation between IL-23 and the severity of the disease was observed.[31] Blood levels of tryptophan were negatively correlated with the severity of the disease. In contrast, blood levels of tryptophan were positively correlated with the levels of sHLA-G, a marker of proinflammatory cytokines. These results suggest that tryptophan metabolism along the kynurenine pathway is related to the severity of clinical symptoms of HD.

The IkB kinase B (IKKB) is a regulator of inflammation in the brain. Proinflammatory cytokines accumulate in the serum and brain of asymptomatic and symptomatic HD patients, and the levels of proinflammatory cytokines correlates with disease progression. Oxidative stress-induced damage to DNA activates IKKB that triggers caspase-dependent cleavage of HD protein to increase the accumulation of oligomeric fragments.[32] The N-terminal fragments of HD protein directly bind to and activate IKKB which cleave HD protein to form insoluble oligomeric fragments. Inhibitors of IKKB prevented the toxicity of HD protein fragments in the striatum.[32] Thus, increased accumulation of HD protein fragments is one of the factors that contribute to the death of striatal neurons.

Treatment of HD rat model (quinolinic acid-induced HD) with a selective inhibitor of cyclooxygenase-2 (COX-2) celecoxib markedly improved behavior and biochemical changes in the brain of HD rats, suggesting that activation of immune cells like microglia may contribute to the pathogenesis of HD.[33] Treatment with verapamil or diltiazem FDA drugs approved for other conditions in humans for 21 days improved motor functions as well as reduced oxidative damage and markers of proinflammatory cytokines (TNF-alpha [tumor necrosis factor-alpha], IL-6, and caspase-3) in HD rat model (quinolinic acid-induced HD phenotype).[34]

GLUTAMATE-INDUCED NEUROTOXICITY IN HD

Glutamate-mediated excitotoxicity is one of the mechanisms involved in the loss of striatal neurons in patients with HD. Treatment of striatal precursor cell line expressing full-length wild-type huntington gene (STHdh (Q7/Q7) or HD gene (STHdh (Q111/Q111) with NMDA agonist caused early death in cells expressing HD gene compared to that in cells expressing wild-type huntington gene.[35] The cells expressing HD gene had higher levels of calcineurin A, a calcium-dependent phosphatase-3, the activity of which was increased after NMDA receptor stimulation. The results suggested that higher levels of calcineurin A in cells expressing HD gene may account for an early death of striatal neurons. This suggestion was confirmed by the fact that transfection of striatal precursor cells (STHdh (Q7/Q7) with calcineurin A increased cell death compared to that observed in green fluorescent protein-transfected cells after NMDA agonist treatment. In addition, treatment with a calcineurin inhibitor FK-506 reduced cell death more in cells expressing HD gene than in cells expressing wild-type huntington gene. These results suggest that high levels of calcineurin A in cells expressing HD gene may increase the sensitivity of striatal to excitotoxicity.

GLUTAMATE TRANSPORTER PROTEINS IN HD

The two major glutamate transporter proteins, glutamate transporter-1 (GLT-1) and glutamate-aspartate transporter (GLAST), are primarily located in the astrocytes of adult brain and play an important role in maintaining physiological extracellular levels of glutamate. Release of vitamin C (ascorbate) from the striatum into the extracellular fluid is reduced together with the reduction in GLT-1 dependent uptake of glutamate in mouse HD model (R6/2). Consequently, the levels of vitamin C decrease and the levels of glutamate increase in the extracellular fluid of striatal neuron. The reduction in vitamin C levels and enhancement of glutamate would contribute to degeneration and death of the striatal neurons. In order to demonstrate the role of GLT-1 in the release of vitamin C, treatment of R6/2 mice with ceftriaxone, an elevator of functional expression of GLT-1, on evoked release of vitamin C into the striatal extracellular fluid was measured.[36] The results showed that evoked release of vitamin C was markedly reduced in R6/2 mice compared to that in wild-type; however, treatment with ceftriaxone restored the levels of striatal vitamin C in R6/2 mice to the same levels as in wild-type mice. Thus, it appears that reduction in the function of glutamate transporter proteins contribute to degeneration of striatal neurons by decreasing the levels of vitamin C and increasing the levels of glutamate. It has been reported that injection of vitamin C restored extracellular levels of vitamin C in R6/2 mice to the levels in wild-type mice and normalized neuronal function in striatum of HD mice.[37]

NEUROTRANSMITTER RECEPTORS

Extensive studies have been performed on the release and transmission of various neurotransmitters, using primarily chemical-induced rodent HD models or transgenic rodent HD models. Impaired neurotransmitters release and their respective receptors contribute to the pathophysiology of HD and associated symptoms. The exact mechanisms are not known.

GLUTAMATE RECEPTORS

Excitotoxicity has been implicated in the selective sensitivity of striatal neurons in HD. Evidence for the role of excitotoxicity was evident by the early presence of increased levels of quinolinate, a NMDA receptor agonist, in patients with HD. This change was associated with increased density of spiny striatal neurons and dendritic length; however, in later stages of HD, degenerative changes, such as loss of dendritic arborization, a reduction in spine density, and reduced levels of 3-hydroxykynurerenine and quinolinate in the brain, were observed. Using a HD mouse model (YAC128), it was demonstrated that the striatal neurons exhibited enhanced sensitivity to excitotoxicity before the onset of HD phenotypes in the brain.[38]

Stimulation of NMDA receptor by glutamate has been implicated in neuronal damaged observed in HD. Neurons expressing high levels of NMDA receptors are lost from the striatum of individuals at their early stage of the disease because of the toxicity of glutamate. This is substantiated by the observations which showed that administration of NMDA receptor agonist into the striatum of rodents or nonhuman primates induced HD phenotypes in the brain.[39]

Glutamate release contributes to pathogenesis of HD. Corticostriatal terminals possess mGluR2/3 autoreceptors, whose activation reduces the release of glutamate. In HD mouse model (R6/2), the efficacy of an mGluR2/3 receptor agonist LY379268 on the HD phenotype was evaluated. The results showed that daily subcutaneous injection of LY379268 produced no adverse effects in wild-type mice; however, in HD mice, it increased the survival by 11%, improved motor functions (activity, speed, endurance, and gait), and enhanced the survival of cortical and striatal neurons by 15–20% (1). Furthermore, deficits of motor neuron function were greater in male HD mice than in female, and beneficial effect of LY379268 was greater in male than in female.[40] The protective effect of LY379268 is mediated via upregulating the expression of brain-derived growth factor (BDNF) in the cerebral cortex and hippocampus of mice.

As the diseases progresses, reduced dopamine and glutamate transmission were observed.[41] Loss of dopaminergic and glutamatergic neurons may account for the loss of their transmission in HD. Impairment of dopamine and glutamate transmission in HD suggests that restoring the balance between dopamine and glutamate transmission to a normal level may be useful in improving some of the symptoms of HD.[41]

GABA Receptors

GABA receptors were elevated in symptomatic and asymptomatic patients with HD.[42] In a chemical (quinolinic acid)-induced rat model of HD, elevated levels of GABA (B1) and GABA (B2) receptors were present in the striatal neurons as well as in the astrocytes.[43] Using transgenic HD model mice (R6/1 and R6/2), it was demonstrated that increases in spontaneous GABAergic synaptic currents and postsynaptic receptor function occurred in parallel to progressive decreases in glutamatergic inputs to GABAergic medium-sized spiny projection neurons.[44] Such changes may lead to impaired control of movement. In transgenic HD mouse model, it was found that GABA (A) receptor trafficking and function is impaired probably due to loss of GABA receptors.[45] The reduced inhibitory synaptic transmission may contribute to the loss of the excitatory/inhibitory balance, causing increased excitotoxicity in neurons in the brain of patients with HD.

Dopamine and Dopamine Receptors

It appears that striatal neuron expressing dopamine receptors primarily degenerate in patients with HD. Using neuroblastoma (NB) cells with dopamine D1 receptor expressing huntington protein with 25 triplet repeat of CAG or HD protein with 103 triplet repeats of CAG, it was demonstrated that nuclear and cytoplasmic HD protein aggregates were present in NB cells expressing HD gene.[46] Low doses of selective dopamine D1 receptors agonist increased the aggregation of HD protein in the nucleus but decreased the number of aggregates in the cytoplasm.[46]

Using primary culture of striatal neurons expressing HD gene, it was demonstrated that low doses of dopamine act synergistically with HD gene in activating the proapoptotic transcriptional factor c-JUN and in increasing the number of aggregates of HD proteins in both the nucleus and the cytoplasm.[47] Furthermore, the effect of dopamine was reversed by vitamin C and SP-600125, a selective inhibitor of the c-JUN N-terminal kinase (JNK) pathway. This would suggest the involvement of free radicals in the dopamine-induced degenerative changes in the striatal neurons expressing HD gene. Dopamine D2 receptors agonist also increased HD protein aggregation which was blocked by a dopamine D2 receptors antagonist. The combination of vitamin C and dopamine D2 antagonist was more effective in reducing the formation of HD protein aggregates and neuronal death in the striatum than the individual agents.

In transgenic rats expressing HD gene, it was observed that chronic treatment with haloperidol, an antagonist of dopamine D2 receptor, protected striatal neurons, suggesting that activation of dopamine D2 receptors contribute to HD protein aggregation and neurodegeneration in the brain.[48]

Cortical dopamine dysfunction has been observed in both symptomatic and asymptomatic patients with HD. Using a radioactive dopamine D2 receptor agonist ^{11}C-raclopride in PET on 16 symptomatic and 11 asymptomatic patients with HD, it was demonstrated that 62.5% of symptomatic and 64.5% of asymptomatic patients showed reduced binding of dopamine D2 receptors, suggesting the loss of dopamine neurons. Furthermore, symptomatic patients with HD showed increased deficits in attention and executive functions.[49] This study was confirmed by another study in which a reduction in binding of dopamine D2 receptors in the striatum of patients with HD; however, the binding of dopamine D2 receptors was not significantly changed in the thalamic and cortical subregions compared to that in control subjects. The severity of clinical symptoms of the disease, such as chorea and cognitive test performance, were correlated with degree of reduction in the binding of dopamine D2 receptors.[50] Another study utilizing PET technology using a radioactive ^{11}C-raclopride (RAC), a specific dopamine D2 receptor agonist, and [11]C(R)-PK11195, a marker of microglia activation in asymptomatic and symptomatic HD patients, revealed that significant loss of dopamine D2 receptors occurred in the hypothalamus of patients with HD.[51]

Impairments of dopamine release and uptake progressed as a function of age in transgenic HD model mice (R6/1).[52] Dopamine release was also reduced in transgenic HD model rats, and this contributed to the motor deficiency as evidenced by gait disturbances in these animals.[53]

Using immortalized striatal neuronal progenitor cell lines Q7 expressing wild-type huntington protein with 7 triplet repeats of glutamine and cell line Q111 expressing HD protein with 111 triplet repeats of glutamine, it was demonstrated that treatment with dopaminergic stabilizers pridopidine and (-)-OSU6162 improved survival and mitochondrial function in the striatal Q111 neurons and increased resistance to certain neurotoxins, such as H_2O_2, rotenone, and 3-nitropropionic acid.[54]

CANNABINOID RECEPTORS

Cannabinoid receptors in adult human brain are primarily located in the forebrain areas associated with cognitive functions; in the forebrain, midbrain, and hindbrain that regulate movement; and in hindbrain areas that control motor and sensory function of the autonomic nervous system.[55]

Cannabinoid receptors CB1 and CB2 are reduced in the key areas of HD brain, such as the striatum and cortex. Loss of CB1 receptors were observed at the early stage of HD in the autopsied brain samples of patients with HD.[56] This was confirmed by the PET, using a novel CB1 ligand N-[2-(3-cyanophenyl)-3-(4-(2-^{18}F-fluorethoxy)phenyl)-1-methylpropyl]-2-(5-methyl-2-pyridyloxyl)-2-methylproponamide in 20 symptomatic HD patients and 14 healthy subjects. The results showed that the levels of CB1 receptors decreased throughout the gray matter of the cerebellum, cerebellum, and brain stem in the early stage of disease compared to healthy controls.[57] This suggested that upregulation of CB1 receptors may be of protective value. Indeed, it was observed that upregulation of CB1 receptors slowed progression of the disease in R6/1 transgenic HD mice.[58] Deletion of CB1 receptors aggravated the symptoms, neurodegeneration, and molecular pathology in transgenic HD mice.[59] Furthermore, administration of an endogenous cannabinoid receptor agonist delta-9-tetrahydrocannabinol prevented the effect of deletion of CB1 receptors in these mice. There data suggest that agonists of CB1 receptors may be useful in improving the symptoms of HD. Indeed, administration of CB1 agonist WIN 55,212-2 prevented the development of HD phenotype in rat model of HD (induced by quinolinic acid, an elevator of glutamate). This effect of CB1 receptor agonist was prevented by the CB1 receptor antagonist AM251.[60]

Using rat model of HD in which the disease phenotype is produce by intrastriatal injection of malonate, an inhibitor of mitochondrial complex II, it was demonstrated that an agonist of CB2 receptor prevented the death of striatal neuron in these animals, and CB2 receptor antagonist increased the sensitivity of neuron to malonate.[61] Furthermore, it was demonstrated that CB2 receptors are present in small amounts in the stratum, but they are abundantly located in microglia and astrocytes, suggesting that protective effects of agonist of CB2 receptor are mediated by glia cells. Activation of CB2 receptors also reduced malonate-induced elevation of TNF-alpha. Activated peripheral immune cells and brain microglia are present in asymptomatic HD patients, and they progressively increased with the progression of disease. Activation of cannabinoid receptor CB2 reduced immune activation. This is shown by the fact that deletion of CB2 receptor in HD mouse model accelerated the onset of motor deficits and increased their severity. Treatment of mice with a CB2 receptor agonist extended lifespan and suppressed motor deficits, synapse loss, and brain inflammation, while a peripherally restricted CB2 receptor antagonist block these effects.[62] Furthermore, treatment with a CB2 receptor agonist reduced blood levels of IL-6 which was elevated in HD mice. Treatment with an antibody against IL-6 also improved motor function in these mice. In contrast to the beneficial effects of activation of cannabinoid receptors on improving some symptoms of HD in animal HD models, a study reported that in mouse model of HD (R6/1) treatment with a CB1 receptor agonist delta (-tetrahydrocannabinol [THC] or CB2 receptor agonist HU210) did not alter the progression of motor deficits. As a matter of fact, HU210 treated HD animals exhibited increased seizure events and in the number of ubiq-uitinated aggregates in the striatum. In addition, treatment with THC or HU210 had no significant effect on the ligand binding of CB1, dopamine D1 and D2 receptors, serotonin 5HT2A, or GABA (A) receptors in R6/1 mice.[63]

OTHER RECEPTORS

It has been reported that treatment with an adenosine A(2A) receptors (A2ARs) ago-nist improved some of the symptoms of HD in mouse HD model (R6/2 mice).[64] This suggests that activation of A2ARs may be a protective value in at least mouse model of HD. If this is the case, then deletion of A2ARs should enhance the symptoms of HD. Indeed, genetic deletion of A2ARs aggravated motor performance and reduced survival of transgenic HD mouse model (N171-82Q mice).[65] Although extensive degeneration and loss of striatal neurons are observed in HD, somatostatin neurons are spared. Similar observations were made in quinolinic acid- and NMDA-induced excitotoxicity in HD animal models. These results suggest that somatostatin through its receptors (SSTR 1–5) plays a protective role against excitotoxicity. Deletion of SSTR-1 and SSTR-5 from wild-type mice produced neurochemical changes, such as loss of dopamine and cyclic AMP-dependent phosphorylation of 32 DA protein (DARPP-32) in the brain similar to those observed in the brain of HD mouse model (R6/2 mice).[66]

KYNURENINE PATHWAY IN HD

Activation of kynurenine pathway in microglia cells may play a role in the pathogen-esis of HD. It has been reported that levels of neurotoxic metabolites, such as free radical generator 3-hydroxyanthranilic acid (an excitotoxin) and NMDAR agonist quinolinic acid in kynurenine pathway of tryptophan degradation, were elevated in mouse HD model. Histone deacetylase appears to be involved in the regulation of the kynurenine pathway. An inhibitor of histone deacetylase blocked activation of the kynurenine pathway in microglia cells and provided neuroprotection in mouse HD model.[67]

PROTECTION BY GROWTH FACTORS IN HD

Immortalized striatal neuronal progenitor cell lines (STHdhQ7/Q7) expressing wild-type huntington protein with 7 triplet repeats of glutamine, also referred to as Q7, acted as a normal control, whereas the same cell line (STHdhQ111/Q111) expressing HD protein with 111 triplets repeats of glutamine, also referred to as Q111, acted as a model for HD. Using these cell lines, the efficacy of various growth factors, such as fetal and postnatal glia-condition medium (GCM), beta-fibroblastic growth factor (bFGF), BDNF, glia cell-derived neurotrophic factor (GDNF) in protecting against

H_2O_2-, glutamate-, and 3-nitropropionic acid-induced toxicity was evaluated. The results showed that GCM was most effective in protecting Q111 cells against the above neurotoxins. Fetal GCM also reduced the caspases-induced fragmentation of the protein PARP, the expression of Hsp70, and accumulation of ROS and polyubiquitinated proteins.[68] BDNF is essential for the survival of brain neurons. In addition, this neurotrophic factor is needed for the correct synaptic activity of corticostriatal neurons as well as the survival of GABAergic medium-sized spiny striatal neurons that are lost in HD. Indeed, analysis of the autopsied samples of HD brain showed a major loss of BDNF protein from the striatum. Thus, loss of BDNF may contribute to the degeneration of striatal neurons associated with HD.[69]

TRANSCRIPTIONAL DEREGULATION IN HD

HISTONE DEACETYLATION

Histone acetylation and deacetylation regulate gene transcriptions. Acetylation of histone at specific residues increases transcription of genes, whereas deacetylation of histones suppresses transcriptional activity. Transcriptional deregulation has been implicated in the pathogenesis of HD. In animal models of HD, HD gene expression decreases the activity of histone acetyl transferase (HAT) activity causing deacetylation of histone. Deacetylation of histone inhibits the transcriptional activity that causes neurodegeneration in the brain. Inhibitors of histone deacetylase (HDAC) produce some beneficial effects in several animal models of HD[70]; however, their therapeutic value is limited by their toxicity. Chronic oral administration of a novel pimelic diphenylamide HDAC inhibitor, HDACi 4b, beginning and after the onset of motor deficits, significantly improved motor performance, overall appearance, and body weight in transgenic HD mice model. These changes were associated with improvement in brains size and reduction in striatal atrophy. In addition, alterations in gene expression caused by HD protein were prevented by the treatment with HDACi 4b.[71]

Wild-type huntington protein is present primarily in the cytoplasm, whereas N-terminal fragments produced by the cleavage of HD protein are present in both the cytoplasm and the nucleus. These HD protein fragments are insoluble. The nuclear deposits of insoluble HD protein fragments may cause transcriptional deregulation that may contribute to the degeneration and death of neurons.[72] Furthermore, repressor element-1-silencing transcription factor (REST) is considered an inhibitory regulator of genes through the transcriptional regulation of miRNAs in the nerve cells. In HD, REST was translocated from the cytoplasm to the nucleus causing repression of genes, such as BDNF.[73] Reduced transcription of BDNF may contribute to the progression of HD.

DEFECTS IN PALMITOYLATION IN HD

Posttranslational modification of proteins by the lipid palmitate is important for the correct targeting and functions of certain proteins, such as huntington protein. Palmitoylation of proteins is regulated by two functionally opposing enzymes palmitoyl acyltransferases (PATs) which add palmitate to proteins and acyl protein thioesterases which remove palmitate from proteins. This process is particularly important for the development of synapses and synaptic activity in the brain. It has been reported that wild-type huntington protein is palmitoylated by huntington-interacting protein-14 (HIP-14) which exhibits palmitate acyltransferase activity.[74] The interaction between HD protein and HIP-14 is reduced causing a reduction in palmitoylation of HD proteins resulting in increased rate of protein aggregations and neuronal toxicity. On the other hand, overexpression of HIP-14 can increase palmitoylation that markedly reduced HD protein aggregations. This study suggests that palmitoylation by HIP-14 plays a role in the pathogenesis of HD. This was further supported by the study in which deletion of HIP-14 caused development of HD phenotype and behavioral features in mice.[75] Huntington-interacting protein-14 like (HIP-14L) is a paralog (as a result of gene duplication that may acquire different functions) of HIP-14. Both HIP-14 and HIP-14L are essential for palmitoylation of huntington protein. It has been shown that HIP-14L-deficient mice exhibited reduced palmitoylation of novel HIP-14L substrate: SNAP25 (synaptosomal-associated protein-25), early onset of motor deficits, and widespread and progressive neurodegenerative in the brain.[76]

CALRETININ PROTEIN PROTECTS NEURONS IN HD

It was found that Calretinin, a member of the EF-hand family of calcium-binding proteins, was associated with the HD protein as well as wild-type huntington protein. Overexpression of Calretinin reduced HD protein-induced cytotoxicity in both neuronal and nonneuronal cells in cultures, whereas deletion of Calretinin enhanced HD protein-induced neuronal death. In addition, overexpression of Calretinin reduced free intracellular calcium and activation of Akt involved in apoptosis of neurons.[77] These results suggest that Calretinin protein could be of neuroprotective value in HD.

REDUCED ACETYLCHOLINE RELEASE IN HD

Although progressive loss of projection neurons in the cortex and striatum occurs in HD, striatal cholinergic interneurons remain relatively intact. However, there is evidence that striatal acetylcholine is reduced in HD. It has been reported that spontaneous release of acetylcholine (Ach) in the striatal neurons is reduced in R6/2 mouse transgenic model of HD compared to that in wild-type mice (control). The reduction in Ach release in HD mice was due to an excessive release of GABA. This was supported by the observation in which intrastriatal application of GABA antagonist bicuculline methiodide increased Ach levels more in R6/2 mice than in wild-type mice. In contrast, systemic administration of dopamine D (1) receptor partial agonist, SKF-38393, failed to increase Ach levels in R6/2 mice, but it did increase in wild-type mice. These results showed that GABA-mediated inhibition of Ach release remains functional in R6/2 mice; however, dopamine-D 1 receptor-dependent activation of excitatory inputs to striatal cholinergic interneurons is dysfunctional.[78]

The studies discussed in the above sections suggest that increased oxidative stress and chronic inflammation play a central role in the initiation and progression of HD.

Therefore, attenuation of these biochemical defects may delay the onset of HD, and in combination with standard therapy, may reduce the progression and improve the symptoms of the disease. Because of the complexity of regulation of oxidative stress and chronic inflammation in humans, it is not possible to reduce these biochemical defects by the use of a single antioxidant.

HOW TO REDUCE OXIDATIVE STRESS OPTIMALLY

Oxidative stress in the body occurs when the antioxidant system fails to provide adequate protection against damage produced by free radicals (reactive oxygen species and reactive nitrogen species). Increased oxidative stress in the body is reduced by upregulating antioxidant enzymes as well as by existing levels of dietary and endogenous antioxidant chemicals, because they work by different mechanisms. For example, antioxidant enzymes reduce free radicals by catalysis, whereas dietary and endogenous antioxidant chemicals reduce free radicals by directly scavenging them. In response to ROS, a nuclear transcriptional factor, Nrf2 (nuclear factor-erythroid 2-related factor 2) is translocated from the cytoplasm to the nucleus where it binds with ARE (antioxidant response element) which increases the levels of antioxidant enzymes (gamma-glutamylcysteine ligase, glutathione peroxidase, glutathione reductase, and heme oxygenase-1) and phase 2 detoxifying enzymes (NAD(P)H: quinine oxidoreductase 1 and glutathione-S-transferase) in order to reduce oxidative damage.[79–81] In response to increased oxidative stress, existing levels of dietary and endogenous antioxidant chemical levels cannot be elevated without supplementation.

FACTORS REGULATING RESPONSE OF NRF2

Antioxidant enzymes are elevated by activation of Nrf2 which depends upon ROS-dependent and ROS-independent mechanisms. In addition, elevated levels of antioxidant enzymes are also dependent upon the binding ability of Nrf2 with ARE in the nucleus. These studies are described here.

ROS-Dependent Regulation of Nrf2

Normally, Nrf2 is associated with Kelch-like ECH associated protein 1 (Keap1) protein which acts as an inhibitor of Nrf2 (INrf2).[82] INrf2 protein serves as an adaptor to link Nrf2 to the ubiquitin ligase CuI-Rbx1 complex for degradation by proteasomes and maintains the steady levels of Nrf2 in the cytoplasm. INrf2 acts as a sensor for ROS/electrophilic stress. In response to increased ROS, Nrf2 dissociates itself from INrf2-CuI-Rbx1 complex and translocates into the nucleus where it binds with ARE that increases antioxidant genes. It has been demonstrated that Nrf2 regulates INrf2 levels by controlling its transcription, whereas INrf2 regulates Nrf2 levels by controlling its degradation by proteasome.[83]

ROS-Independent Regulation of Nrf2

Antioxidants such as vitamin E, genistein (a flavonoid),[84] allicin, a major organosulfur compound found in garlic,[85] sulforaphane, a organosulfur compound found in cruciferous vegetables,[86] kavalactones (methysticin, kavain, and yangonin),[87] and dietary restriction[88] activate Nrf2 without stimulation by ROS.

Reduced Binding of Nrf2 with ARE

Age-related decline in antioxidant enzymes in the liver of older rats compared to that in younger rats was due to reduction in the binding ability of Nrf2 with ARE; however, treatment with alpha-lipoic acid restored this defect, increased the levels of antioxidant enzymes, and restored the loss of glutathione from the liver of older rats.[89]

DIFFERENTIAL RESPONSE OF Nrf2 TO ROS STIMULATION DURING ACUTE AND CHRONIC OXIDATIVE STRESS

It appears that Nrf2 responds to ROS generated during acute and chronic oxidative stress differently. For example, acute oxidative stress during strenuous exercise translocates Nrf2 from the cytoplasm to the nucleus where it binds with ARE to upregulate antioxidant genes. However, during chronic oxidative stress commonly observed in older individuals and in neurodegenerative diseases, such as Parkinson's disease and Alzheimer's disease, Nrf2/ARE pathway becomes unresponsive to ROS. A reduction in the binding ability of Nrf2 with ARE was demonstrated in older rats.[89] The reasons for Nrf2/ARE pathway to become unresponsive to ROS during chronic oxidative stress are unknown.

Nrf2 IN HD

Using striatal neurons expressing HD gene and wild type huntington gene, it was demonstrated that HD protein disrupted Nrf2 signaling pathway which contributes to mitochondrial dysfunction and enhanced sensitivity to oxidative stress.[90] Treatment of rats with 3-NP caused a reduction in Nrf2 levels in the cytoplasm and the nucleus. Transcranial magnetic stimulation (TMS) applied to 3-NP-treated rats increased the levels of Nrf2 in the cytoplasm and the nucleus.[91] The efficacy of fumaric acid ester dimethylfumarate (DMF) in transgenic HD mouse models (R6/2 mice and YAC128 mice) was evaluated. The results showed that treatment of these mice with DMF prevented weight loss, improved motor function, and protected neurons in the striatum and motor cortex. These effects appear to be mediated via Nrf2 signaling pathway.[92] It has been demonstrated that Nrf2-deficient cells and Nrf2 knockout mice (Nrf2−/Nrf2−) are very sensitive to complex II inhibitors (3-NP and malonate) in causing degeneration of the striatal neurons. Intrastriatal transplantation of Nrf2 overexpressing astrocytes before treatments with 3-NP or malonate provided significant protection against damage produced by inhibitors of complex II.[93] It has been demonstrated that treatment of rat striatal slices with quinolinic acid (Quin) induce oxidative damage. During the early phase of treatment, Nrf2 pathway is upregulated as an adaptive response to acute increase in oxidative stress; whereas down regulation of Nrf2 contributes to increased oxidative damage to the neurons. Furthermore, striatal slices obtained from Nrf2−/− mice were more sensitive to oxidative damage than those obtained from Nrf2[+]/[+] mice.[94] These studies suggest that Nrf2/ARE pathway plays an important role in the pathogenesis of HD and that an elevation of this pathway would be of neuroprotective value.

The following groups of selected nontoxic agents in combination may be useful in reducing oxidative stress optimally:

1. *Agents that can reduce oxidative stress by directly scavenging free radicals*: Some examples are dietary antioxidants, such as vitamin A, beta-carotene, vitamin C, and vitamin E, and endogenous antioxidants, such as glutathione, alpha-lipoic acid, and coenzyme Q_{10}.

2. *Agents which can reduce oxidative stress by activating Nrf2-regulated antioxidant genes without ROS stimulation*: Some examples are organosulfur compound sulforaphane found in cruciferous vegetables, kavalactones, found in Kava shrubs, and Puerarin, a major flavonoid from the root of *Pueraria lobata*,[86,87,95] genistein and vitamin E,[84] and coenzyme Q_{10}[96] activate Nrf2 without ROS stimulation.

3. *Agents which can reduce oxidative stress directly by scavenging free radicals as well as indirectly by activating Nrf2/ARE pathway*: Some examples are vitamin E,[84] alpha-lipoic acid,[89] curcumin,[97] resveratrol,[98,99] omega-3 fatty acids,[100,101] and NAC.[102]

4. *Agents reducing oxidative stress by ROS-dependent mechanism*: They include L-carnitine which generates transient ROS.[103]

A combination of selected agents from the above groups may reduce oxidative stress optimally, and thereby, may reduce the risk of developing HD, and in combination with standard therapy, may improve the management of this disease.

A study on the aged mouse hippocampus revealed that supplementation with allicin, a major organosulfur compound found in garlic, which has an electrophilic center (electron deficient) prevented age-related decline in cognitive function. This effect of allicin was due to enhancement of antioxidant enzymes via Nrf2-ARE pathway.[85] This study suggests that INrf2/Nrf2 complex and binding of Nrf2 with ARE remain responsive to allicin. Repeated administration of another organosulfur compound, sulforaphane, found in cruciferous vegetables, simulated Nrf2-dependent increase of Nqo1 gene which codes for NAD(P)H: quinone oxidoreductase, and Hmox1 gene which codes for HO-1 enzyme in astrocytes in culture, and reduced oxidative damage.[86] It appears that sulforaphane-induced activation of Nrf2 does not require ROS stimulation. Indeed, kavalactones (methysticin, kavain and yangonin)-induced activation of Nrf2 is not dependent upon ROS stimulation in neuronal cells and astroglia cells in culture.[87]

In a study on murine alveolar cells in culture, NAC, which directly scavenges free radicals via increasing intracellular glutathione levels, requires the presence of Nrf2 for an optimal reduction in oxidative stress.[104] For example, cigarette smoking produces greater damage in alveolar cells obtained from Nrf2-deleted mice (Nrf2[-]/[-]) than in cells obtained from wild-type mice.[104] Pretreatment of alveolar cells with NAC reduced cigarette smoke induce damage more in cells obtained from the wild-type mice than in cells from Nrf2 deleted mice. In another study on rat liver, pretreatment with NAC prevents the ROS-induced activation of Nrf2.[105] If NAC scavenged all ROS, then ROS was not available for activating Nrf2/ARE pathway.

How to Reduce Chronic Inflammation and Glutamate

Some individual antioxidants from the above groups have been shown to reduce chronic inflammation and prevent the release[114] and toxicity[115,116] of glutamate.

A combination of selected agents from the above groups may reduce chronic inflammation and release of glutamate and its toxicity optimally, and thereby, may reduce the risk of developing HD, and in combination with standard therapy, may improve the management of this disease.

LABORATORY AND CLINICAL STUDIES ON ANTIOXIDANTS AND POLYPHENOLIC COMPOUNDS

Alpha-Tocopherol (Vitamin E)

In a clinical study on 73 patients with HD, it was found that treatment with D-alpha-tocopherol had no effect on neurological or neuropsychiatric symptoms; however, some beneficial effects on neurological symptoms were observed during the early course of the disease.[117]

Vitamin C

Using transgenic mouse HD model R6/2, it was shown that injection of vitamin C (ascorbate) at the beginning of the onset of symptoms restored striatal release of ascorbate and improved neurological motor signs without altering overall motor activity.[118]

N-Acetylcysteine (NAC)

Since mitochondrial dysfunction is present in HD, the efficacy of NAC in improving mitochondrial function in rat HD model (induced by the treatment with 3-nitropropionic acid) was tested.[119] Rats treated with 3-NP exhibited inhibition of brain mitochondrial complexes II, IV, and V but not of complex I in the striatum. As expected, increased production of ROS and lipid peroxidation were observed in brain mitochondria of 3-NP treated rats. In addition, increased cytosolic cytochrome c levels, mitochondrial swelling, and increased expression of caspase-3 and p53 were observed in the brain of NP-3 treated animals. Neuropathological changes included neurodegeneration and gliosis and were associated with motor and cognitive deficits. Treatment with NAC reversed 3-NP-induced mitochondrial dysfunctions and deficits in motor and cognitive functions.

Alpha-Lipoic Acid

Treatment with alpha-lipoic acid increased the survival of transgenic mouse HD models (R6/2 and N171-82Q).[120]

COENZYME Q_{10}

Using transgenic mice HD model (expression of HD protein with approximately 120 trinucleotide repeats), it was demonstrated that mice fed with 0.2 and 0.6% of coenzyme Q_{10} in chow improved early behavior deficits and normalized some transcriptional deficits without altering the levels of HD protein aggregates in the striatum.[121] It was noted that coenzyme Q_{10} at a low dose was more effective than that observed at a high dose. Treatment of wild-type mice with a low-dose coenzyme Q_{10} (0.2%) induced motor deficits. This deleterious effect of coenzyme Q_{10} may be unique to mice since no harmful effects of even high doses of coenzyme Q_{10} have been observed in humans.

In another study using transgenic mouse model of HD (R6/2), it was demonstrated that the brain levels of coenzyme Q_9 and coenzyme Q_{10} were lower in R6/2 mice than in wild-type mice. Oral administration of coenzyme Q_{10} increased the levels of coenzyme Q_{10} in plasma and of coenzyme Q_9 and coenzyme Q_{10} and adenosine triphosphate (ATP) in the brain of R6/2 mice. Treatment with high doses of coenzyme Q_{10} significantly extended survival of R6/2 mice in a dose-dependent manner and improved motor deficits and reduced weight loss, brain atrophy, and HD protein aggregates.[122] A combination of coenzyme Q_{10} and creatine produced an additive protective effect in improving motor performance and extending survival of transgenic R6/2 HD mice.[123]

L-CARNITINE

Using chemical-induced HD animal models (rats treated with quinolinic acid or 3-NP), it was demonstrated that treatment with L-carnitine prevented quinolinic acid-induced motor deficits and 3-NP-induced hypokinetic pattern (impaired movements).[124] L-Carnitine treatment also reduced quinolinic acid-induced gliosis and 3-NP-induced brain damage. Using transgenic mouse HD model (N171-82Q), it was shown that administration of L-carnitine increased survival of HD mice and improved motor function as well as reduced neuronal loss and the number of intranuclear mutated protein aggregates. It was suggested that protective effect of L-carnitine was due to a reduction in oxidative damage.[125]

LYCOPENE AND EPIGALLOCATECHIN

Using 3-NP-induced rat HD model, it was demonstrated that treatment with lycopene or epigallocatechin improved memory deficits and restored the levels of glutathione and glutathione-S-transferase in the striatum, hippocampus, and cortex areas of the brain. Furthermore, pretreatment with arginine increases the effectiveness of lycopene and epigallocatechin in protecting neuronal damage.[126]

MELATONIN

This hormone is secreted by the pineal gland and is necessary for sleep. Melatonin also exhibits antioxidant activity. A study has reported that supplementation with melatonin delayed the onset and mortality in a transgenic mouse model of HD.[127] Loss of type 1 melatonin receptors (MT1) has been found in human HD as well as in the transgenic mouse HD model. It has been reported that high levels of MT1 receptors are present in the mitochondria from the brain of wild-type mice; however, in the transgenic mouse HD model, reduced levels of MT1 receptors were present in the brain.[127] Treatment with melatonin inhibited mutated huntington protein-induced caspase activation and protected MT1 receptors expression, suggesting that protective effect of melatonin may be mediated through activation of MT1 receptors.

Curcumin

Curcumin is a naturally occurring polyphenolic compound with the ability to enter the blood–brain barrier. The efficacy of curcumin in improving the symptoms of HD was tested in the transgenic mouse HD model (expressing 140 repeats of trinucleotide). The results showed that HD mice fed with curcumin-containing diet since conception showed decreased aggregates of mutated huntington protein and increased striatal dopamine- and cAMP-regulated neuronal phosphoprotein (DARPP-32) and dopamine D1 receptor mRNAs and prevented rearing deficits.[128] Curcumin treatment improved impaired motor function in transgenic HD mice and wild-type mice in early study; however, in this study, curcumin treatment did not affect motor function, behavioral deficits, and muscle strength or food utilization in transgenic mice.

Resveratrol

Using rat HD model (3-NP-induced HD phenotype), it was demonstrated that treatment with resveratrol before and after 3-NP treatment improved motor and cognitive functions by reducing oxidative stress.[129] Reduction in mitogen-activated protein kinase signaling pathway, particularly the Ras-extracellular signal-regulated kinase (ERK) cascade has been implicated in the pathogenesis of HD. Therefore, activation of ERK may be of therapeutic value in the management of HD. This hypothesis was tested in three HD models (PC-12, a neuronal cell line expressing HD gene, Drosophila expressing HD gene, and R6/2 mouse HD model), using polyphenols, such as fisetin and resveratrol, which activate ERK. The results showed that these activators of ERK reduced the harmful effects effects of HD protein in all three models.[130]

Ginkgo biloba Extract and Olive Oil

Pretreatment with *Ginkgo biloba* extract (EGb761) prevented 3-NP-induced motor deficits and elevated strital MDA levels in rats.[131] Treatment with 3-NP upregulated the expression of striatal Bax gene and downregulated the expression of striatal Bcl-xl gene, upregulated the expression of striatal glyceraldehyde-3-pohosphate dehydrogenase (GAPDH), and inhibited succinate dehydrogenase enzyme activity. Pretreatment with (EGb-761) reversed the above changes in gene expression and enzyme involved in energy metabolism.

Treatment with extra-virgin olive oil prevented 3-NP-induced elevated levels of lipid peroxides and depletion of glutathione in the striatum of rats.[132] In addition, olive oil treatment also reversed 3-NP-induced inhibition of succinate dehydrogenase activity.

PROBUCOL

Probucol is known to exhibit antioxidant activity. Treatment with probucol prevented ROS formation and lipid peroxidationin in all chemical-induced HD models (quinolinic acid, as an excitotoxic model; 3-NP, as an inhibitor of mitochondrial succinate dehydrogenase model; and combined model of quinolinic acid and 3-NP treatment), but it did not protect against 3-NP-induced mitochondrial dysfunctions.[133] Treatment with sodium succinate protected striatal slices only against 3-NP-induced mitochondrial dysfunctions. Treatment with a NMDA receptor antagonist MK-801 (also called Dizocilpine) protected mitochondrial dysfunctions in all HD models used in this study. These data suggest that a combination of NMDA receptor antagonist and antioxidants may be more useful in reducing oxidative stress and mitochondrial dysfunction than the individual agents.

B VITAMINS

Nicotinamide, a water soluble B_3 vitamin, is an inhibitor of sirtuin 1/class III NAD^+-dependent histone deacetylase activity. Using the B6.HDR6/1 transgenic mouse model, it was demonstrated that treatment with nicotinamide increased mRNA levels of BDNF and PGC-1 alpha. In addition, nicotinamide treatment enhanced protein levels of BDNF and activation of PGC-1 alpha in HD mice. Furthermore, the above treatment improved motor function in HD mice even though there was no reduction in the levels of HD protein aggregates in the striatum or in the weight loss.[134]

Examination of the autopsied samples of human HD striatum showed increased levels in carbonylation of proteins (a marker of protein oxidation). Oxidation of mitochondrial enzymes decreased catalytic activities which reduced energy levels in HD, whereas oxidation of pyridoxal kinase and antiquitin-1 decreased the levels of pyridoxal 5-phosphate (vitamin B_6). Using the Tet/HD94 conditional mouse HD model, it was shown that carbonylation (oxidation) of proteins in the striatum was dependent upon the expression of HD protein.[135] Vitamin B_6 acts as a cofactor for several biological processes including transaminases, and synthesis of glutathione, GABA, and dopamine; therefore, the reduction in the levels of vitamin B_6 in HD may be responsible for reduction in the levels of dopamine and GABA in this disease.

PROBLEMS OF USING A SINGLE ANTIOXIDANT IN HD PATIENTS

Laboratory studies consistently showed that supplementation with certain individual antioxidants may reduce the symptoms and improve neurochemical changes in animal models of HD. Administration of a single antioxidant in HD patients may not be effective, because this antioxidant may be oxidized in the presence of a high internal oxidative environment and then acts as a pro-oxidant.

Previous studies in other chronic diseases, such as beta-carotene in male heavy smokers for reducing the risk of lung cancer, vitamin E in AD for improving cognitive function, and vitamin E in PD for improving the symptoms and as expected, produced inconsistent results varying from no effect as in PD,[136] to modest beneficial[137] or no effect effects as in AD,[138] and harmful effects as in heavy male smokers.[139] Because of the failure to obtain consistent beneficial effects with individual agents, I recommend a preparation of micronutrients such as proposed in the section of Secondary Prevention for prevention and/or delaying the onset of HD.

RATIONALE FOR USING MULTIPLE ANTIOXIDANTS IN A MICRONUTRIENT PREPARATION

Based on the consistency of laboratory data on the beneficial effects of the individual dietary and endogenous antioxidants or B vitamins alone, it is tempting to suggest that a similar beneficial effect of individual dietary or endogenous antioxidants can also be obtained in asymptomatic individuals carrying the HD gene or in patients with HD symptoms. The fact that these individuals may have increased oxidative stress and chronic inflammation suggests that administration of single antioxidants may be ineffective. This is due to the fact that administered antioxidants would be oxidized and an oxidized antioxidant acts as a pro-oxidant rather than as an antioxidant. Additional rationales are described here.

Different antioxidants are distributed differently in various cellular compartments and various organs, and their affinity to various types of free radicals are different. In addition, the levels of oxygenations are different within the same cells and in various organs. It has been shown that beta-carotene (BC) is more effective in quenching oxygen radicals than most other antioxidants.[140] BC can perform certain biological functions that cannot be produced by its metabolite vitamin A and vice versa.[141,142] It has been reported that BC treatment enhances the expression of the connexin gene which codes for a gap junction protein in mammalian fibroblasts in culture, whereas vitamin A treatment does not produce such an effect.[142] Vitamin A can induce differentiation in certain normal and cancer cells, whereas BC and other carotenoids do not.[143,144] Thus, BC and vitamin A have, in part, different biological functions. The gradient of oxygen pressure varies within cells. Some antioxidants, such as vitamin E, are more effective as quenchers of free radicals in reduced oxygen pressure, whereas BC and vitamin A are more effective in higher atmospheric pressures.[145] Vitamin C is necessary to protect cellular components in aqueous environments, whereas carotenoids and vitamins A and E protect cellular components in lipid environments. Vitamin C also plays an important role in maintaining cellular levels of vitamin E by recycling vitamin E radical (oxidized) to the reduced (antioxidant) form.[146]

The form of vitamin E used is also important in any clinical trial. It has been established that D-alpha-tocopheryl succinate (vitamin E succinate) is the most effective form of vitamin E both *in vitro* and *in vivo*.[147,148] This form of vitamin E is more soluble than alpha-tocopherol or alpha-tocopheryl acetate and enters cells more readily than other forms of vitamin E. Therefore, it is expected to cross the blood–brain barrier in greater amounts than alpha-tocopherol or alpha-tocopheryl acetate. However, this has not yet been demonstrated in animals or in humans. We have reported that an oral ingestion of alpha-TS (800 IU/day) in humans increased plasma levels of not only alpha-tocopherol, but also alpha-TS, suggesting that a portion of alpha-TS can be absorbed from the intestinal tract before hydrolysis.[149] It is possible that increased levels of vitamin E succinate in the plasma occur only after the pool for alpha-tocopherol becomes saturated. This observation is important because the conventional assumption based on rodents has been that esterified forms of vitamin E, such as alpha-tocopheryl succinate, alpha-tocopheryl nicotinate, and alpha-tocopheryl acetate, can be absorbed from the intestinal tract only after they are hydrolyzed to alpha-tocopherol. Our preliminary data showed that this assumption may not be true for the absorption of vitamin E succinate in humans.

An endogenous antioxidant, glutathione, is effective in catabolizing H_2O_2 and anions. However, oral supplementation with glutathione failed to significantly increase plasma levels of glutathione in human subjects,[150] suggesting that this tripeptide is completely hydrolyzed in the G.I. tract. Therefore, I propose to utilize N-acetylcysteine (NAC) and alpha-lipoic acid that increase the cellular levels of glutathione by different mechanisms in a multiple micronutrient preparation.

Another endogenous antioxidant, coenzyme Q_{10}, may have some potential value in prevention and improved treatment of HD. Since mitochondrial dysfunction is associated with HD and since coenzyme Q_{10} is needed for the generation of ATP by mitochondria, it is essential to add this antioxidant in multiple micronutrient preparation. A study has shown that coenzyme Q_{10} scavenges peroxy radicals faster than alpha–tocopherol,[151] and like vitamin C, can regenerate vitamin E in a redox cycle.[152] However, it is a weaker antioxidant than alpha-tocopherol. Coenzyme Q_{10} administration has been shown to improve clinical symptoms in patients with mitochondrial encephalomyopathies[153] and PD.[154]

Selenium is a cofactor of glutathione peroxidase, and Se-glutathione peroxidase acts as an antioxidant by increasing the intracellular level of glutathione. There may be some other mechanisms of selenium. Therefore, selenium in the form of seleno-L-methionine should be added to a multiple micronutrient preparation.

Nicotinamide (vitamin B_3), a precursor of NAD^+ also attenuated glutamate-induced toxicity and preserved cellular levels of NAD^+ to support the activity of SIRT1.[155] It is also a competitive inhibitor of histone deacetylase activity and has been helpful in improving some of the symptoms of HD in animal model. These preclinical data suggest that oral supplementation with higher doses of nicotinamide should be added in a micronutrient preparation.

In addition to dietary and endogenous antioxidants and vitamin B_3, other B vitamins, vitamin D, and certain minerals should be added to a multiple micronutrient preparation, because they are also important neuronal functions and vital to general health. Two recent studies of supplementation with multiple vitamin preparations reduced cancer incidence by 10 percent in men[156] and improved clinical outcomes in patients with HIV/AIDS who were not taking medication.[157]

CAN HD BE PREVENTED OR DELAYED?

It is often believed that the genetic basis of neurodegenerative diseases such as HD cannot be prevented or delayed by any pharmacological and/or physiological means.

Laboratory experiments on the genetic basis of another disease model (cancer) in *Drosophila melanogaster* (fruit fly) show that it may be possible to prevent or at least delay the onset of the genetic basis of human diseases.

The gene HOP (TUM-1) is essential for the development of fruit flies. A mutation in this gene markedly increases the risk of developing a leukemia-like tumor in female flies (unpublished observation in collaboration with Dr. Bhattacharya et al. of NASA, Moffat Field, CA). Proton radiation is a powerful cancer-causing agent. Whole-body irradiation of these flies with proton radiation dramatically increased the incidence of cancer compared to that in unirradiated flies. The question arose as to whether or not a preparation of multiple antioxidants can reduce the incidence of cancer which is due to a specific gene defect. To test this possibility, a mixture of multiple dietary and endogenous antioxidants were fed to these flies through diet 7 days before proton irradiation and continued throughout the experimental period of 7 days. The results showed that antioxidant treatment before and after irradiation totally blocked the proton radiation-induced cancer in fruit flies. This finding on fruit flies is of particular interest, because to my knowledge, this is a first demonstration in which genetic basis of a disease can be prevented by antioxidant treatment. This observation made on fruit flies cannot readily be extrapolated to humans. It is not known whether daily supplementation with antioxidants in women of reproductive age carrying the HD gene without HD symptoms before conception, during entire pregnancy and throughout the postnatal growth can prevent or delay the onset of HD in their children. It is also unknown whether daily supplementation with antioxidants at the age of 5 years or earlier for the entire lifespan could prevent or delay the onset of HD. The results on fruit flies suggest that daily supplementation with multiple antioxidants could potentially prevent or delay the onset of HD in humans. A clinical study is needed to evaluate the effectiveness of multiple antioxidants in prevention of or delayed onset of HD in humans.

PREVENTION AND/OR DELAYING THE ONSET OF HD

Before discussing the strategies for HD prevention, it is essential to define primary and secondary prevention. The purpose of primary prevention is to protect healthy individuals from developing PD. This prevention strategy may not be applicable to HD, because the disease has a genetic basis. The purpose of secondary prevention is to prevent or delay the onset of HD. Individuals who carry the HD gene, but have not developed any signs or symptoms of the disease, would be suitable for the study on secondary prevention.

SECONDARY PREVENTION

Since increased oxidative stress, mitochondrial dysfunction, and chronic inflammation play important roles in the development of HD, attenuation of oxidative stress and chronic inflammation may be one of the rational choices for secondary prevention of HD. A preparation of multiple dietary and endogenous antioxidants, certain phenolic compounds (curcumin and resveratrol), vitamin D, selenium, L-carnitine, and B vitamin including high-dose vitamin B_3 is recommended. These agents would reduce oxidative stress indirectly by increasing the levels of antioxidant enzymes through activation of the Nrf2/ARE pathway and directly by scavenging free radicals. The same preparation of micronutrients would also reduce chronic inflammation and release the toxicity of glutamate.

PROPOSED PREVENTION AND/OR DELAYING STRATEGIES FOR THE ONSET OF HD

Increased oxidative stress may induce aggregations of HD proteins that are neurotoxic. Increased oxidative stress can also induce chronic inflammation that releases toxic proinflammatory cytokines and ROS. Among various etiological factors that initiate HD include increased oxidative stress, chronic inflammation, and an excitotoxic process represent early events in the development of HD. Therefore, decreasing oxidative stress, chronic inflammation, and excitatory events may delay the onset of this disease. Antioxidants decrease oxidative stress, inflammation,[107,108,158] and release and toxicity of glutamate, an excitatory neurotransmitter.[114,115] Therefore, daily oral supplementation with a preparation of micronutrients proposed in the Secondary Prevention Section right from childhood may prevent or at least delay the onset of HD and if combined with standard therapy, may reduce the rate of progression of this fatal disease more than that produced by standard therapy alone. If the patients have difficulty in swallowing solid food, micronutrients from the capsules can be mixed in a liquid diet, such as juice.

UNIQUENESS OF MICRONUTRIENT PREPARATION

The proposed micronutrient formulations have some unique properties that are not found in other multiple vitamin preparations currently sold. For example, the proposed micronutrient formulations have no iron, copper, manganese, and heavy metals (vanadium, zirconium, and molybdenum). Iron and copper are not added because they are known to interact with vitamin C and generate excessive amounts of free radicals. In addition, iron and copper are absorbed more in the presence of antioxidants than in the absence of antioxidants. Therefore, it is possible that prolonged consumption of these trace minerals in the presence of antioxidants may increase the levels of free iron or copper stores in the body, because there are no significant mechanisms of excretion of iron among men of all ages and women after menopause. Increased stores of free iron may enhance the progression of HD. Heavy metals are not added because prolonged consumption of these metals may increase their levels in the body, because there is no significant mechanism for excretion of these metals from the body. High levels of these metals are considered neurotoxic. The efficacy of the proposed micronutrient preparations should be tested in clinical studies.

DOSE SCHEDULE

Most clinical studies have utilized a once-a-day dose schedule. Taking vitamins and antioxidants once-a-day can create large fluctuations in their levels in the body. This is due to the fact that the biological half-lives of vitamins and antioxidants markedly vary, depending upon their lipid or water solubility. A twofold difference in the levels of vitamin E succinate can produce marked alterations in the expression profiles of several genes in neuroblastoma cells in culture. Therefore, taking a multiple vitamin preparation once-a-day may produce large fluctuation in the levels of micronutrients in the body which could potentially cause genetic stress in cells that may compromise the effectiveness of the vitamin supplementation after long-term consumption. I recommend taking a preparation of micronutrients containing multiple dietary and endogenous antioxidants twice-a-day in order to reduce fluctuations in the levels of gene expressions. Such a dose schedule may improve the effectiveness of a multiple vitamin preparation in reducing the development and progression of HD.

TOXICITY OF ANTIOXIDANTS PRESENT IN THE MICRONUTRIENT PREPARATION

Antioxidants and B vitamins used in proposed micronutrient preparation are considered safe. Antioxidants at doses higher than those that are recommended for the proposed micronutrient preparations have been consumed by the U.S. population for decades without significant toxicity. However, a few of them could produce harmful effects at certain high doses in some individuals when consumed daily for a long period of time. For example, vitamin A at doses of 10,000 IU or more per day can cause birth defects in pregnant women, and beta-carotene at doses 50 mg or more can produce bronzing of the skin that is reversible on discontinuation. Vitamin C as ascorbic acid at high doses (10 g or more per day) can cause diarrhea in some individuals. Vitamin E at high doses (2000 IU or more per day) can induce clotting defects after long-term consumption. Vitamin B_6 at high doses (50 mg or more per day) may produce peripheral neuropathy, and selenium at doses 400 mcg or more per day can cause skin and liver toxicity after long-term consumption. Coenzyme Q_{10} has no known toxicity, and recommended daily doses are 30–400 mg. N-acetylcysteine doses of 250–1500 mg and alpha-lipoic acid doses of 600 mg are used in humans without toxicity at these recommended doses. All ingredients present in the proposed micronutrient preparations are safe and come under the category of "Food Supplement" and therefore do not require FDA approval for their use.

CURRENT TREATMENTS OF HD

The purpose of treatment is to improve the symptoms and reduce the progression of the HD. The contents of this section are based on publication by the Mayo Clinic Foundation for Medical Education and Research. At present, a combination of medications, psychotherapy, speech therapy, and physical therapy is used to manage the symptoms of HD. There are no drug treatments that can alter the course of HD in humans. The following groups of drugs are used in the treatment of HD in humans.

MOVEMENT DISORDERS DRUGS

Tetrabenazine (Xenazine), a FDA approved drug, suppresses chorea (jerking movements) associated with HD; however, serious side effects include the risk of worsening or triggering depression or other psychiatric problems, insomnia, drowsiness, nausea, and restlessness. These side effects of this drug limit its value in the management of the symptoms of HD.

ANTIPSYCHOTIC DRUGS

Haloperidol (Haldol) and Clozapine can suppress chorea movements, but they can worsen involuntary contraction (dystonia) and muscle rigidity; therefore, they are not adequate for improving the symptoms of HD.

OTHER MEDICATIONS

Other drugs that can suppress chorea, dystonia, and muscle rigidity include anti-seizure drugs, such as clonazepam (klonopin), and anti-anxiety medications, such as diazepam (valium). These drugs can alter consciousness and induce addiction and dependency.

MEDICATIONS FOR PSYCHIATRIC DISORDERS

Drugs to treat psychiatric disorders may vary depending upon the disorders and symptoms. Possible treatment drugs include the following:

ANTIDEPRESSANTS

Commonly used drugs include escitalopram (Lexapro), fluoxetine (Prozac, Sarafem), and sertraline (Zoloft). These drugs may also be useful in treating obsessive-compulsive disorder associated with HD. Some adverse side effects may include nausea, diarrhea, insomnia, and sexual problems.

MOOD-STABILIZING DRUGS

Drugs including lithium (Lithobid) and anticonvulsants, such as valporic acid (Depakene), divalproex (Depakote), and lamotrigine (Lamictal), may be useful in the treatment of highs and lows associated with bipolar disorder. Common side effects include weight gain, tremor, and gastrointestinal problems. Periodic blood tests are needed because of toxicity of lithium on the thyroid and kidney.

CLINICAL STUDIES WITH ADDITIONAL DRUGS IN HD

In a clinical study involving six patients with HD, the efficacy of Aripiprazole (AP), a dopamine D2 receptor partial agonist that is used to reduce schizophrenic symptoms was compared with Tetrabenazine (TBZ), a dopamine depletor that is used to treat hyperkinesia in HD, on chorea, motor function, and functional disability. The results showed that both drugs reduce chorea in a similar manner; however, AP caused less sedation and sleepiness than TBZ.[159] This study is too small to make any conclusion. It is interesting to note that two drugs that have an opposite effect on the level of dopamine are used in this study.

In a randomized, double-blind, placebo-controlled trial involving multicenters from 32 European countries, the efficacy of pridopidine, a dopaminergic stabilizer, was evaluated on motor function in patients with HD. The results showed that this drug did not affect nonmotor endpoints, but some improvements in motor function were detected.[160] The drug at the dose of 90 mg/day was considered safe. A similar study with pridopidine was performed utilizing outpatients from neurological clinics at 27 sites in the USA and Canada on HD patients receiving 20 mg (N = 56), 45 mg (N = 55), 90 mg (N = 58), or placebo (N = 58) for a period of 12 weeks. The results showed that pridopidine treatment at a dose of 90 mg/day may improve some motor functions.[161]

PSYCHOTHERAPY

This type of therapy can be provided by a psychiatrist, psychologist, or social worker. It is important to help a person with HD to manage behavioral problems, develop coping strategies, manage expectations during progression of the disease, and facilitate effective communication among family members.

SPEECH THERAPY

HD can markedly impair control of muscles of the mouth and throat that are essential for speech, eating, and swallowing. A speech therapist can help in improving the ability of patients with HD to speak clearly and to use communication devices correctly.

PHYSICAL THERAPY

A physical therapist can teach HD patients how to exercise safely and correctly in order to enhance muscle strength, flexibility, balance, and coordination. These exercises can help in maintaining mobility as long as possible and may reduce the risk of falls. The physical therapist can also provide instruction on appropriate posture and the use of supports to improve posture that may reduce the severity of some movement disorders. For those patients who may require a wheel chair or walker, a physical therapist can teach how to use these devices appropriately.

RECOMMENDED MICRONUTRIENTS IN COMBINATION WITH STANDARD THERAPY

None of the standard therapeutic agents affect oxidative stress, chronic inflammation, or release and toxicity of glutamate which play a central role in the progression of HD. Therefore, a combination of the preparation of micronutrients recommended for the Secondary Prevention with the standard therapy may reduce the progression and improve the symptoms of the disease more than those produced by standard therapy alone by reducing oxidative stress, chronic inflammation, and preventing the release and toxicity of glutamate.

RECOMMENDATIONS FOR DIET AND LIFESTYLE CHANGES

ASYMPTOMATIC INDIVIDUALS CARRYING HD GENE

I recommend daily consumption of a low-fat and high-fiber diet with plenty of fruits (especially grapes and berries) and leafy vegetables. Whenever oil is used for cooking, virgin olive oil is preferred. For nonvegetarians, fish (especially salmon) twice-a-week and chicken (or other meat not more than 4 oz. per meal) is recommended. For the vegetarians, increased intake of lima beans and soy/soy products is recommended.

Changes in lifestyle recommendations include maintaining normal weight, reducing overweight or obesity, increasing physical activity, stopping tobacco smoking, reducing stress (vacation, yoga, and/or meditation), and performing moderate exercise four to five times a week. Moderate exercise includes walking 20–25 min per day at least 5 days per week or using a treadmill (25 min at a moderate speed) and weight lifting for 30 min three to four times a week. The level of exercise depends upon the age of the individual. Younger individuals can usually do more strenuous exercise than the older individuals.

SYMPTOMATIC INDIVIDUALS WITH HD

Depending upon the severity of symptoms, patients with HD have difficulty in swallowing; they may take a long time to eat. There is a risk of choking, if proper attention is not given. The patients with HD should have enough calories to maintain adequate body weight. Care givers are often trained how to deal with eating-related problems. It is also important for the patients to maintain sufficient hydration. Physical activity is essential for HD patients, but this should be performed under the supervision of a physical therapist and/or care giver.

CONCLUSIONS

HD caused by a mutation in the wild-type huntington gene is a rare fatal hereditary disease of the brain in which neurons (primarily in striatum and cortex) involved in movement, intellect, and emotions are gradually destroyed. The mutated huntington gene is referred to as the HD gene. It has repeated expansion of trinucleotide CAG that codes for glutamine more than the wild-type gene. HD is characterized by jerking, uncontrollable movements of the limbs, trunk, and face (chorea); progressive loss of mental abilities; and the development of psychiatric problems. Each child of HD parents has a 50–50 chance of inheriting a mutated HD gene. There is no cure for this disease, and there are no strategies for preventing or delaying the onset of this disease.

It appears that increased oxidative stress mitochondrial dysfunction and chronic inflammation are early events in the initiation of HD. Damaged mitochondria produce more free radicals. Later increased release of glutamate together with increased oxidative stress and chronic inflammation participate in the progression of the disease.

Treatment with BDNF, individual antioxidants, such as vitamin E, vitamin C, alpha-lipoic acid, N-acetylcysteine, coenzyme Q_{10}, L-carnitine, lycopene, melatonin, curcumin, resveratrol, epigallocatechin, *Ginkgo biloba* extract, and probucol or nicotinamide (vitamin B_3) improved some symptoms of HD in animal models of HD.

At present, there are no effective strategies to prevent or delay the onset of HD symptoms. It is proposed that a combination of agents which can increase antioxidant enzymes by activating Nrf2-ARE pathway without ROS stimulation, and which can directly scavenge free radicals may be necessary to reduce oxidative stress and chronic inflammation optimally in HD. Dietary and endogenous antioxidants, curcumin, resveratrol, and omega-3 fatty acids can fulfill the above requirements for reducing oxidative stress and chronic inflammation optimally. The same multiple antioxidants and phenolic compounds may also prevent release and toxicity of glutamate on the nerve cells. All the agents described here are of low toxicity, which would allow their prolonged safe usage among individuals carrying the HD gene.

The current treatment of HD is not satisfactory. The medications used in the treatment of HD do not affect increased oxidative stress, chronic inflammation, or glutamate release and its toxicity. Therefore, the proposed preparation of micronutrients in combination with standard medications may reduce the progression and improve the symptoms of the disease more than those produced by medications alone. Separate clinical studies using the proposed micronutrient recommendations for secondary prevention and treatment should be initiated. In the meantime, those individuals carrying HD gene interested in micronutrient approach in delaying the onset of the disease or improving the efficacy of standard therapy in the treatment of HD may like to adopt these recommendations in consultation with their physicians or health professionals.

REFERENCES

1. Pringsheim T, Wiltshire K, Day L, Dykeman J, Steeves T, Jette N. The incidence and prevalence of Huntington's disease: A systematic review and meta-analysis. *Mov Disord.* Aug 2012; 27(9): 1083–1091.
2. Hoffner G, Soues S, Djian P. Aggregation of expanded huntingtin in the brains of patients with Huntington disease. *Prion.* Jan–Mar 2007; 1(1): 26–31.
3. Hands S, Sajjad MU, Newton MJ, Wyttenbach A. In vitro and in vivo aggregation of a fragment of huntingtin protein directly causes free radical production. *J Biol Chem.* Dec 30 2011; 286(52): 44512–44520.
4. Sadri-Vakili G, Cha JH. Mechanisms of disease: Histone modifications in Huntington's disease. *Nat Clin Pract Neurol.* Jun 2006; 2(6): 330–338.
5. Maldonado PD, Molina-Jijon E, Villeda-Hernandez J, Galvan-Arzate S, Santamaria A, Pedraza-Chaverri J. NAD(P)H oxidase contributes to neurotoxicity in an excitotoxic/prooxidant model of Huntington's disease in rats: Protective role of apocynin. *J Neurosci Res.* Feb 15 2010; 88(3): 620–629.
6. Perez-De La Cruz V, Gonzalez-Cortes C, Galvan-Arzate S et al. Excitotoxic brain damage involves early peroxynitrite formation in a model of Huntington's disease in rats: Protective role of iron porphyrinate 5,10,15,20-tetrakis (4-sulfonatophenyl)porphyrinate iron (III). *Neuroscience.* 2005; 135(2): 463–474.
7. Tunez I, Santamaria A. (Model of Huntington's disease induced with 3-nitropropionic acid). *Revista de neurologia.* Apr 16–30 2009; 48(8): 430–434.
8. Kuhn A, Goldstein DR, Hodges A et al. Mutant huntingtin's effects on striatal gene expression in mice recapitulate changes observed in human Huntington's disease brain and do not differ with mutant huntingtin length or wild-type huntingtin dosage. *Hum Mol Genet.* Aug 1 2007; 16(15): 1845–1861.

9. Browne SE, Beal MF. Oxidative damage in Huntington's disease pathogenesis. *Antioxid Redox Signal.* Nov–Dec 2006; 8(11–12): 2061–2073.

10. Browne SE. Mitochondria and Huntington's disease pathogenesis: Insight from genetic and chemical models. *Ann N Y Acad Sci.* Dec 2008; 1147: 358–382.

11. Hickey MA, Kosmalska A, Enayati J et al. Extensive early motor and non-motor behavioral deficits are followed by striatal neuronal loss in knock-in Huntington's disease mice. *Neuroscience.* Nov 11 2008; 157(1): 280–295.

12. del Hoyo P, Garcia-Redondo A, de Bustos F et al. Oxidative stress in skin fibroblasts cultures of patients with Huntington's disease. *Neurochem Res.* Sep 2006; 31(9): 1103–1109.

13. Chen CM, Wu YR, Cheng ML et al. Increased oxidative damage and mitochondrial abnormalities in the peripheral blood of Huntington's disease patients. *Biochem Biophys Res Commun.* Jul 27 2007; 359(2): 335–340.

14. Browne SE, Bowling AC, MacGarvey U et al. Oxidative damage and metabolic dysfunction in Huntington's disease: Selective vulnerability of the basal ganglia. *Ann Neurol.* May 1997; 41(5): 646–653.

15. Goswami A, Dikshit P, Mishra A, Mulherkar S, Nukina N, Jana NR. Oxidative stress promotes mutant huntingtin aggregation and mutant huntingtin-dependent cell death by mimicking proteasomal malfunction. *Biochem Biophys Res Commun.* Mar 31 2006; 342(1): 184–190.

16. Sanchez Mejia RO, Friedlander RM. Caspases in Huntington's disease. The Neuroscientist: A review journal bringing neurobiology, neurology, and psychiatry. Dec 2001; 7(6): 480–489.

17. Hermel E, Gafni J, Propp SS et al. Specific caspase interactions and amplification are involved in selective neuronal vulnerability in Huntington's disease. *Cell Death Differ.* Apr 2004; 11(4): 424–438.

18. Rivera-Mancia S, Perez-Neri I, Rios C, Tristan-Lopez L, Rivera-Espinosa L, Montes S. The transition metals copper and iron in neurodegenerative diseases. *Chem Biol Interact.* Jul 30 2010; 186(2): 184–199.

19. Fox JH, Kama JA, Lieberman G et al. Mechanisms of copper ion mediated Huntington's disease progression. *PLoS One.* 2007; 2(3): e334.

20. Kim J, Moody JP, Edgerly CK et al. Mitochondrial loss, dysfunction, and altered dynamics in Huntington's disease. *Hum Mol Genet.* Oct 15 2010; 19(20): 3919–3935.

21. Damiano M, Galvan L, Deglon N, Brouillet E. Mitochondria in Huntington's disease. *Biochim Biophys Acta.* Jan 2010; 1802(1): 52–61.

22. McGill JK, Beal MF. PGC-1 alpha, a new therapeutic target in Huntington's disease? *Cell.* Nov 3 2006; 127(3): 465–468.

23. Cui L, Jeong H, Borovecki F, Parkhurst CN, Tanese N, Krainc D. Transcriptional repression of PGC-1 alpha by mutant huntingtin leads to mitochondrial dysfunction and neurodegeneration. *Cell.* Oct 6 2006; 127(1): 59–69.

24. Tsunemi T, Ashe TD, Morrison BE et al. PGC-1 alpha rescues Huntington's disease proteotoxicity by preventing oxidative stress and promoting TFEB function. *Sci Translat Med.* Jul 11 2012; 4(142): 142ra197.

25. Martin E, Betuing S, Pages C et al. Mitogen- and stress-activated protein kinase 1-induced neuroprotection in Huntington's disease: Role on chromatin remodeling at the PGC-1-alpha promoter. *Hum Mol Genet.* Jun 15 2011; 20(12): 2422–2434.

26. Pavese N, Gerhard A, Tai YF et al. Microglial activation correlates with severity in Huntington disease: A clinical and PET study. *Neurology.* Jun 13 2006; 66(11): 1638–1643.

27. Tai YF, Pavese N, Gerhard A et al. Microglial activation in presymptomatic Huntington's disease gene carriers. *Brain.* Jul 2007; 130(Pt 7): 1759–1766.

28. Politis M, Pavese N, Tai YF et al. Microglial activation in regions related to cognitive function predicts disease onset in Huntington's disease: A multimodal imaging study. *Hum Brain Mapp.* Feb 2011; 32(2): 258–270.

29. Kraft AD, Kaltenbach LS, Lo DC, Harry GJ. Activated microglia proliferate at neurites of mutant huntingtin-expressing neurons. *Neurobiol Aging.* Mar 2012; 33(3): 621 e617–633.

30. Bjorkqvist M, Wild EJ, Thiele J et al. A novel pathogenic pathway of immune activation detectable before clinical onset in Huntington's disease. *J Exp Med.* Aug 4 2008; 205(8): 1869–1877.

31. Forrest CM, Mackay GM, Stoy N et al. Blood levels of kynurenines, interleukin-23, and soluble human leucocyte antigen-G at different stages of Huntington's disease. *J Neurochem.* Jan 2010; 112(1): 112–122.

32. Khoshnan A, Patterson PH. The role of IkappaB kinase complex in the neurobiology of Huntington's disease. *Neurobiol Dis.* Aug 2011; 43(2): 305–311.

33. Kalonia H, Kumar A. Suppressing inflammatory cascade by cyclo-oxygenase inhibitors attenuates quinolinic acid induced Huntington's disease-like alterations in rats. *Life Sci.* Apr 25 2011; 88(17–18): 784–791.

34. Kalonia H, Kumar P, Kumar A. Attenuation of proinflammatory cytokines and apoptotic process by verapamil and diltiazem against quinolinic acid induced Huntington like alterations in rats. *Brain Res.* Feb 4 2011; 1372: 115–126.

35. Xifro X, Garcia-Martinez JM, Del Toro D, Alberch J, Perez-Navarro E. Calcineurin is involved in the early activation of NMDA-mediated cell death in mutant huntingtin knock-in striatal cells. *J Neurochem.* Jun 2008; 105(5): 1596–1612.

36. Miller BR, Dorner JL, Bunner KD et al. Up-regulation of GLT1 reverses the deficit in cortically evoked striatal ascorbate efflux in the R6/2 mouse model of Huntington's disease. *J Neurochem.* May 2012; 121(4): 629–638.

37. Rebec GV, Conroy SK, Barton SJ. Hyperactive striatal neurons in symptomatic Huntington R6/2 mice: Variations with behavioral state and repeated ascorbate treatment. *Neuroscience.* 2006; 137(1): 327–336.

38. Graham RK, Pouladi MA, Joshi P et al. Differential susceptibility to excitotoxic stress in YAC128 mouse models of Huntington disease between initiation and progression of disease. *J Neurosci.* Feb 18 2009; 29(7): 2193–2204.

39. Fan MM, Raymond LA. N-methyl-D-aspartate (NMDA) receptor function and excitotoxicity in Huntington's disease. *Prog Neurobiol.* Apr 2007; 81(5–6): 272–293.

40. Reiner A, Lafferty DC, Wang HB, Del Mar N, Deng YP. The group 2 metabotropic glutamate receptor agonist LY379268 rescues neuronal, neurochemical, and motor abnormalities in R6/2 Huntington's disease mice. *Neurobiol Dis.* Jul 2012; 47(1): 75–91.

41. Andre VM, Cepeda C, Levine MS. Dopamine and glutamate in Huntington's disease: A balancing act. *CNS Neurosci Ther.* Jun 2010; 16(3): 163–178.

42. Kunig G, Leenders KL, Sanchez-Pernaute R et al. Benzodiazepine receptor binding in Huntington's disease: [11C] flumazenil uptake measured using positron emission tomography. *Ann Neurol.* May 2000; 47(5): 644–648.

43. Rekik L, Daguin-Nerriere V, Petit JY, Brachet P. gamma-Aminobutyric acid type B receptor changes in the rat striatum and substantia nigra following intrastriatal quinolinic acid lesions. *J Neurosci Res.* Apr 2011; 89(4): 524–535.

44. Cepeda C, Starling AJ, Wu N et al. Increased GABAergic function in mouse models of Huntington's disease: Reversal by BDNF. *J Neurosci Res.* Dec 15 2004; 78(6): 855–867.

45. Yuen EY, Wei J, Zhong P, Yan Z. Disrupted GABAAR trafficking and synaptic inhibition in a mouse model of Huntington's disease. *Neurobiol Dis.* May 2012; 46(2): 497–502.

46. Robinson P, Lebel M, Cyr M. Dopamine D1 receptor-mediated aggregation of N-terminal fragments of mutant huntingtin and cell death in a neuroblastoma cell line. *Neuroscience.* May 15 2008; 153(3): 762–772.

47. Charvin D, Vanhoutte P, Pages C, Borrelli E, Caboche J. Unraveling a role for dopamine in Huntington's disease: The dual role of reactive oxygen species and D2 receptor stimulation. *Proc Natl Acad Sci U S A.* Aug 23 2005; 102(34): 12,218–12,223.

48. Charvin D, Roze E, Perrin V et al. Haloperidol protects striatal neurons from dysfunction induced by mutated huntingtin *in vivo. Neurobiol Dis.* Jan 2008; 29(1): 22–29.
49. Pavese N, Politis M, Tai YF et al. Cortical dopamine dysfunction in symptomatic and premanifest Huntington's disease gene carriers. *Neurobiol Dis.* Feb 2010; 37(2): 356–361.
50. Esmaeilzadeh M, Farde L, Karlsson P et al. Extrastriatal dopamine D(2) receptor binding in Huntington's disease. *Hum Brain Mapp.* Oct 2011; 32(10): 1626–1636.
51. Politis M, Pavese N, Tai YF, Tabrizi SJ, Barker RA, Piccini P. Hypothalamic involvement in Huntington's disease: An in vivo PET study. *Brain.* Nov 2008; 131(Pt 11): 2860–2869.
52. Ortiz AN, Kurth BJ, Osterhaus GL, Johnson MA. Impaired dopamine release and uptake in R6/1 Huntington's disease model mice. *Neurosci Lett.* Mar 29 2011; 492(1): 11–14.
53. Ortiz AN, Osterhaus GL, Lauderdale K et al. Motor function and dopamine release measurements in transgenic Huntington's disease model rats. *Brain Res.* Apr 23 2012; 1450: 148–156.
54. Ruiz C, Casarejos MJ, Rubio I et al. The dopaminergic stabilizer, (-)-OSU6162, rescues striatal neurons with normal and expanded polyglutamine chains in huntingtin protein from exposure to free radicals and mitochondrial toxins. *Brain Res.* Jun 12 2012; 1459: 100–112.
55. Glass M, Dragunow M, Faull RL. Cannabinoid receptors in the human brain: A detailed anatomical and quantitative autoradiographic study in the fetal, neonatal, and adult human brain. *Neuroscience.* Mar 1997; 77(2): 299–318.
56. Glass M, Dragunow M, Faull RL. The pattern of neurodegeneration in Huntington's disease: A comparative study of cannabinoid, dopamine, adenosine, and GABA(A) receptor alterations in the human basal ganglia in Huntington's disease. *Neuroscience.* 2000; 97(3): 505–519.
57. Van Laere K, Casteels C, Dhollander I et al. Widespread decrease of type 1 cannabinoid receptor availability in Huntington disease *in vivo. J Nucl Med.* Sep 2010; 51(9): 1413–1417.
58. Glass M, van Dellen A, Blakemore C, Hannan AJ, Faull RL. Delayed onset of Huntington's disease in mice in an enriched environment correlates with delayed loss of cannabinoid CB1 receptors. *Neuroscience.* 2004; 123(1): 207–212.
59. Blazquez C, Chiarlone A, Sagredo O et al. Loss of striatal type 1 cannabinoid receptors is a key pathogenic factor in Huntington's disease. *Brain.* Jan 2011; 134(Pt 1): 119–136.
60. Pintor A, Tebano MT, Martire A et al. The cannabinoid receptor agonist WIN 55,212-2 attenuates the effects induced by quinolinic acid in the rat striatum. *Neuropharmacology.* Oct 2006; 51(5): 1004–1012.
61. Sagredo O, Gonzalez S, Aroyo I et al. Cannabinoid CB2 receptor agonists protect the striatum against malonate toxicity: Relevance for Huntington's disease. *Glia.* Aug 15 2009; 57(11): 1154–1167.
62. Bouchard J, Truong J, Bouchard K et al. Cannabinoid receptor 2 signaling in peripheral immune cells modulates disease onset and severity in mouse models of Huntington's disease. *J Neurosci.* Dec 12 2012; 32(50): 18259–18268.
63. Dowie MJ, Howard ML, Nicholson LF, Faull RL, Hannan AJ, Glass M. Behavioural and molecular consequences of chronic cannabinoid treatment in Huntington's disease transgenic mice. *Neuroscience.* Sep 29 2010; 170(1): 324–336.
64. Martire A, Calamandrei G, Felici F et al. Opposite effects of the A2A receptor agonist CGS21680 in the striatum of Huntington's disease versus wild-type mice. *Neurosci Lett.* Apr 24 2007; 417(1): 78–83.
65. Mievis S, Blum D, Ledent C. A2A receptor knockout worsens survival and motor behaviour in a transgenic mouse model of Huntington's disease. *Neurobiol Dis.* Feb 2011; 41(2): 570–576.

66. Rajput PS, Kharmate G, Norman M et al. Somatostatin receptor 1 and 5 double knockout mice mimic neurochemical changes of Huntington's disease transgenic mice. *PLoS One.* 2011; 6(9): e24467.

67. Giorgini F, Moller T, Kwan W et al. Histone deacetylase inhibition modulates kynurenine pathway activation in yeast, microglia, and mice expressing a mutant huntingtin fragment. *J Biol Chem.* Mar 21 2008; 283(12): 7390–7400.

68. Ruiz C, Casarejos MJ, Gomez A, Solano R, de Yebenes JG, Mena MA. Protection by glia-conditioned medium in a cell model of Huntington disease. *PLoS Curr.* 2012; 4: e4fbca54a2028b.

69. Zuccato C, Cattaneo E. Role of brain-derived neurotrophic factor in Huntington's disease. *Prog Neurobiol.* Apr 2007; 81(5–6): 294–330.

70. Sadri-Vakili G, Cha JH. Histone deacetylase inhibitors: A novel therapeutic approach to Huntington's disease (complex mechanism of neuronal death). *Curr Alzheimer Res.* Sep 2006; 3(4): 403–408.

71. Thomas EA, Coppola G, Desplats PA et al. The HDAC inhibitor 4b ameliorates the disease phenotype and transcriptional abnormalities in Huntington's disease transgenic mice. *Proc Natl Acad Sci U S A.* Oct 7 2008; 105(40): 15564–15569.

72. Bithell A, Johnson R, Buckley NJ. Transcriptional dysregulation of coding and noncoding genes in cellular models of Huntington's disease. *Biochem Soc Trans.* Dec 2009; 37(Pt 6): 1270–1275.

73. Buckley NJ, Johnson R, Zuccato C, Bithell A, Cattaneo E. The role of REST in transcriptional and epigenetic dysregulation in Huntington's disease. *Neurobiol Dis.* Jul 2010; 39(1): 28–39.

74. Yanai A, Huang K, Kang R et al. Palmitoylation of huntingtin by HIP14 is essential for its trafficking and function. *Nat Neurosci.* Jun 2006; 9(6): 824–831.

75. Young FB, Butland SL, Sanders SS, Sutton LM, Hayden MR. Putting proteins in their place: Palmitoylation in Huntington disease and other neuropsychiatric diseases. *Prog Neurobiol.* May 2012; 97(2): 220–238.

76. Sutton LM, Sanders SS, Butland SL et al. Hip14l-deficient mice develop neuropathological and behavioural features of Huntington disease. *Hum Mol Genet.* Feb 1 2013; 22(3): 452–465.

77. Dong G, Gross K, Qiao F et al. Calretinin interacts with huntingtin and reduces mutant huntingtin-caused cytotoxicity. *J Neurochem.* Nov 2012; 123(3): 437–446.

78. Farrar AM, Callahan JW, Abercrombie ED. Reduced striatal acetylcholine efflux in the R6/2 mouse model of Huntington's disease: An examination of the role of altered inhibitory and excitatory mechanisms. *Exp Neurol.* Dec 2011; 232(2): 119–125.

79. Itoh K, Chiba T, Takahashi S et al. An Nrf2/small Maf heterodimer mediates the induction of phase II detoxifying enzyme genes through antioxidant response elements. *Biochem Biophys Res Commun.* Jul 18 1997; 236(2): 313–322.

80. Hayes JD, Chanas SA, Henderson CJ et al. The Nrf2 transcription factor contributes both to the basal expression of glutathione S-transferases in mouse liver and to their induction by the chemopreventive synthetic antioxidants, butylated hydroxyanisole and ethoxyquin. *Biochem Soc Trans.* Feb 2000; 28(2): 33–41.

81. Chan K, Han XD, Kan YW. An important function of Nrf2 in combating oxidative stress: Detoxification of acetaminophen. *Proc Natl Acad Sci U S A.* Apr 10 2001; 98(8): 4611–4616.

82. Williamson TP, Johnson DA, Johnson JA. Activation of the Nrf2-ARE pathway by siRNA knockdown of Keap 1 reduces oxidative stress and provides partial protection from MPTP-mediated neurotoxicity. *Neurotoxicology.* Jun 2012; 33(3): 272–279.

83. Niture SK, Kaspar JW, Shen J, Jaiswal AK. Nrf2 signaling and cell survival. *Toxicol Appl Pharmacol.* Apr 1 2010; 244(1): 37–42.

84. Xi YD, Yu HL, Ding J et al. Flavonoids protect cerebrovascular endothelial cells through Nrf2 and PI3K from beta-aamyloid peptide-induced oxidative damage. *Curr Neurovasc Res.* Feb 2012; 9(1): 32–41.

85. Li XH, Li CY, Lu JM, Tian RB, Wei J. Allicin ameliorates cognitive deficits ageing-induced learning and memory deficits through enhancing of Nrf2 antioxidant signaling pathways. *Neurosci Lett.* Apr 11 2012; 514(1): 46–50.

86. Bergstrom P, Andersson HC, Gao Y et al. Repeated transient sulforaphane stimulation in astrocytes leads to prolonged Nrf2-mediated gene expression and protection from superoxide-induced damage. *Neuropharmacology.* Feb–Mar 2011; 60(2–3): 343–353.

87. Wruck CJ, Gotz ME, Herdegen T, Varoga D, Brandenburg LO, Pufe T. Kavalactones protect neural cells against amyloid beta peptide-induced neurotoxicity via extracellular signal-regulated kinase 1/2-dependent nuclear factor erythroid 2-related factor 2 activation. *Mol Pharmacol.* Jun 2008; 73(6): 1785–1795.

88. Hine CM, Mitchell JR. NRF2 and the phase II response in acute stress resistance induced by dietary restriction. *J Clin Exp Pathol.* Jun 19 2012; S4(4).

89. Suh JH, Shenvi SV, Dixon BM et al. Decline in transcriptional activity of Nrf2 causes age-related loss of glutathione synthesis, which is reversible with lipoic acid. *Proc Natl Acad Sci U S A.* Mar 9 2004; 101(10): 3381–3386.

90. Jin YN, Yu YV, Gundemir S et al. Impaired mitochondrial dynamics and Nrf2 signaling contribute to compromised responses to oxidative stress in striatal cells expressing full-length mutant huntingtin. *PLoS One.* 2013; 8(3): e57932.

91. Tasset I, Perez-Herrera A, Medina FJ, Arias-Carrion O, Drucker-Colin R, Tunez I. Extremely low-frequency electromagnetic fields activate the antioxidant pathway Nrf2 in a Huntington's disease-like rat model. *Brain Stimul.* Jan 2013; 6(1): 84–86.

92. Ellrichmann G, Petrasch-Parwez E, Lee DH et al. Efficacy of fumaric acid esters in the R6/2 and YAC128 models of Huntington's disease. *PLoS One.* 2011; 6(1): e16172.

93. Calkins MJ, Jakel RJ, Johnson DA, Chan K, Kan YW, Johnson JA. Protection from mitochondrial complex II inhibition *in vitro* and *in vivo* by Nrf2-mediated transcription. *Proc Natl Acad Sci U S A.* Jan 4 2005; 102(1): 244–249.

94. Bahramisharif A, van Gerven MA, Aarnoutse EJ et al. Propagating neocortical gamma bursts are coordinated by traveling alpha waves. *J Neurosci.* Nov 27 2013; 33(48): 18849–18854.

95. Zou Y, Hong B, Fan L et al. Protective effect of puerarin against beta-amyloid-induced oxidative stress in neuronal cultures from rat hippocampus: Involvement of the GSK-3beta/Nrf2 signaling pathway. *Free Radic Res.* Jan 2013; 47(1): 55–63.

96. Choi HK, Pokharel YR, Lim SC et al. Inhibition of liver fibrosis by solubilized coenzyme Q_{10}: Role of Nrf2 activation in inhibiting transforming growth factor-beta1 expression. *Toxicol Appl Pharmacol.* Nov 1 2009; 240(3): 377–384.

97. Trujillo J, Chirino YI, Molina-Jijon E, Anderica-Romero AC, Tapia E, Pedraza-Chaverri J. Renoprotective effect of the antioxidant curcumin: Recent findings. *Redox biology.* 2013; 1(1): 448–456.

98. Steele ML, Fuller S, Patel M, Kersaitis C, Ooi L, Munch G. Effect of Nrf2 activators on release of glutathione, cysteinylglycine and homocysteine by human U373 astroglial cells. *Redox Biol.* 2013;1(1): 441–445.

99. Kode A, Rajendrasozhan S, Caito S, Yang SR, Megson IL, Rahman I. Resveratrol induces glutathione synthesis by activation of Nrf2 and protects against cigarette smoke-mediated oxidative stress in human lung epithelial cells. *Am J Physiol Lung Cell Mol Physiol.* Mar 2008; 294(3): L478–488.

100. Gao L, Wang J, Sekhar KR et al. Novel n-3 fatty acid oxidation products activate Nrf2 by destabilizing the association between Keap1 and Cullin3. *J Biol Chem.* Jan 26 2007; 282(4): 2529–2537.

101. Saw CL, Yang AY, Guo Y, Kong AN. Astaxanthin and omega-3 fatty acids individually and in combination protect against oxidative stress via the Nrf2-ARE pathway. *Food Chem Toxicol.* Dec 2013; 62: 869–875.
102. Ji L, Liu R, Zhang XD et al. N-acetylcysteine attenuates phosgene-induced acute lung injury via upregulation of Nrf2 expression. *Inhal Toxicol.* Jun 2010; 22(7): 535–542.
103. Zambrano S, Blanca AJ, Ruiz-Armenta MV et al. The renoprotective effect of L-carnitine in hypertensive rats is mediated by modulation of oxidative stress-related gene expression. *Eur J Nutr.* Sep 2013; 52(6): 1649–1659.
104. Messier EM, Day BJ, Bahmed K et al. N-acetylcysteine protects murine alveolar type II cells from cigarette smoke injury in a nuclear erythroid 2-related factor-2-independent manner. *Am J Respir Cell Mol Biol.* May 2013; 48(5): 559–567.
105. Romanque P, Cornejo P, Valdes S, Videla LA. Thyroid hormone administration induces rat liver Nrf2 activation: Suppression by N-acetylcysteine pretreatment. *Thyroid.* Jun 2011; 21(6): 655–662.
106. Abate A, Yang G, Dennery PA, Oberle S, Schroder H. Synergistic inhibition of cyclo-oxygenase-2 expression by vitamin E and aspirin. *Free Radic Biol Med.* Dec 2000; 29(11): 1135–1142.
107. Devaraj S, Tang R, Adams-Huet B et al. Effect of high-dose alpha-tocopherol supplementation on biomarkers of oxidative stress and inflammation and carotid atherosclerosis in patients with coronary artery disease. *Am J Clin Nutr.* Nov 2007; 86(5): 1392–1398.
108. Fu Y, Zheng S, Lin J, Ryerse J, Chen A. Curcumin protects the rat liver from CCl4-caused injury and fibrogenesis by attenuating oxidative stress and suppressing inflammation. *Mol Pharmacol.* Feb 2008; 73(2): 399–409.
109. Lee HS, Jung KK, Cho JY et al. Neuroprotective effect of curcumin is mainly mediated by blockade of microglial cell activation. *Pharmazie.* Dec 2007; 62(12): 937–942.
110. Peairs AT, Rankin JW. Inflammatory response to a high-fat, low-carbohydrate weight loss diet: Effect of antioxidants. *Obesity (Silver Spring).* May 1 2008.
111. Rahman S, Bhatia K, Khan AQ et al. Topically applied vitamin E prevents massive cutaneous inflammatory and oxidative stress responses induced by double application of 12-O-tetradecanoylphorbol-13-acetate (TPA) in mice. *Chem Biol Interact.* Apr 15 2008; 172(3): 195–205.
112. Suzuki YJ, Aggarwal BB, Packer L. Alpha-lipoic acid is a potent inhibitor of NF-kappaB activation in human T cells. *Biochem Biophys Res Commun.* Dec 30 1992; 189(3): 1709–1715.
113. Zhu J, Yong W, Wu X et al. Antiinflammatory effect of resveratrol on TNF-alpha-induced MCP-1 expression in adipocytes. *Biochem Biophys Res Commun.* May 2 2008; 369(2): 471–477.
114. Barger SW, Goodwin ME, Porter MM, Beggs ML. Glutamate release from activated microglia requires the oxidative burst and lipid peroxidation. *J Neurochem.* Jun 2007; 101(5): 1205–1213.
115. Schubert D, Kimura H, Maher P. Growth factors and vitamin E modify neuronal glutamate toxicity. *Proc Natl Acad Sci U S A.* Sep 1 1992; 89(17): 8264–8267.
116. Sandhu JK, Pandey S, Ribecco-Lutkiewicz M et al. Molecular mechanisms of glutamate neurotoxicity in mixed cultures of NT2-derived neurons and astrocytes: Protective effects of coenzyme Q_{10}. *J Neurosci Res.* Jun 15 2003; 72(6): 691–703.
117. Peyser CE, Folstein M, Chase GA et al. Trial of d-alpha-tocopherol in Huntington's disease. *Am J Psychiatry.* Dec 1995; 152(12): 1771–1775.
118. Rebec GV, Barton SJ, Marseilles AM, Collins K. Ascorbate treatment attenuates the Huntington behavioral phenotype in mice. *Neuroreport.* Jul 1 2003; 14(9): 1263–1265.

119. Sandhir R, Sood A, Mehrotra A, Kamboj SS. N-Acetylcysteine reverses mitochondrial dysfunctions and behavioral abnormalities in 3-nitropropionic acid-induced Huntington's disease. *Neurodegener Dis.* 2012; 9(3): 145–157.

120. Andreassen OA, Ferrante RJ, Dedeoglu A, Beal MF. Lipoic acid improves survival in transgenic mouse models of Huntington's disease. *Neuroreport.* Oct 29 2001; 12(15): 3371–3373.

121. Hickey MA, Zhu C, Medvedeva V, Franich NR, Levine MS, Chesselet MF. Evidence for behavioral benefits of early dietary supplementation with coenzyme Q_{10} in a slowly progressing mouse model of Huntington's disease. *Mol Cell Neurosci.* Feb 2012; 49(2): 149–157.

122. Smith KM, Matson S, Matson WR et al. Dose ranging and efficacy study of high-dose coenzyme Q_{10} formulations in Huntington's disease mice. *Biochim Biophys Acta.* Jun 2006; 1762(6): 616–626.

123. Yang L, Calingasan NY, Wille EJ et al. Combination therapy with coenzyme Q_{10} and creatine produces additive neuroprotective effects in models of Parkinson's and Huntington's diseases. *J Neurochem.* Jun 2009; 109(5): 1427–1439.

124. Silva-Adaya D, Perez-De La Cruz V, Herrera-Mundo MN et al. Excitotoxic damage, disrupted energy metabolism, and oxidative stress in the rat brain: Antioxidant and neuroprotective effects of L-carnitine. *J Neurochem.* May 2008; 105(3): 677–689.

125. Vamos E, Voros K, Vecsei L, Klivenyi P. Neuroprotective effects of L-carnitine in a transgenic animal model of Huntington's disease. *Biomed Pharmacother.* Apr 2010; 64(4): 282–286.

126. Kumar P, Kumar A. Effect of lycopene and epigallocatechin-3-gallate against 3-nitropropionic acid induced cognitive dysfunction and glutathione depletion in rat: A novel nitric oxide mechanism. *Food Chem Toxicol.* Oct 2009; 47(10): 2522–2530.

127. Wang X, Sirianni A, Pei Z et al. The melatonin MT1 receptor axis modulates mutant Huntingtin-mediated toxicity. *J Neurosci.* Oct 12 2011; 31(41): 14,496–14,507.

128. Hickey MA, Zhu C, Medvedeva V et al. Improvement of neuropathology and transcriptional deficits in CAG 140 knock-in mice supports a beneficial effect of dietary curcumin in Huntington's disease. *Mol Neurodegener.* 2012; 7: 12.

129. Kumar P, Padi SS, Naidu PS, Kumar A. Effect of resveratrol on 3-nitropropionic acid-induced biochemical and behavioural changes: Possible neuroprotective mechanisms. *Behav Pharmacol.* Sep 2006; 17(5–6): 485–492.

130. Maher P, Dargusch R, Bodai L, Gerard PE, Purcell JM, Marsh JL. ERK activation by the polyphenols fisetin and resveratrol provides neuroprotection in multiple models of Huntington's disease. *Hum Mol Genet.* Jan 15 2011; 20(2): 261–270.

131. Mahdy HM, Tadros MG, Mohamed MR, Karim AM, Khalifa AE. The effect of Ginkgo biloba extract on 3-nitropropionic acid-induced neurotoxicity in rats. *Neurochem Int.* Nov 2011; 59(6): 770–778.

132. Tasset I, Pontes AJ, Hinojosa AJ, de la Torre R, Tunez I. Olive oil reduces oxidative damage in a 3-nitropropionic acid-induced Huntington's disease-like rat model. *Nutr Neurosci.* May 2011; 14(3): 106–111.

133. Colle D, Hartwig JM, Soares FA, Farina M. Probucol modulates oxidative stress and excitotoxicity in Huntington's disease models *in vitro*. *Brain Res Bull.* Mar 10 2012; 87(4–5): 397–405.

134. Hathorn T, Snyder-Keller A, Messer A. Nicotinamide improves motor deficits and upregulates PGC-1 alpha and BDNF gene expression in a mouse model of Huntington's disease. *Neurobiol Dis.* Jan 2011; 41(1): 43–50.

135. Sorolla MA, Rodriguez-Colman MJ, Tamarit J et al. Protein oxidation in Huntington disease affects energy production and vitamin B_6 metabolism. *Free Radic Biol Med.* Aug 15 2010; 49(4): 612–621.

136. Shoulson I. DATATOP: A decade of neuroprotective inquiry. Parkinson Study Group. Deprenyl and tocopherol antioxidative therapy of Parkinsonism. *Ann Neurol.* Sep 1998; 44(3 Suppl 1): S160–S166.

137. Sano M, Ernesto C, Thomas RG et al. A controlled trial of selegiline, alpha-tocopherol, or both as treatment for Alzheimer's disease. The Alzheimer's Disease Cooperative Study. *N Engl J Med.* Apr 24 1997; 336(17): 1216–1222.

138. Farina N, Isaac MG, Clark AR, Rusted J, Tabet N. Vitamin E for Alzheimer's dementia and mild cognitive impairment. *Cochrane Database Syst Rev.* 2012; 11: CD002854.

139. Albanes D, Heinonen OP, Huttunen JK et al. Effects of alpha-tocopherol and beta-carotene supplements on cancer incidence in the Alpha-Tocopherol Beta-Carotene Cancer Prevention Study. *Am J Clin Nutr.* Dec 1995; 62(6 Suppl): 1427S–1430S.

140. Krinsky NI. Antioxidant functions of carotenoids. *Free Radic Biol Med.* 1989; 7(6): 617–635.

141. Hazuka MB, Edwards-Prasad J, Newman F, Kinzie JJ, Prasad KN. Beta-carotene induces morphological differentiation and decreases adenylate cyclase activity in melanoma cells in culture. *J Am Coll Nutr.* Apr 1990; 9(2): 143–149.

142. Zhang LX, Cooney RV, Bertram JS. Carotenoids up-regulate connexin 43 gene expression independent of their provitamin A or antioxidant properties. *Cancer Res.* Oct 15 1992; 52(20): 5707–5712.

143. Carter CA, Pogribny M, Davidson A, Jackson CD, McGarrity LJ, Morris SM. Effects of retinoic acid on cell differentiation and reversion toward normal in human endometrial adenocarcinoma (RL95-2) cells. *Anticancer Res.* Jan–Feb 1996; 16(1): 17–24.

144. Meyskens Jr FL. Role of vitamin A and its derivatives in the treatment of human cancer. In: Prasad KN, Santamaria L, Williams RM, eds. *Nutrients in Cancer Prevention and Treatment.* New Jersey: Humana Press. 1995; 349–362.

145. Vile GF, Winterbourn CC. Inhibition of adriamycin-promoted microsomal lipid peroxidation by beta-carotene, alpha-tocopherol, and retinol at high and low oxygen partial pressures. *FEBS Lett.* Oct 10 1988; 238(2): 353–356.

146. McCay PB. Vitamin E: Interactions with free radicals and ascorbate. *Annu Rev Nutr.* 1985; 5: 323–340.

147. Prasad KN, Kumar B, Yan XD, Hanson AJ, Cole WC. Alpha-tocopheryl succinate, the most effective form of vitamin E for adjuvant cancer treatment: A review. *J Am Coll Nutr.* Apr 2003; 22(2): 108–117.

148. Schwartz JL. Molecular and biochemical control of tumor growth following treatment with carotenoids or tocopherols. In: Prasad KN, Santamaria L, Williams RM, eds. *Nutrients in Cancer Prevention and Treatment.* New Jersey: Humana Press. 1995; 287–316.

149. Prasad KN, Edwards-Prasad J. Vitamin E and cancer prevention: Recent advances and future potentials. *J Am Coll Nutr.* Oct 1992; 11(5): 487–500.

150. Witschi A, Reddy S, Stofer B, Lauterburg BH. The systemic availability of oral glutathione. *Eur J Clin Pharmacol.* 1992; 43(6): 667–669.

151. Niki E. Mechanisms and dynamics of antioxidant action of ubiquinol. *Mol Aspects Med.* 1997; 18 Suppl: S63–S70.

152. Hiramatsu M, Velasco RD, Wilson DS, Packer L. Ubiquinone protects against loss of tocopherol in rat liver microsomes and mitochondrial membranes. *Res Commun Chem Pathol Pharmacol.* May 1991; 72(2): 231–241.

153. Chen RS, Huang CC, Chu NS. Coenzyme Q_{10} treatment in mitochondrial encephalomyopathies. Short-term double-blind, crossover study. *Eur Neurol.* 1997; 37(4): 212–218.

154. Shults CW, Oakes D, Kieburtz K et al. Effects of coenzyme Q_{10} in early Parkinson disease: Evidence of slowing of the functional decline. *Arch Neurol.* Oct 2002; 59(10): 1541–1550.

155. Liu D, Pitta M, Mattson MP. Preventing NAD$^{(+)}$ depletion protects neurons against excitotoxicity: Bioenergetic effects of mild mitochondrial uncoupling and caloric restriction. *Ann NY Acad Sci.* Dec 2008; 1147: 275–282.

156. Gaziano JM, Sesso HD, Christen WG et al. Multivitamins in the prevention of cancer in men: The Physicians' Health Study II randomized controlled trial. *JAMA.* Nov 14 2012; 308(18): 1871–1880.

157. Baum MK, Campa A, Lai S et al. Effect of micronutrient supplementation on disease progression in asymptomatic, antiretroviral-naive, HIV-infected adults in Botswana: A randomized clinical trial. *JAMA.* Nov 27 2013; 310(20): 2154–2163.

158. Albini A, Morini M, D'Agostini F et al. Inhibition of angiogenesis-driven Kaposi's sarcoma tumor growth in nude mice by oral N-acetylcysteine. *Cancer Res.* Nov 15 2001; 61(22): 8171–8178.

159. Brusa L, Orlacchio A, Moschella V, Iani C, Bernardi G, Mercuri NB. Treatment of the symptoms of Huntington's disease: Preliminary results comparing aripiprazole and tetrabenazine. *Mov Disord.* Jan 15 2009; 24(1): 126–129.

160. de Yebenes JG, Landwehrmeyer B, Squitieri F et al. Pridopidine for the treatment of motor function in patients with Huntington's disease (MermaiHD): A phase 3, randomised, double-blind, placebo-controlled trial. *Lancet Neurol.* Dec 2011; 10(12): 1049–1057.

161. Investigators THSGH. A randomized, double-blind, placebo-controlled trial of pridopidine in Huntington disease. *Mov Disord.* 2013.

6 Etiology of Post-traumatic Stress Disorders

Prevention and Improved Management by Micronutrients

INTRODUCTION

Post-traumatic stress disorder (PTSD) is a complex mental disorder often resulting from exposure to sudden or repeatedly extreme traumatic events such as war, terrorism, natural or human-caused disaster, as well as violent personal assault, such as rape, mugging, domestic violence, and accidents. There is also a strong direct relationship between mild traumatic brain injury (mTBI) and PTSD.[1,2] The symptoms of PTSD often appear within 3 months of the exposure to traumatic stressors, and they include unwanted reexperiencing of the trauma in memory (flashbacks, nightmares, and triggered emotional responses), passive and active avoidance (emotional numbing and avoidance of discussions about the traumatic event), and hyperarousal.[3] In addition, PTSD is usually accompanied by other psychiatric and medical comorbidities, including depression, substance abuse, cognitive dysfunction, and other problems of physical and mental health, and in some cases, it can lead to suicide. It has been reported that PTSD is associated with general learning and memory impairment.[4] These problems may lead to impairment of the ability to function in social life or family life including occupational instability, marital stress, and family problems. Some of the symptoms of PTSD overlap with other diseases including chronic fatigue syndrome, fibromyalgia, and multiple chemical sensitivities.[5]

At present, there are no prevention strategies for the onset of PTSD. The current gold standard management of PTSD involves antidepressant medications that rarely yield better than 40% reduction in the Clinician Administered PTSD Scale (CAPS) scores, but most patients still exhibit PTSD symptoms at the end of any treatment trial.[6] Therefore, additional approaches that attenuate some biochemical events that contribute to the development and progression of PTSD should be developed.

This chapter briefly describes the incidence, prevalence, cost, and some biochemical events that initiate and promote PTSD. In addition, this chapter discusses the role of increased oxidative stress, chronic inflammation, and glutamate release in the initiation and progression of PTSD. This chapter also proposes that supplementation with a preparation of micronutrients containing dietary and endogenous antioxidants, and certain polyphenolic compounds (curcumin and resveratrol), would reduce oxidative stress indirectly by enhancing the levels of antioxidant enzymes through a nuclear transcription factor (Nrf2)/ARE (antioxidant response element), and directly by scavenging free radicals. The same preparation of micronutrients may also reduce chronic inflammation and the release and toxicity of glutamate.

PREVALENCE, INCIDENCE, AND COST OF PTSD

The U.S. National Comorbidity Survey Replication (NCS-R) estimated that the lifetime prevalence of PTSD among adult Americans is 6.8%.[7] The lifetime prevalence of PTSD among men was 3.6% and among women was 9.7%. The 1-year prevalence of PTSD was estimated to be 1.8% in men and 5.2% in women.

Children and adolescents, who are exposed to at least one specific traumatic event, such as abuse or natural disaster, have higher prevalence of PTSD than adults in the general population. The 6-month prevalence of PTSD among adolescents between the ages of 13–17 years was estimated to be 3.7% for boys and 6.3% for girls.[7]

PTSD affects about 7.7 million Americans over the ages of 18 or about 3.5% of people in this age group in a given year.[8] In a recent large-scale study of military personnel in the current combat theatres, it was demonstrated that U.S. Army and Marine Corps personnel returning from duty in Iraq exhibited PTSD rates of 18% and 20%, respectively.[9] Before deployment, only 5% of soldiers showed PTSD symptoms, but after a full year of deployment, about 17% of soldiers exhibited PTSD symptoms. The rate of increase in PTSD was proportional to the length of their stay in Iraq[10] (Table 6.1). The number of soldiers with PTSD may further increase due to repeated combat deployments.[11]

In 2007, the National Center for Post-traumatic Disorder estimated that the incidence of PTSD among Vietnam veterans is about 30.9% for men and 26.9% for women. An additional 22.5% of men and 21.2% of women have had partial PTSD. This constitutes about 1.7 million Vietnam veterans, who have experienced clinically

TABLE 6.1
Incidence of Partial and Fully Established PTSD in U.S. Military Personnel after Deployment

Source	Incidence (%)
Veterans from Iraq, 2006	18–20
Veterans from Vietnam, 2007	30.9 in men
	26.9 in women
	22.5 partial PTSD in men
	21.2 partial PTSD in women

Note: The incidence of PTSD in U.S. troops before deployment was 5%. The incidence of PTSD appears to increase with time as well as with repeated combat deployment.

significant combat-related stress disorder. Among the total Gulf War veterans, the prevalence of PTSD was estimated to be 10.1%.[7]

The estimated societal cost of PTSD and depression among returning troops for 2 years varied from about $6000 to more than $25,000 per case. The total cost including direct medical treatment and care, lost productivity, and suicide for 2 years ranges from $4 billion to $6.2 billion (Rand Corporation analysis, 2008). In 2010, Veteran Health Administration (VHA) spent $2 billion (in 2011 dollars) to treat veterans with PTSD.

NEUROPATHOLOGY

The neuropathology of patients with PTSD is not well defined, possibly due to the lack of sufficient autopsied brain tissues. Most data on neuropathology have been obtained by examining the brain tissue by MRI (magnetic resonance imaging). The reduction in the volume of certain areas of the brain, particularly in the hippocampus, has been consistently observed. For example, reduction in the hippocampal volume was found in patients with PTSD.[12–14] The loss of hippocampal volume may account for cognitive dysfunction commonly observed in patients with PTSD. MRI scanning of the brains of patients with PTSD revealed that accelerated brain atrophy occurred throughout the brain, particularly in the brain stem and frontal and temporal lobes. Accelerated brain atrophy was associated with increased severity of the PTSD symptoms.[15] In addition, it was observed that greater rates of brain atrophy were associated with greater rates of decline in verbal memory and delayed facial recognition. Another MRI study showed that the cortical gray matter abnormalities, particularly in the frontal and occipital lobes, decreased in patients with PTSD compared to that in healthy controls.[16] Using MRI technique, it was shown that the reduction of gray matter volume in the left anterior cingulate cortex was associated with the development of PTSD, whereas the reduction of gray matter volume in the right pulvinar and left pallidus was associated with severe trauma without PTSD.[17] In addition, the atrophy of the frontal and limbic cortices was associated with the severity of the PTSD symptoms. MRI study on the brains of twins with or without PTSD revealed that significant reduction in gray matter volume occurred in four brain regions: right hippocampus, pregenual anterior cingulate cortex, and left and right insulae in twins with PTSD compared to that in twins without PTSD.[18]

The cerebellum of the brain is involved in fear perception, anticipation, and recollection. Examination of the brain by the MRI technique showed that the reduction in volume of the cerebellum was associated with mood change, anxiety, and PTSD symptoms, whereas the reduction in the volume of the vermis was associated with an early traumatic life experiences, and may be considered as a risk factor for future development of PTSD.[19] Examination of the brain by MRI revealed that the volume of the left amygdala, right amygdala. and left hippocampus was reduced in patients with PTSD compared to trauma exposed individuals without PTSD; however, the right hippocampus was not reduced in patients with PTSD.[20] Studies on the scanning of brain with MRI suggested that greater reexperiencing score predicted reduced volume of the middle temporal and inferior occipital cortices, whereas increased reports of flashback predicted reduced volume of the insula/parietal operculum and inferior temporal gyrus in patients with PTSD.[21]

A review of nine studies with 319 subjects revealed that the reduction in gray matter in the anterior cingulate cortex, ventromedial prefrontal cortex, left temporal pole/middle temporal gyrus, and left hippocampus occurred in patients with PTSD compared to individuals exposed to trauma without PTSD.[22]

Serotonin transporter (5-HTT) located in the amygdala regulates stress response. Therefore, deficient 5-HTT function and abnormal amygdala activity may contribute to the development of PTSD. This was shown by the fact that patients with PTSD exhibited reduced amygdala expression of 5-HTT, as measured by PET (positron emission tomography) using a radioactive tracer of 5-HTT[11] (C-AFM). It was observed that reduced amygdala 5-HTT binding was associated with higher anxiety and depression symptoms in patients with PTSD.[23]

MAJOR BIOCHEMICAL EVENTS

The biochemical events responsible for initiation and progression of PTSD are not fully understood; however, some that contribute to the initiation and progression of PTSD include increased oxidative stress and chronic inflammation, and the release of glutamate. These biochemical events can provide a basis for developing an effective strategy for reducing the risk of developing PTSD and improving its current management (Table 6.2).

INCREASED OXIDATIVE STRESS IN PTSD

There are some studies which show that increased oxidative stress may be involved in the initiation and progression of some human chronic neurological disorders, including psychiatric disorders and PTSD.[24] Stress evokes a sustained increase in nitric oxide synthase (NOS) activity that can generate excessive amounts of nitric oxide.[25,26] The oxidation of nitric oxide produces peroxynitrite that is very toxic to nerve cells.[27] It has been proposed that the deficiency of tetrahydrobioptrin causes NOS to produce superoxide,[28] which can oxidize nitric oxide to produce peroxynitrite. Peroxynitrite can then damage vital molecules, thus repeating a vicious cycle of producing increased levels of peroxynitrite. The combination of high-NOS activity and low levels of tetrahydrobioptrin

TABLE 6.2
Biochemical Events Responsible for Initiation and Progression of PTSD

Biochemical Events	Status
Markers of oxidative stress	Increases
Markers of chronic inflammation	Increases
Glutamate release	Increases
Certain gene expression profiles	Altered
Extinction of conditioned fear	Impaired

can produce a sustainable increase in peroxynitrite levels. Indeed, elevated levels of peroxynitrite and its precursor nitric oxide have been observed in patients with PTSD.[29]

Platelet monoamine oxidase, which generates excessive amounts of free radicals while degrading catecholamines, is also elevated in patients with PTSD.[30] This is further confirmed by the fact that the depletion of catecholamines has been observed in patients with PTSD.[31] Peroxynitrite and other free radicals increase the level of oxidative damage in the brain tissue of patients with PTSD, causing cognitive and other brain dysfunction. The above studies in humans support the view that the increased levels of oxidative stress may contribute to the development of PTSD and associated cognitive dysfunctions. This was confirmed in animal models of PTSD.

Severe life stresses can induce PTSD-like symptoms. A review has described the impact of severe life stress in animals, which includes sleep deprivation and social isolation.[32] Rats exposed to single prolonged stress exhibit symptoms of PTSD. It has been demonstrated that rats exposed to single prolonged stress showed apoptosis in the hippocampus region of the brain and impaired spatial memory. These effects were mediated by Bcl2 (B-cell lymphoid-2) and *Bax* genes.[33] Rats exposed to foot shock and maternal separation (forms of stress) exhibited impaired spatial memory and increased number of DNA breaks in the hippocampus.[34] It is interesting to point out that increased oxidative stress has also been observed in other neurodegenerative diseases, such as Alzheimer's disease.[35] Thus, the attenuation of oxidative stress appears to be one of the rational choices for reducing the risk of onset and progression of PTSD.

INCREASED CHRONIC INFLAMMATION IN PTSD

In addition to increased oxidative stress, increased chronic inflammation due to activation of microglia may be associated with PTSD. For example, serum levels of interleukin-6 (IL-6) are elevated in patients with PTSD.[36] Increased levels of IL-6, and IL-6 receptors, were found in patients with PTSD.[37] High levels of tumor necrosis factor-alpha (TNF-alpha) and IL-1-beta were elevated in patients with PTSD in comparison to control subjects.[38] Psychological stress also induces chronic inflammation.[39] Chronic fear of terror in women, but not in men, is associated with elevated levels of C-reactive protein (CRP) that may contribute to increased risk of cardiovascular disease in patients with PTSD.[40] The levels of CRP and receptor to IL-6 were elevated in patients with PTSD.[41] A study has reported that in men, but not in women, the episodes of depression is associated with increased levels of CRP[42]; however, others have reported no such association.[43]

In a clinical study on 35 severely traumatized patients with PTSD and 25 healthy controls, it was demonstrated that spontaneous production of proinflammatory cytokines IL-1β, IL-6, and TNF-alpha by peripheral blood mononuclear cells (PBMCs) was significantly higher in patients with PTSD than in healthy individuals. Furthermore, the increased levels of these proinflammatory cytokines correlated with the severity of symptoms.[44] However, circulating plasma levels of proinflammatory and anti-inflammatory cytokines, such as IL-6, IL-8, IL-10, TNF-alpha, or monocyte chemotactic protein (MCP)-1 were not significantly changed either in patients with PTSD or in healthy controls. These studies suggest the presence of low-grade inflammation in patients with PTSD.

In a clinical study on 48 patients with an established pain disorder or PTSD and 48 age- and gender-matched healthy controls, it was found that the levels of proinflammatory cytokines were detectable in the serum of 87% of anxiety patients (men and women), but only 25% of healthy controls showed such changes.[45] Another clinical study on 50 patients with PTSD and 50 age- and gender-matched healthy control, it was shown that the levels of proinflammatory cytokines (IL-2, IL-4, IL-6, IL-8, and TNF-alpha) were elevated in the serum of patients with PTSD compared to healthy controls.[46]

The above studies suggest that increased levels of chronic inflammation may also contribute to the development of PTSD and associated behavior and cognitive dysfunctions. Enhanced chronic inflammation is also associated with certain neurodegenerative diseases such as Alzheimer's disease.[35] Thus, the attenuation of chronic inflammation may be one of the rational strategies for reducing the risk of onset and progression of PTSD.

Excess Release of Glutamate and Inhibition of Gamma-Aminobutyric Acid in PTSD

The glutamatergic systems appear to play an important role in the pathophysiology of PTSD.[47] The effect of glutamate is mediated by increasing the release of corticotropin-releasing factor (CRF) and subsequently activating the stress-response hormone cascade, which increases the extracellular levels of glutamate and NMDA receptor expression. Increased levels of CRF have been found in the cerebral spinal fluid (CSF) of patients with PTSD.[48] Stress-induced glutamate release and glucocorticoids have been implicated to cause hippocampal atrophy in patients with PTSD. This observation is not unexpected because glutamate in high doses is known to be neurotoxic. Glutamate and nitric oxide (NO) released during stress play a central role in maintaining anxiety disorders.[25,47,49,50] Stress activates glutamate-NMDA receptors and decreases brain-derived neurotrophic factors and excessive amounts of glutamate can cause death to cholinergic neurons that may account for the cognitive dysfunction associated with PTSD. Therefore, blocking the release of glutamate and reducing the toxicity of glutamate would be useful in reducing the risk and progression of PTSD symptoms. Indeed, antiglutamatergic agents such as lamotrigine improve some of the symptoms of PTSD (reexperiencing hyperarousal and avoidance).

The levels of gamma-aminobutyric acid (GABA) in the insular cortex were lower in patients with PTSD than in matched healthy control subjects. Lower levels of GABA were associated with higher state of anxiety.[51] Plasma levels of GABA were lower in patients with PTSD than in control subjects.[52] Lower levels of GABA can enhance the action of glutamate on PTSD symptoms.

Changes in Gene Expression Profiles

The expression profiles of certain genes in the mitochondria of autopsied samples of dorsolateral prefrontal cortex from patients with PTSD are altered in comparison to healthy control.[53] This study is important because the activity of the dorsolateral prefrontal cortex region of the brain that regulates working memory and fear responses is decreased in patients with PTSD.[53] The DNA microarray analysis of postmortem samples of prefrontal cortex from patients with major depression revealed that the expression profiles of some specific genes are altered in comparison to those from normal control.[54] The alterations in expression profile of certain genes are very interesting observations, but they have not been confirmed by real time polymerase chain reaction (PCR); therefore, additional studies would be needed to establish changes in the levels of specific genes that are associated with PTSD.

HOW TO REDUCE OXIDATIVE STRESS, CHRONIC INFLAMMATION, AND GLUTAMATE RELEASE

Significant studies discussed in this chapter suggest that increased oxidative stress, chronic inflammation, and the release of glutamate are involved in the initiation and progression of PTSD.

How to Reduce Oxidative Stress

Oxidative stress in the body occurs when the antioxidant system fails to provide adequate protection against damage produced by free radicals (reactive oxygen species and reactive nitrogen species). Increased oxidative stress in the body can be most effectively reduced by up-regulating antioxidant enzymes as well as by existing levels of dietary and endogenous antioxidant chemicals, because they work by different mechanisms. For example, antioxidant enzymes reduce free radicals by catalysis, whereas dietary and endogenous antioxidant chemicals reduce free radicals by directly scavenging them. In response to reactive oxygen species (ROS), a nuclear transcriptional factor, Nrf2 (nuclear factor-erythroid 2-related factor 2), was translocated from the cytoplasm to the nucleus, where it binds with ARE, which increases the levels of antioxidant enzymes (gamma-glutamylcysteine ligase, glutathione peroxidase, glutathione reductase, and heme oxygenase-1) and phase 2 detoxifying enzymes (NAD(P)H: quinine oxidoreductase 1 and glutathione-S-transferase), in order to reduce oxidative damage.[55–57] In response to increased oxidative stress, existing levels of dietary and endogenous antioxidant chemical levels cannot be elevated without supplementation.

Factors Regulating Response of Nrf2 and Its Action

Several studies suggest that antioxidant enzymes are elevated by Nrf2 activation, which depends upon ROS-dependent[58] and -independent[59–63] mechanisms. In addition, the levels of antioxidant enzymes are also dependent upon the binding ability of Nrf2 with ARE in the nucleus.[64]

DIFFERENTIAL RESPONSE OF Nrf2 TO ROS GENERATED DURING ACUTE AND CHRONIC OXIDATIVE STRESS

It appears that Nrf2 responds to ROS, generated during acute and chronic oxidative stress differently. For example, the excessive amounts of ROS are generated during acute oxidative stress observed during strenuous exercise. In response to ROS, Nrf2 translocates to the nucleus, where it binds with ARE to up-regulate antioxidant genes.

Excessive amounts of ROS are also present during chronic oxidative stress commonly observed in older individuals and neurological diseases, such as Parkinson's disease, Alzheimer's disease, and PTSD, suggesting that the Nrf2/ARE regulatory system has become unresponsive to ROS in these diseases. Age-related decline in antioxidant enzymes in the liver of older rats compared to that in younger rats was due to the reduction in the binding ability of Nrf2 with ARE; however, treatment with alpha-lipoic acid restored this defect, increased the levels of antioxidant enzymes, and restored the loss of glutathione from the liver of older rats.[64] The exact reasons for the Nrf2/ARE regulatory system to become unresponsive to ROS during chronic oxidative stress are unknown; however, defects in the binding ability of Nrf2 with ARE may be one of the reasons.

Nrf2 IN PTSD

No studies have been performed to evaluate the role of Nrf2 in PTSD. Since increased oxidative stress plays an important role in the initiation and progression of PTSD, the following groups of agents in combination may be useful in the prevention and improved management of PTSD:

1. *Agents that can reduce oxidative stress by directly scavenging free radicals without activating Nrf2-regulated antioxidant enzymes*: Some examples are dietary antioxidants, such as vitamin A, beta-carotene, vitamin C, and vitamin E, and endogenous antioxidants, such as glutathione, alpha-lipoic acid, and coenzyme Q_{10}.
2. *Agents that can reduce oxidative stress by activating Nfr2-regulated antioxidant genes without ROS stimulation*: Some examples are organosulfur compound sulforaphane found in cruciferous vegetables, kavalactones found in Kava shrubs, and Puerarin, a major flavonoid from the root of *Pueraria lobata*.[61,62,65] Genistein vitamin E[59] and coenzyme Q_{10}[66] also activate Nrf2 without ROS.
3. *Agents that can reduce oxidative stress directly by scavenging free radicals as well as indirectly by activating Nrf2/ARE pathway*: Some examples are vitamin E,[59] alpha-lipoic acid,[64] curcumin,[67] resveratrol,[68,69] omega-3-fatty acids,[70,71] and NAC.[72]
4. *Agents that can reduce oxidative stress by ROS stimulation*: They include L-carnitine which generates transient ROS.[73]

ACTIVATION OF Nrf2 BY DIET RESTRICTION

A review has revealed that dietary restriction also reduces oxidative stress by activating Nrf2-ARE pathways.[63] It appears that dietary restriction-induced Nrf2 activation does not require ROS stimulation. Dietary restriction-induced reduction in oxidative stress would be difficult to implement for a long period of time. Prolonged activation of Nrf2 by dietary restriction can produce unacceptable serious side effects.[74] Therefore, dietary restriction may not be suitable for reducing oxidative stress for the prevention or improved management of PTSD.

How to Reduce Chronic Inflammation and Glutamate

Some individual antioxidants from the above groups have been shown to reduce chronic inflammation[75-87] and prevent the release[88] and toxicity[89,90] of glutamate. A combination of selected agents from the above groups may reduce chronic inflammation and release of glutamate and its toxicity optimally, and thereby, may reduce the risk of developing PTSD, and in combination with standard therapy, may improve the management of this disease.

STUDIES ON ANTIOXIDANTS IN PTSD

The role of antioxidants in the prevention or improved management of PTSD has not been evaluated in humans. A few studies on the effects of antioxidants on PTSD as well as on other neurological disorders are described here.

Omega-3-Fatty Acids

It has been reported that daily supplementation with omega-3-fatty acids reduced some of the symptoms of PTSD in critically injured patients during the earthquake in Japan in 2011.[91] The question arose whether or not the supplementation with omega-3-fatty acids during maturation of brain can protect the adult brain against trauma, which increase the risk of developing PTSD. To answer this, rats were fed diets enriched or deficient in omega-3-fatty acids during the period of brain maturation. After attaining adulthood, rats were switched to a western diet and then subjected to mTBI, which increases the risk of developing PTSD. The result showed the following: animals fed with omega-3-fatty acid-rich diet exhibited an increase in anxiety behavior and neuropeptide Y receptor type 1 (NPY1R), which is a characteristic of PTSD.[92] These symptoms were aggravated in rats that were fed with omega-3-fatty acid-deficient diet during brain maturation, suggesting that a diet deficient in omega-3-fatty acids during the development may lower the threshold for developing certain neurological disorders, such as PTSD, in response to trauma or accident. These preliminary animal and human studies suggest that omega-3-fatty acids may reduce the risk of developing PTSD; however, additional studies are needed to substantiate the role of omega-3-fatty acids in the prevention of PTSD.

Curcumin

The administration of curcumin increased hippocampal neurogenesis in chronically stressed rats, similar to the effect of antidepressant imipramine treatment. New hippocampal cells mature and become neurons. In addition, curcumin treatment prevented stress-induced decline in serotonin receptor-1A (5-HT-1A) mRNA and brain-derived neurotrophic factor (BDNF) protein levels in the hippocampal regions.[93]

Flavonoids

Xiaobuxin-Tang (XBXT), a traditional Chinese herbal product, has been used for the treatment of depressive disorders for centuries in China. Flavonoids (XBXT-2) isolated from the extract of XBXT increased neurogenesis in the hippocampus of chronically stressed rats. In addition, this treatment with flavonoids prevented stress-induced decrease in BDNF.[94]

Effect of Multiple Micronutrients in Troops Returning from Iraq and Afghanistan

A commercial formulation of multiple micronutrients was tested in a clinical study on troops returning from Iraq and Afghanistan with mild to moderate TBI. Thirty-four patients with post-traumatic dizziness were admitted to the Naval Medical Center San Diego Clinic over a 2-month period and agreed to participate in the study under the supervision of Dr. Michael Hoffer and his colleagues.[95] All patients had received their injury 3–20 weeks prior to admission, and they received identical treatment consisting of medical therapy (for any migraines), supportive care, steroids, and vestibular rehabilitation therapy. Fifteen of the 34 patients also received a dose of an antioxidant and micronutrient formula (two capsules by mouth twice a day). At the onset of therapy, all patients were evaluated in outcome measures, which included the Sensory Organization Test (SOT) by Computerized Dynamic Posturography (CDP), the Dynamic Gait Index (DGI), the Activities Balance Confidence (ABC) scale, the Dizziness Handicap Index (DHI), the Vestibular Disorders Activities of Daily Living (VADL) score, and the Balance Scoring System (BESS) test. The study was carried out for 12 weeks. The therapist, who graded these outcomes and performed the testing, was blinded as to whether the patient was receiving antioxidant therapy or not. The pretrial test scores did not differ significantly between the two groups on any of the tests.

Both groups of patients showed trends toward significant improvement on all tests after the 12 weeks of therapy, but the combination treatment trend was stronger than that of the standard therapy alone group. After only 4 weeks, the SOT score by CDP was 78 for the antioxidant group as compared to 63 for the nonantioxidant group. This difference was statistically significant at the level $P < 0.05$. The improvement noted by the antioxidant group on the other tests was also greater than the nonantioxidant group, although these differences did not reach statistical significance because of the short trial period and small sample size. This study should be expanded using a randomized, double-blind, and placebo-control clinical study design, in which the efficacy of the proposed multiple micronutrient preparation should be tested in soldiers returning from combat theaters, exhibiting mild to moderate traumatic brain injury, or any sign of mental disorders such as anxiety, fear, and depression.

Effects of Individual Antioxidants and B Vitamins on Other Neurodegenerative Diseases

The values of antioxidants in reducing the risk of cognitive dysfunction have been evaluated in other neurological diseases such as Alzheimer's disease and Parkinson's disease. It has been reported that beta-amyloid fragments, which are associated with neurodegeneration in Alzheimer's disease, mediate their actions by free radicals.[96] This is supported by the fact that vitamin E protects neuronal cells in culture against beta-amyloid-induced toxicity.[97] Vitamin E at a dose of 2000 IU per day produced some beneficial effects in patients with Alzheimer's disease.[98] Patients consuming antioxidants showed reduced risk of vascular dementia and slower decline of cognitive function in cases of dementia and Alzheimer's disease.[99] Glutathione deficiency has been consistently found in the autopsied brain samples from patients with neurological diseases such as Alzheimer's disease[100] and Parkinson's disease.[101,102]

Administration of coenzyme Q_{10} has been shown to improve clinical symptoms of mitochondrial encephalomyopathies[103] and only modest improvement in Parkinson's disease.[104] Others have reported inconsistent results with coenzyme Q_{10}.[105]

We have reported that PGE2, a product of inflammatory reactions, is very toxic to mature neurons, and a mixture of antioxidants reduces this toxicity.[106] In MPTP rat model of Parkinson's disease, an administration of a mixture of dietary and endogenous antioxidants before treatment with MPTP blocked MPTP-induced depletion of tyrosine hydroxylase (TH), a rate limiting enzyme in the biosynthesis of Dopa, as well as enhanced the expression of TH.[107] Antioxidants also blocked MPTP-induced hypokinesia. In addition, intravenous injection of vitamin B_{12} improved cognitive function in Alzheimer's disease.[108]

The studies discussed above suggest that a preparation of micronutrients containing antioxidant and other polyphenolic compounds, such as curcumin and resveratrol, which would reduce oxidative stress, chronic inflammation, and glutamate release, may be useful in reducing the risk of developing PTSD, and in combination with standard therapy, in reducing the progression, and improving the management of this disease.

PROPOSED PTSD PREVENTION STUDIES

PRIMARY PREVENTION

The purpose of primary prevention is to protect healthy individuals from developing PTSD. In case of PTSD, it is not possible to develop a primary prevention strategy, because some traumatic events that increase the risk of developing PTSD may occur suddenly. However, in some cases such as troops to be deployed in a military conflict, it is possible to develop primary prevention strategy, which can increase the threshold for developing PTSD following exposure to PTSD-related risk factors, such as blast and other traumatic events. Since exposure to PTSD-related risk factors generates excessive amounts of free radicals and inflammation, and since antioxidants and certain polyphenolic compounds reduce free radicals and inflammation, supplementation with a preparation of micronutrients containing dietary and endogenous antioxidants and polyphenolic compounds (curcumin and resveratrol) may be one of the rational choices for primary PTSD prevention. We will discuss it in detail later.

SECONDARY PREVENTION

The purpose of secondary prevention is to stop or delay the progression of PTSD in those individuals who are exposed to blast and other traumatic events, but have not developed clinical signs of PTSD and are not on PTSD-related medications.

Following exposure to PTSD-related risk factors, excessive amounts of free radicals and inflammation, which play an important role in the development and progression of PTSD, are produced. Therefore, supplementation with a preparation of micronutrients containing dietary and endogenous antioxidants and certain polyphenolic compounds may be one of the rational choices for reducing the risk of developing PTSD as well as for reducing the progression of the disease. Secondary prevention strategy should be implemented 24–48 h after exposure to PTSD-related risk factors. This is due to the fact that following exposure to PTSD-related risk factors, both anti-inflammatory and proinflammatory cytokines are released. Anti-inflammatory cytokines help repair cellular damage. Since antioxidants reduce inflammation, supplementation with antioxidants soon after exposure to PTSD-related risk factors may interfere with the repair processes.

PROBLEMS OF USING SINGLE MICRONUTRIENT IN PTSD

The use of single agents, such as curcumin, omega-3-fatty acids, and flavonoids, produced some benefits in a few animal models and human PTSD. These studies are not sufficient to draw any conclusion regarding the value of multiple micronutrients in reducing the risk of developing PTSD. Previous studies on the effect of single antioxidants in chronic diseases have produced inconsistent results. For example, the study on beta-carotene in male heavy smokers for reducing the risk of lung cancer, vitamin E in patients with Alzheimer's disease (AD) for improving cognitive function, and vitamin E in patients with Parkinson's disease (PD) for improving the symptoms, as expected, produced inconsistent results varying from no effect[109] to modest beneficial[98] as in PD, no effect as in AD,[110] or harmful effect as in heavy male smokers.[111] This is due to the fact that patients with the above diseases have high internal oxidative environments, in which individual antioxidant is oxidized and then acts as a pro-oxidant rather than as an antioxidant. An oxidized antioxidant is likely to increase the risk of chronic diseases after long-term consumption. Because of the failure to obtain consistent results with individual antioxidants in other neurodegenerative diseases, I recommend a preparation of micronutrients containing dietary and endogenous antioxidants, vitamin D, B vitamins, certain minerals, and polyphenolic compounds (resveratrol and curcumin), and omega-3-fatty acids for reducing the risk of developing PTSD.

RATIONALE FOR USING MULTIPLE MICRONUTRIENTS IN PTSD PREVENTION

The references for this section are described in a review.[35] The mechanisms of action of micronutrients and polyphenolic compounds in the proposed formulation are in part different; their distribution in various organs and cells, their affinity to various types of free radicals, and their biological half-lives are also different. Beta-carotene (BC) is more effective in quenching oxygen radicals than most other antioxidants. BC can perform certain biological functions that cannot be produced by its metabolite vitamin A, and vice versa. It has been reported that BC treatment enhances the expression of the connexin gene, which codes for a gap junction protein in mammalian fibroblasts in culture, whereas vitamin A treatment does not produce such an effect. Vitamin A can induce differentiation in certain normal and cancer cells, whereas BC and other carotenoids do not. Thus, BC and vitamin A have, in part, different biological functions in the body. The gradient of oxygen pressure varies within cells. Some antioxidants, such as vitamin E, are more effective as quenchers of free radicals in reduced oxygen pressure, whereas BC and vitamin A are more effective in higher atmospheric pressures. Vitamin C is necessary to protect cellular components in aqueous environments, whereas carotenoids and vitamins A and E protect cellular components in lipid environments. Vitamin C also plays an important role in maintaining the cellular levels of vitamin E by recycling vitamin E radical (oxidized) to the reduced (antioxidant) form.

The form of vitamin E, used in preparation of micronutrients, is also important. It has been established that D-alpha-tocopheryl succinate (vitamin E succinate) is the most effective form of vitamin in both in vitro and in vivo. This form of vitamin E is more soluble than alpha-tocopherol and enters cells more readily, and therefore, it is expected that vitamin E succinate would cross the blood–brain barrier in greater amounts than alpha-tocopherol. However, this idea has not yet been tested in animals or humans. We have reported that an oral ingestion of vitamin E succinate (800 IU/day) in humans increased plasma levels of not only alpha-tocopherol but also of vitamin E succinate, suggesting that a portion of this form of vitamin E can be absorbed from the intestinal tract before hydrolysis to alpha-tocopherol, provided that the plasma pool of alpha-tocopherol is saturated. This observation is important, because the conventional assumption, based on the studies in rodents, has indicated that esterified forms of vitamin E, such as alpha-tocopheryl succinate, alpha-tocopheryl nicotinate, and alpha-tocopheryl acetate, can be absorbed from the intestinal tract only after they are hydrolyzed to alpha-tocopherol. Our preliminary data showed that this assumption may not be true for the absorption of vitamin E succinate in humans, provided that the plasma pool of alpha-tocopherol is saturated.

An endogenous antioxidant, glutathione, is effective in catabolizing H_2O_2 and anions. However, oral supplementation with glutathione failed to significantly increase plasma levels of glutathione in human subjects, suggesting that this tripeptide is completely hydrolyzed in the GI tract. Therefore, I propose to utilize N-acetylcysteine and alpha-lipoic acid, which increases the cellular levels of glutathione by different mechanisms in a multiple micronutrient preparation.

Another endogenous antioxidant, coenzyme Q_{10}, may have some potential value in the prevention of PTSD. Since coenzyme Q_{10} is needed for the generation of ATP by mitochondria, it is essential to add this antioxidant in a multiple micronutrient preparation. A study has shown that coenzyme Q_{10} scavenges peroxy radicals faster than alpha-tocopherol, and like vitamin C, can regenerate vitamin E in a redox cycle. However, it is a weaker antioxidant than alpha-tocopherol. Coenzyme Q_{10} administration has been shown to improve clinical symptoms in patients with mitochondrial encephalomyopathies.[103]

Since memory loss occurs in PTSD, nicotinamide, a precursor of NAD+ attenuated glutamate-induced toxicity and preserved cellular levels of NAD+, to support the activity of SIRT-1. It is also a competitive inhibitor of histone deacetylase activity and restored memory deficits in AD transgenic mice. These preclinical data suggest that oral supplementation with nicotinamide may be safe and useful in preventing memory deficits.

Selenium is a cofactor of glutathione peroxidase, and Se-glutathione peroxidase acts as an antioxidant by increasing the intracellular level of glutathione. Therefore, selenium should be added to multiple micronutrient preparation for the prevention of PTSD.

In addition to dietary and endogenous antioxidants, all B vitamins with high doses of vitamin B_3 (nicotinamide) and vitamin D should be added to a multiple micronutrient preparation for maintaining normal health. Curcumin and omega-3-fatty acids were also added because they appear to produce some benefits in PTSD. Resveratrol is also added because it has produced some beneficial effects in other neurodegenerative diseases.

Dietary and endogenous antioxidants and polyphenolic compounds derived from herbs, fruits, and vegetables inhibit chronic inflammation.[75-87]

Fear and anxiety that are associated with PTSD release excessive amounts of glutamate. In addition, animal studies have suggested that increased proinflammatory stimuli and oxidative stress cause microglia to release excessive amounts of glutamate, which not only maintain anxiety disorders through NMDA receptor but also contributes to neurodegeneration.[88] The release of glutamate was blocked by vitamin E,[88] and this could help in improving anxiety disorders. Indeed, an inhibitor of the NMDA receptor reduces anxiety,[112] but is toxic. Both vitamin E[89] and coenzyme Q_{10}[90] also protect against glutamate-induced neurotoxicity in cell culture models.

PROPOSED MICRONUTRIENTS FOR PRIMARY PTSD PREVENTION

Studies on primary prevention can be performed on individuals, such as combat troops, who are going to be deployed in a military conflict, where they are likely to be exposed to PTSD-related risk factors, such as blast, mild traumatic brain injury, and other traumatic events. A preparation of multiple micronutrients may include vitamin A (retinyl palmitate), vitamin E (both D-alpha-tocopherol and D-alpha-TS), natural mixed carotenoids, vitamin C (calcium ascorbate), coenzyme Q_{10}, R-alpha-lipoic acid, n-acetylcysteine, L-carnitine, vitamin D, all B-vitamins, selenium, zinc, chromium, omega-3 fatty acids, and certain polyphenolic compounds (curcumin and resveratrol). No iron, copper, or manganese would be included, because these trace minerals are known to interact with vitamin C to produce free radicals. These trace minerals are absorbed from the intestinal tract more in the presence of antioxidants than in their absence that could result in increased body stores of free forms of these minerals. Increased iron stores have been linked to increased risk of some neurodegenerative diseases.[113] No heavy metals such as zirconium and molybdenum were added because of their potential neurotoxicity after long-term consumption.

The recommended micronutrient supplements should be taken daily, orally divided into two doses, one half in the morning and the other half in the evening with meal. This is because the biological half-lives of micronutrients are highly variable, which can create high levels of fluctuations in the tissue levels of micronutrients if they are consumed once a day. A twofold difference in the levels of certain micronutrients such as alpha-tocopheryl succinate can cause a marked difference in the expression of gene profiles.[114] In order to maintain relatively consistent levels of micronutrients in the brain, the proposed micronutrients should be taken twice a day.

The efficacy of proposed micronutrient formulation in troops to be deployed in military conflicts should be tested by well-designed clinical studies. Meanwhile, the proposed micronutrient recommendations may be adopted by individuals who are in combat theater or who have suffered from concussive injury during deployment in consultation with their physicians or health professionals. It is expected that the proposed recommendations would reduce the risk of developing PTSD.

TOXICITY OF INGREDIENTS IN PROPOSED MICRONUTRIENT PREPARATION

Antioxidants and B vitamins used in proposed micronutrient preparation are considered safe. Antioxidants at doses higher than those that are recommended for the proposed micronutrient preparation have been consumed by the U.S. population for decades without significant toxicity. However, a few of them could produce harmful effects at certain high doses in some individuals when consumed daily for a long period of time. For example, vitamin A at doses of 10,000 IU or more per day can cause birth defects in pregnant women, and beta-carotene at a 50 mg dose or more can produce bronzing of the skin, which is reversible on discontinuation. Vitamin C as ascorbic acid at high doses (10 g or more per day) can cause diarrhea in some individuals. Vitamin E at high doses (2000 IU or more per day) can induce clotting defects after long-term consumption. Vitamin B_6 at high doses (50 mg or more per day) may produce peripheral neuropathy, and selenium at doses 400 mcg or more per day can cause skin and liver toxicity after long-term consumption. Coenzyme Q_{10} has no known toxicity, and recommended daily doses are 30–400 mg. N-acetylcysteine doses of 250–1500 mg and alpha-lipoic acid doses of 600 mg are used in humans without toxicity at these doses. All ingredients present in the proposed micronutrient preparations are safe and come under the category of "Food Supplement" and therefore do not require FDA approval for their use.

PROPOSED MICRONUTRIENTS FOR SECONDARY PREVENTION IN HIGH-RISK POPULATIONS

High-risk populations for developing PTSD include troops or individuals who have already been exposed to PTSD-related risk factors, but have not developed any symptoms of the disease, and are not on PTSD-related medications. They provide an excellent opportunity to study the efficacy of a multiple micronutrient preparation in reducing the risk of developing PTSD. The efficacy of the proposed micronutrients preparation should be tested by well-designed clinical studies. Meanwhile, the proposed micronutrient recommendations may be adopted by the troops or individuals who have already been exposed PTSD-related risk factors, but have not developed any symptoms in consultation with their physicians or health professionals. It is expected that the proposed recommendations would reduce the risk of developing PTSD.

CURRENT STANDARD THERAPY FOR PTSD

The purpose of the treatment is to delay the progression of disease and improve the symptoms of the disease. Standard therapy includes drugs and psychological/psychiatric treatment. The drug therapy is primarily based on the symptoms rather than the causes of PTSD. The standard therapy has produced very limited success in the treatment of PTSD. None of the drugs used in the treatment of PTSD affect the levels of increased oxidative stress and chronic inflammation, which play an important role in the progression of PTSD. Therefore, additional approaches that could improve the management of PTSD and reduce the progression of the disease should be developed. Some examples of commonly used medications to improve the symptoms of PTSD are described below. Details can be found in the website of the United States Department of Veterans Affairs (National Center for PTSD, 2013).

SELECTIVE SEROTONIN REUPTAKE INHIBITORS

Serotonin is important in regulating several bodily functions including mood, anxiety, appetite, and sleep. Examples of selective serotonin reuptake inhibitors are sertraline (Zoloft), paroxetine (Paxil), and fluoxetine (Prozac).

ANTIDEPRESSANTS

Examples of antidepressants are mirtazapine (Remeron), venlafaxine (Effexor), and nefazodone (Serzone).

MOOD STABILIZERS

These medications are also called anticonvulsants or antiepileptic drugs. They block glutamate release or enhance GABA release or both. Mood stabilizer drugs include carbamazepine (Tegretol), divalproex (Depakote), lamotrigine (Lamictal), and topiramate (Topimax).

OTHER MEDICATIONS

Some examples are prazosin (Minipress), tricyclic antidepressants (imipramine), and monoamine oxidase inhibitors (Phenelzine).

BENZODIAZEPINES

These drugs directly act on the GABA system, which produces calming effects on the central nervous system, but they are potentially addictive and not very effective in core symptoms of PTSD. Examples of benzodiazepines are lorazepam (Ativan), clonazepam (klonopin), and alprazolam (Xanax).

D-SERINE

In a 6-week randomized, double-blind, placebo-controlled trial using 22 chronic PTSD outpatients, it was found that D-serine, an endogenous agonist of NMDA receptor at the site of glycine, may improve some of the symptoms of PTSD.[115] Antiglutamatergic agents, such as lamotrigine, was effective in reducing some of the symptoms of PTSD.[47] Selective serotonin reuptake inhibitors also were useful in improving the symptoms of PTSD.[116] The efficacy of other drugs in the treatment of PTSD, such as antidepressants, antiadrenergic agents, anticonvulsants, benzodiazepines, and atypical antipsychotics yielding variable degrees of improvement, has been reviewed.[117]

CYCLOSERINE

The extinction of conditioned fear appears to be defective in patients with PTSD. D-cycloserine, a partial agonist of NMDA receptor, was useful in enhancing the extinction of learned fear in rats.[118] This was achieved when D-cycloserine was administered shortly before or after the extinction training of rats.[119]

CORTISOL

Persistent retrieval and maintenance of traumatic memories is a biological process that keeps these memories vivid and thereby maintains the symptoms of PTSD. It has been demonstrated that elevated glucocorticoid levels inhibit the memory retrieval process in animals and humans.[120] In patients with PTSD, low-dose cortisol treatment for 1 month reduced symptoms of traumatic memories without causing adverse health effects, probably by preventing recall of traumatic memories.[120,121]

None of the drugs that are currently used in the treatment of PTSD addressed the issue of increased oxidative stress and chronic inflammation, which play an important role in the progression of PTSD. Therefore, I propose a novel micronutrient strategy, which in combination with standard therapy may reduce the progression and further improve the symptoms of PTSD.

RECOMMENDED MICRONUTRIENTS IN COMBINATION WITH STANDARD THERAPY IN PTSD

Increased oxidative stress and chronic inflammation, and glutamate release appear to play an important role in the progression of PTSD. The fact that antioxidants can reduce oxidative stress, chronic inflammation, and the release and toxicity of glutamate suggests that they may reduce the progression of the disease. The current standard therapies are not considered sufficient in the management of PTSD. The addition of a preparation of multiple micronutrients described in the section of primary prevention may improve the management of PTSD more than that produced by the standard therapy alone. In addition, supplementation with a preparation of micronutrients may reduce the progression of the disease. The efficacy of this micronutrient preparation in combination with standard therapy should be tested in patients with PTSD by well-designed clinical studies. Meanwhile, the proposed micronutrient recommendations may be adopted by individuals who are suffering from PTSD in consultation with their physicians or health professionals.

DIET AND LIFESTYLE RECOMMENDATIONS FOR PTSD

In addition to supplementation with the proposed micronutrient preparation, a balanced diet, low in fat, and high in fiber and rich in fruits and vegetables is very necessary for reducing the risk of developing PTSD, as well as for improving the efficacy of standard therapy in the management of PTSD. Lifestyle recommendations include daily moderate exercise, reduced stress, no tobacco smoking, and reduced intake of caffeine or alcoholic beverages.

CONCLUSIONS

In summary, PTSD is a complex mental disorder resulting from exposure to blast, sudden or repeated extreme traumatic events, and possibly other stressful environmental stressors. At present, there are no strategies to reduce the risk of developing PTSD. The current standard therapy of PTSD that includes drug therapy and psychological counseling is considered unsatisfactory. The major biochemical events that contribute to the initiation and progression of PTSD include increased oxidative stress, chronic inflammation, and the release of glutamate. Standard therapy does not influence these biochemical events; consequently, the disease continues to progress despite medication and other therapies. Oxidative stress can be optimally reduced by antioxidants and certain polyphenolic compounds, which increase antioxidant enzymes by activating Nrf2-ARE-regulated pathways as well as directly scavenging free radicals. These antioxidants and phenolic compounds also reduce inflammation and inhibit the release and toxicity of glutamate on neurons. Therefore, daily supplementation with these agents may be useful in reducing the risk of developing PTSD when administered orally before exposure to traumatic events. In addition, these agents, when combined with standard therapies, may reduce the progression and improve the symptoms of PTSD more than those produced by the standard therapy alone. A well-designed clinical study to test the efficacy of proposed micronutrient preparation in reducing the risk of PTSD in individuals, such as troops who are scheduled to be employed in military conflict should be initiated. Another clinical study to test the efficacy of proposed micronutrient preparation in combination with standard therapy in patients who have well-established PTSD should be initiated.

REFERENCES

1. Hoge CW, McGurk D, Thomas JL, Cox AL, Engel CC, Castro CA. Mild traumatic brain injury in U.S. Soldiers returning from Iraq. *N Engl J Med.* Jan 31 2008; 358(5): 453–463.
2. Schneiderman AI, Braver ER, Kang HK. Understanding sequelae of injury mechanisms and mild traumatic brain injury incurred during the conflicts in Iraq and Afghanistan: Persistent postconcussive symptoms and posttraumatic stress disorder. *Am J Epidemiol.* Jun 15 2008; 167(12): 1446–1452.

3. King DL, Leskin GA, Weathers, FW. Confirmatory factor analysis of the clinician-administered PTSD scale: Evidence for the dimensionality of postraumatic stress disorder. *Psychol Assess.* 1998; 10: 90–96.
4. Burriss L, Ayers E, Ginsberg J, Powell DA. Learning and memory impairment in PTSD: Relationship to depression. *Depress Anxiety.* 2008; 25(2): 149–157.
5. Stander VA, Merrill LL, Thomsen CJ, Milner JS. Posttraumatic stress symptoms in Navy personnel: Prevalence rates among recruits in basic training. *J Anxiety Disord.* 2007; 21(6): 860–870.
6. Hamner MB, Robert S, Frueh BC. Treatment-resistant posttraumatic stress disorder: Strategies for intervention. *CNS Spectr.* Oct 2004; 9(10): 740–752.
7. Gradus JL. *Epidemiology of PTSD.* National Center for PTSD. 2011.
8. Kessler RC, Chiu WT, Demler O, Merikangas KR, Walters EE. Prevalence, severity, and comorbidity of 12-month DSM-IV disorders in the National Comorbidity Survey Replication. *Arch Gen Psychiatry.* Jun 2005; 62(6): 617–627.
9. Hoge CW, Castro CA, Messer SC, McGurk D, Cotting DI, Koffman RL. Combat duty in Iraq and Afghanistan, mental health problems, and barriers to care. *N Engl J Med.* Jul 1 2004; 351(1): 13–22.
10. Castro C, Hoge CW. Building psychological resiliency and mitigating the risks of combat and deplyment stressors faced by soldiers. Presented at *NATO Human Factors and Medicine Panel Symposium, Prague, Czech Republic, October 3–5, 2005.*
11. Friedman MJ. Veterans' mental health in the wake of war. *N Engl J Med.* Mar 31 2005; 352(13): 1287–1290.
12. Bremner JD, Scott TM, Delaney RC et al. Deficits in short-term memory in posttraumatic stress disorder. *Am J Psychiatry.* Jul 1993; 150(7): 1015–1019.
13. Tischler L, Brand SR, Stavitsky K et al. The relationship between hippocampal volume and declarative memory in a population of combat veterans with and without PTSD. *Ann N Y Acad Sci.* Jul 2006; 1071: 405–409.
14. Villarreal G, Hamilton DA, Petropoulos H et al. Reduced hippocampal volume and total white matter volume in posttraumatic stress disorder. *Biol Psychiatry.* Jul 15 2002; 52(2): 119–125.
15. Cardenas VA, Samuelson K, Lenoci M et al. Changes in brain anatomy during the course of posttraumatic stress disorder. *Psychiatry Res.* Aug 30 2011; 193(2): 93–100.
16. Tavanti M, Battaglini M, Borgogni F et al. Evidence of diffuse damage in frontal and occipital cortex in the brain of patients with post-traumatic stress disorder. *Neurol Sci.* Feb 2012; 33(1): 59–68.
17. Chen Y, Fu K, Feng C et al. Different regional gray matter loss in recent onset PTSD and non PTSD after a single prolonged trauma exposure. *PloS One.* 2012; 7(11): e48298.
18. Kasai K, Yamasue H, Gilbertson MW, Shenton ME, Rauch SL, Pitman RK. Evidence for acquired pregenual anterior cingulate gray matter loss from a twin study of combat-related posttraumatic stress disorder. *Biol Psychiatry.* Mar 15 2008; 63(6): 550–556.
19. Baldacara L, Jackowski AP, Schoedl A et al. Reduced cerebellar left hemisphere and vermal volume in adults with PTSD from a community sample. *J Psychiatr Res.* Dec 2011; 45(12): 1627–1633.
20. Morey RA, Gold AL, LaBar KS et al. Amygdala volume changes in posttraumatic stress disorder in a large case-controlled veterans group. *Arch Gen Psychiatry.* Nov 2012; 69(11): 1169–1178.
21. Kroes MC, Whalley MG, Rugg MD, Brewin CR. Association between flashbacks and structural brain abnormalities in posttraumatic stress disorder. *Eur Psychiatry.* Nov 2011; 26(8): 525–531.
22. Kuhn S, Gallinat J. Gray matter correlates of posttraumatic stress disorder: A quantitative meta-analysis. *Biol Psychiatry.* Jan 1 2013; 73(1): 70–74.

23. Murrough JW, Huang Y, Hu J et al. Reduced amygdala serotonin transporter binding in posttraumatic stress disorder. *Biol Psychiatry.* Dec 1 2011; 70(11): 1033–1038.

24. Bremner JD. Stress and brain atrophy. *CNS Neurol Disord Drug Targets.* Oct 2006; 5(5): 503–512.

25. Harvey BH, Bothma T, Nel A, Wegener G, Stein DJ. Involvement of the NMDA receptor, NO-cyclic GMP and nuclear factor K-beta in an animal model of repeated trauma. *Hum Psychopharmacol.* Jul 2005; 20(5): 367–373.

26. Harvey BH, Oosthuizen F, Brand L, Wegener G, Stein DJ. Stress-restress evokes sustained iNOS activity and altered GABA levels and NMDA receptors in rat hippocampus. *Psychopharmacology (Berl).* Oct 2004; 175(4): 494–502.

27. Pall ML, Satterlee JD. Elevated nitric oxide/peroxynitrite mechanism for the common etiology of multiple chemical sensitivity, chronic fatigue syndrome, and posttraumatic stress disorder. *Ann N Y Acad Sci.* Mar 2001; 933: 323–329.

28. Pall ML. Nitric oxide synthase partial uncoupling as a key switching mechanism for the NO/ONOO-cycle. *Med Hypotheses.* 2007; 69(4): 821–825.

29. Tezcan E, Atmaca M, Kuloglu M, Ustundag B. Free radicals in patients with posttraumatic stress disorder. *Eur Arch Psychiatry Clin Neurosci.* Apr 2003; 253(2): 89–91.

30. Richardson JS. On the functions of monoamine oxidase, the emotions, and adaptation to stress. *Int J Neurosci.* May 1993; 70(1–2): 75–84.

31. Pivac N, Knezevic J, Kozaric-Kovacic D et al. Monoamine oxidase (MAO) intron 13 polymorphism and platelet MAO-B activity in combat-related posttraumatic stress disorder. *J Affect Disord.* Nov 2007; 103(1–3): 131–138.

32. Schiavone S, Jaquet V, Trabace L, Krause KH. Severe life stress and oxidative stress in the brain: From animal models to human pathology. *Antioxid Redox Signal.* Apr 20 2013; 18(12): 1475–1490.

33. Li X, Han F, Liu D, Shi Y. Changes of Bax, Bcl-2 and apoptosis in hippocampus in the rat model of post-traumatic stress disorder. *Neurol Res.* Jul 2010; 32(6): 579–586.

34. Diehl LA, Alvares LO, Noschang C et al. Long-lasting effects of maternal separation on an animal model of post-traumatic stress disorder: Effects on memory and hippocampal oxidative stress. *Neurochem Res.* Apr 2012; 37(4): 700–707.

35. Prasad KN, Cole WC, Prasad KC. Risk factors for Alzheimer's disease: Role of multiple antioxidants, non-steroidal anti-inflammatory and cholinergic agents alone or in combination in prevention and treatment. *J Am Coll Nutr.* Dec 2002; 21(6): 506–522.

36. Yehuda R. Biology of posttraumatic stress disorder. *J Clin Psychiatry.* 2001; 62 Suppl 17: 41–46.

37. Maes M, Lin AH, Delmeire L et al. Elevated serum interleukin-6 (IL-6) and IL-6 receptor concentrations in posttraumatic stress disorder following accidental man-made traumatic events. *Biol Psychiatry.* Apr 1 1999; 45(7): 833–839.

38. von Kanel R, Hepp U, Kraemer B et al. Evidence for low-grade systemic proinflammatory activity in patients with posttraumatic stress disorder. *J Psychiatr Res.* Nov 2007; 41(9): 744–752.

39. Sutherland AG, Alexander DA, Hutchison JD. Disturbance of pro-inflammatory cytokines in post-traumatic psychopathology. *Cytokine.* Dec 7 2003; 24(5): 219–225.

40. Melamed S, Shirom A, Toker S, Berliner S, Shapira I. Association of fear of terror with low-grade inflammation among apparently healthy employed adults. *Psychosom Med.* Jul–Aug 2004; 66(4): 484–491.

41. Miller RJ, Sutherland AG, Hutchison JD, Alexander DA. C-reactive protein and interleukin 6 receptor in post-traumatic stress disorder: A pilot study. *Cytokine.* Feb 21 2001; 13(4): 253–255.

42. Danner M, Kasl SV, Abramson JL, Vaccarino V. Association between depression and elevated C-reactive protein. *Psychosom Med.* May–Jun 2003; 65(3): 347–356.

43. Douglas KM, Taylor AJ, O'Malley PG. Relationship between depression and C-reactive protein in a screening population. *Psychosom Med.* Sep–Oct 2004; 66(5): 679–683.
44. Gola H, Engler H, Sommershof A et al. Posttraumatic stress disorder is associated with an enhanced spontaneous production of pro-inflammatory cytokines by peripheral blood mononuclear cells. *BMC Psychiatry.* 2013; 13: 40.
45. Hoge EA, Brandstetter K, Moshier S, Pollack MH, Wong KK, Simon NM. Broad spectrum of cytokine abnormalities in panic disorder and posttraumatic stress disorder. *Depress Anxiety.* 2009; 26(5): 447–455.
46. Guo M, Liu T, Guo JC, Jiang XL, Chen F, Gao YS. Study on serum cytokine levels in posttraumatic stress disorder patients. *Asian Pac J Tropic Med.* Apr 2012; 5(4): 323–325.
47. Nair J, Singh Ajit S. The role of the glutamatergic system in posttraumatic stress disorder. *CNS Spectr.* Jul 2008; 13(7): 585–591.
48. Bremner JD, Licinio J, Darnell A et al. Elevated CSF corticotropin-releasing factor concentrations in posttraumatic stress disorder. *Am J Psychiatry.* May 1997; 154(5): 624–629.
49. Joca SR, Ferreira FR, Guimaraes FS. Modulation of stress consequences by hippocampal monoaminergic, glutamatergic and nitrergic neurotransmitter systems. *Stress.* Aug 2007; 10(3): 227–249.
50. Trist DG. Excitatory amino acid agonists and antagonists: Pharmacology and therapeutic applications. *Pharm Acta Helv.* Mar 2000; 74(2–3): 221–229.
51. Rosso IM, Weiner MR, Crowley DJ, Silveri MM, Rauch SL, Jensen JE. Insula and anterior cingulate Gaba levels in posttraumatic stress disorder: Preliminary findings using magnetic resonance spectroscopy. *Depress Anxiety.* Jul 16 2013.
52. Vaiva G, Boss V, Ducrocq F et al. Relationship between posttrauma GABA plasma levels and PTSD at 1-year follow-up. *Am J Psychiatry.* Aug 2006; 163(8): 1446–1448.
53. Su YA, Wu J, Zhang L et al. Dysregulated mitochondrial genes and networks with drug targets in postmortem brain of patients with posttraumatic stress disorder (PTSD) revealed by human mitochondria-focused cDNA microarrays. *Int J Biol Sci.* 2008; 4(4): 223–235.
54. Tochigi M, Iwamoto K, Bundo M, Sasaki T, Kato N, Kato T. Gene expression profiling of major depression and suicide in the prefrontal cortex of postmortem brains. *Neurosci Res.* Feb 2008; 60(2): 184–191.
55. Itoh K, Chiba T, Takahashi S et al. An Nrf2/small Maf heterodimer mediates the induction of phase II detoxifying enzyme genes through antioxidant response elements. *Biochem Biophys Res Commun.* Jul 18 1997; 236(2): 313–322.
56. Hayes JD, Chanas SA, Henderson CJ et al. The Nrf2 transcription factor contributes both to the basal expression of glutathione S-transferases in mouse liver and to their induction by the chemopreventive synthetic antioxidants, butylated hydroxyanisole and ethoxyquin. *Biochem Soc Trans.* Feb 2000; 28(2): 33–41.
57. Chan K, Han XD, Kan YW. An important function of Nrf2 in combating oxidative stress: Detoxification of acetaminophen. *Proc Natl Acad Sci U S A.* Apr 10 2001; 98(8): 4611–4616.
58. Niture SK, Kaspar JW, Shen J, Jaiswal AK. Nrf2 signaling and cell survival. *Toxicol Appl Pharmacol.* Apr 1 2010; 244(1): 37–42.
59. Xi YD, Yu HL, Ding J et al. Flavonoids protect cerebrovascular endothelial cells through Nrf2 and PI3K from beta-amyloid peptide-induced oxidative damage. *Curr Neurovasc Res.* Feb 2012; 9(1): 32–41.
60. Li XH, Li CY, Lu JM, Tian RB, Wei J. Allicin ameliorates cognitive deficits ageing-induced learning and memory deficits through enhancing of Nrf2 antioxidant signaling pathways. *Neurosci Lett.* Apr 11 2012; 514(1): 46–50.

61. Bergstrom P, Andersson HC, Gao Y et al. Repeated transient sulforaphane stimulation in astrocytes leads to prolonged Nrf2-mediated gene expression and protection from superoxide-induced damage. *Neuropharmacology.* Feb–Mar 2011; 60(2–3): 343–353.

62. Wruck CJ, Gotz ME, Herdegen T, Varoga D, Brandenburg LO, Pufe T. Kavalactones protect neural cells against amyloid beta peptide-induced neurotoxicity via extracellular signal-regulated kinase 1/2-dependent nuclear factor erythroid 2-related factor 2 activation. *Mol Pharmacol.* Jun 2008; 73(6): 1785–1795.

63. Hine CM, Mitchell JR. NRF2 and the phase II response in acute stress resistance induced by dietary restriction. *J Clin Exp Pathol.* Jun 19 2012; S4(4).

64. Suh JH, Shenvi SV, Dixon BM et al. Decline in transcriptional activity of Nrf2 causes age-related loss of glutathione synthesis, which is reversible with lipoic acid. *Proc Natl Acad Sci U S A.* Mar 9 2004; 101(10): 3381–3386.

65. Zou Y, Hong B, Fan L et al. Protective effect of puerarin against beta-amyloid-induced oxidative stress in neuronal cultures from rat hippocampus: Involvement of the GSK-3beta/Nrf2 signaling pathway. *Free Radic Res.* Jan 2013; 47(1): 55–63.

66. Choi HK, Pokharel YR, Lim SC et al. Inhibition of liver fibrosis by solubilized coenzyme Q_{10}: Role of Nrf2 activation in inhibiting transforming growth factor-beta1 expression. *Toxicol aAppl Pharmacol.* Nov 1 2009; 240(3): 377–384.

67. Trujillo J, Chirino YI, Molina-Jijon E, Anderica-Romero AC, Tapia E, Pedraza-Chaverri J. Renoprotective effect of the antioxidant curcumin: Recent findings. *Redox Biol.* 2013; 1(1): 448–456.

68. Steele ML, Fuller S, Patel M, Kersaitis C, Ooi L, Munch G. Effect of Nrf2 activators on release of glutathione, cysteinylglycine and homocysteine by human U373 astroglial cells. *Redox Biol.* 2013; 1(1): 441–445.

69. Kode A, Rajendrasozhan S, Caito S, Yang SR, Megson IL, Rahman I. Resveratrol induces glutathione synthesis by activation of Nrf2 and protects against cigarette smoke-mediated oxidative stress in human lung epithelial cells. *Am J Physiol Lung Cell Mol Physiol.* Mar 2008; 294(3): L478–L488.

70. Gao L, Wang J, Sekhar KR et al. Novel n-3 fatty acid oxidation products activate Nrf2 by destabilizing the association between Keap1 and Cullin3. *J Biol Chem.* Jan 26 2007; 282(4): 2529–2537.

71. Saw CL, Yang AY, Guo Y, Kong AN. Astaxanthin and omega-3 fatty acids individually and in combination protect against oxidative stress via the Nrf2-ARE pathway. *Food Chemical Toxicol.* Dec 2013; 62: 869–875.

72. Ji L, Liu R, Zhang XD et al. N-acetylcysteine attenuates phosgene-induced acute lung injury via up-regulation of Nrf2 expression. *Inhal Toxicol.* Jun 2010; 22(7): 535–542.

73. Zambrano S, Blanca AJ, Ruiz-Armenta MV et al. The renoprotective effect of L-carnitine in hypertensive rats is mediated by modulation of oxidative stress-related gene expression. *Eur J Nutr.* Sep 2013; 52(6): 1649–1659.

74. Wakabayashi N, Itoh K, Wakabayashi J et al. Keap1-null mutation leads to postnatal lethality due to constitutive Nrf2 activation. *Nat Genet.* Nov 2003; 35(3): 238–245.

75. Abate A, Yang G, Dennery PA, Oberle S, Schroder H. Synergistic inhibition of cyclooxygenase-2 expression by vitamin E and aspirin. *Free Radic Biol Med.* Dec 2000; 29(11): 1135–1142.

76. Devaraj S, Tang R, Adams-Huet B et al. Effect of high-dose alpha-tocopherol supplementation on biomarkers of oxidative stress and inflammation and carotid atherosclerosis in patients with coronary artery disease. *Am J Clin Nutr.* Nov 2007; 86(5): 1392–1398.

77. Fu Y, Zheng S, Lin J, Ryerse J, Chen A. Curcumin protects the rat liver from CCl4-caused injury and fibrogenesis by attenuating oxidative stress and suppressing inflammation. *Mol Pharmacol.* Feb 2008; 73(2): 399–409.

78. Hori K, Hatfield D, Maldarelli F, Lee BJ, Clouse KA. Selenium supplementation suppresses tumor necrosis factor alpha-induced human immunodeficiency virus type 1 replication in vitro. *AIDS Res Hum Retroviruses.* Oct 10 1997; 13(15): 1325–1332.
79. Jesudason EP, Masilamoni JG, Ashok BS et al. Inhibitory effects of short-term administration of DL-alpha-lipoic acid on oxidative vulnerability induced by Abeta amyloid fibrils (25–35) in mice. *Mol Cell Biochem.* Apr 2008; 311(1–2): 145–156.
80. Kuhlmann MK, Levin NW. Potential Interplay between Nutrition and Inflammation in Dialysis Patients. *Contrib Nephrol.* 2008; 161: 76–82.
81. Lee HS, Jung KK, Cho JY et al. Neuroprotective effect of curcumin is mainly mediated by blockade of microglial cell activation. *Pharmazie.* Dec 2007; 62(12): 937–942.
82. Brinjikji W, Rabinstein AA, Cloft HJ. Hospitalization costs for acute ischemic stroke patients treated with intravenous thrombolysis in the United States are substantially higher than medicare payments. *Stroke.* Apr 2012; 43(4): 1131–1133.
83. Peairs AT, Rankin JW. Inflammatory response to a high-fat, low-carbohydrate weight loss diet: Effect of antioxidants. *Obesity (Silver Spring).* May 1 2008.
84. Rahman S, Bhatia K, Khan AQ et al. Topically applied vitamin E prevents massive cutaneous inflammatory and oxidative stress responses induced by double application of 12-O-tetradecanoylphorbol-13-acetate (TPA) in mice. *Chem Biol Interact.* Apr 15 2008; 172(3): 195–205.
85. Suzuki YJ, Aggarwal BB, Packer L. Alpha-lipoic acid is a potent inhibitor of NF-kappa B activation in human T cells. *Biochem Biophys Res Commun.* Dec 30 1992; 189(3): 1709–1715.
86. Wood LG, Garg ML, Powell H, Gibson PG. Lycopene-rich treatments modify non-eosinophilic airway inflammation in asthma: Proof of concept. *Free Radic Res.* Jan 2008; 42(1): 94–102.
87. Zhu J, Yong W, Wu X et al. Anti-inflammatory effect of resveratrol on TNF-alpha-induced MCP-1 expression in adipocytes. *Biochem Biophys Res Commun.* May 2 2008; 369(2): 471–477.
88. Barger SW, Goodwin ME, Porter MM, Beggs ML. Glutamate release from activated microglia requires the oxidative burst and lipid peroxidation. *J Neurochem.* Jun 2007; 101(5): 1205–1213.
89. Schubert D, Kimura H, Maher P. Growth factors and vitamin E modify neuronal glutamate toxicity. *Proc Natl Acad Sci U S A.* Sep 1 1992; 89(17): 8264–8267.
90. Sandhu JK, Pandey S, Ribecco-Lutkiewicz M et al. Molecular mechanisms of glutamate neurotoxicity in mixed cultures of NT2-derived neurons and astrocytes: Protective effects of coenzyme Q_{10}. *J Neurosci Res.* Jun 15 2003; 72(6): 691–703.
91. Matsuoka Y, Nishi D, Nakaya N et al. Attenuating posttraumatic distress with omega-3 polyunsaturated fatty acids among disaster medical assistance team members after the Great East Japan Earthquake: The APOP randomized controlled trial. *BMC Psychiatry.* 2011; 11: 132.
92. Tyagi E, Agrawal R, Zhuang Y, Abad C, Waschek JA, Gomez-Pinilla F. Vulnerability imposed by diet and brain trauma for anxiety-like phenotype: Implications for post-traumatic stress disorders. *PloS One.* 2013; 8(3): e57945.
93. Xu Y, Ku B, Cui L et al. Curcumin reverses impaired hippocampal neurogenesis and increases serotonin receptor 1A mRNA and brain-derived neurotrophic factor expression in chronically stressed rats. *Brain Res.* Aug 8 2007; 1162: 9–18.
94. Aarsland D, Rongve A, Nore SP et al. Frequency and case identification of dementia with Lewy bodies using the revised consensus criteria. *Dement Geriatr Cogn Disord.* 2008; 26(5): 445–452.
95. Gottshall K, Hoffer, ME, Balough, BJ. Use of antioxidants micronutrient compounds in vestibular rehabilitation after operational head trauma or blast injury. Paper presented at *Barany International Balance Meeting, June, 2006, Stockholm, Sweden.*

96. Schubert D, Behl C, Lesley R et al. Amyloid peptides are toxic via a common oxidative mechanism. *Proc Natl Acad Sci U S A.* Mar 14 1995; 92(6): 1989–1993.

97. Behl C, Davis J, Cole GM, Schubert D. Vitamin E protects nerve cells from amyloid beta protein toxicity. *Biochem Biophys Res Commun.* Jul 31 1992; 186(2): 944–950.

98. Sano M, Ernesto C, Thomas RG et al. A controlled trial of selegiline, alpha-tocopherol, or both as treatment for Alzheimer's disease. The Alzheimer's Disease Cooperative Study. *N Engl J Med.* Apr 24 1997; 336(17): 1216–1222.

99. Maxwell CJ, Hicks MS, Hogan DB, Basran J, Ebly EM. Supplemental use of antioxidant vitamins and subsequent risk of cognitive decline and dementia. *Dement Geriatr Cogn Disord.* 2005; 20(1): 45–51.

100. Liu H, Wang H, Shenvi S, Hagen TM, Liu RM. Glutathione metabolism during aging and in Alzheimer disease. *Ann N Y Acad Sci.* Jun 2004; 1019: 346–349.

101. Chinta SJ, Kumar MJ, Hsu M et al. Inducible alterations of glutathione levels in adult dopaminergic midbrain neurons result in nigrostriatal degeneration. *J Neurosci.* Dec 19 2007; 27(51): 13997–14006.

102. Hsu M, Srinivas B, Kumar J, Subramanian R, Andersen J. Glutathione depletion resulting in selective mitochondrial complex I inhibition in dopaminergic cells is via an NO-mediated pathway not involving peroxynitrite: Implications for Parkinson's disease. *J Neurochem.* Mar 2005; 92(5): 1091–1103.

103. Chen RS, Huang CC, Chu NS. Coenzyme Q_{10} treatment in mitochondrial encephalomyopathies. Short-term double-blind, crossover study. *Eur Neurol.* 1997; 37(4): 212–218.

104. Muller T, Buttner T, Gholipour AF, Kuhn W. Coenzyme Q_{10} supplementation provides mild symptomatic benefit in patients with Parkinson's disease. *Neurosci Lett.* May 8 2003; 341(3): 201–204.

105. Investigators TNN-P. A randomized clinical trial of coenzyme Q_{10} and GPI-1485 in early Parkinson disease. *Neurology.* 2007; 68: 20–28.

106. Yan XD, Kumar B, Nahreini P, Hanson AJ, Prasad JE, Prasad KN. Prostaglandin-induced neurodegeneration is associated with increased levels of oxidative markers and reduced by a mixture of antioxidants. *J Neurosci Res.* Jul 1 2005; 81(1): 85–90.

107. King J, Mackey V, Prasad K, Charlton C. Blockage of the proposed precipitating stage for Parkinson's disease by antioxidants: A potential preventive measure for PD. Paper presented at *FASEB, April, 2008, San Diego.*

108. Ikeda T, Yamamoto K, Takahashi K et al. Treatment of Alzheimer-type dementia with intravenous mecobalamin. *Clin Ther.* May–Jun 1992; 14(3): 426–437.

109. Shoulson, I. DATATOP: A decade of neuroprotective inquiry. Parkinson Study Group. Deprenyl And Tocopherol Antioxidative Therapy Of Parkinsonism. *Ann Neurol.* Sep 1998; 44(3 Suppl 1): S160–S166.

110. Farina N, Isaac MG, Clark AR, Rusted J, Tabet N. Vitamin E for Alzheimer's dementia and mild cognitive impairment. *Cochrane Database Syst Rev.* 2012; 11: CD002854.

111. Albanes D, Heinonen OP, Huttunen JK et al. Effects of alpha-tocopherol and beta-carotene supplements on cancer incidence in the Alpha-Tocopherol Beta-Carotene Cancer Prevention Study. *Am J Clin Nutr.* Dec 1995; 62(6 Suppl): 1427S–1430S.

112. Davis M, Ressler K, Rothbaum BO, Richardson R. Effects of D-cycloserine on extinction: Translation from preclinical to clinical work. *Biol Psychiatry.* Aug 15 2006; 60(4): 369–375.

113. Olanow CW, Arendash GW. Metals and free radicals in neurodegeneration. *Curr Opin Neurol.* Dec 1994; 7(6): 548–558.

114. Prasad KN, Kumar B, Yan XD, Hanson AJ, Cole WC. Alpha-tocopheryl succinate, the most effective form of vitamin E for adjuvant cancer treatment: A review. *J Am Coll Nutr.* Apr 2003; 22(2): 108–117.

115. Heresco-Levy U, Vass A, Bloch B et al. Pilot controlled trial of d-serine for the treatment of post-traumatic stress disorder. *Int J Neuropsychopharmacol.* Apr 15 2009: 1–8.

116. Ipser J, Seedat S, Stein DJ. Pharmacotherapy for post-traumatic stress disorder—A systematic review and meta-analysis. *S Afr Med J.* Oct 2006; 96(10): 1088–1096.
117. Ravindran LN, Stein MB. Pharmacotherapy of PTSD: Premises, principles, and priorities. *Brain Res.* Mar 28 2009.
118. Richardson R, Ledgerwood L, Cranney J. Facilitation of fear extinction by D-cycloserine: Theoretical and clinical implications. *Learn Mem.* Sep–Oct 2004; 11(5): 510–516.
119. Vervliet B. Learning and memory in conditioned fear extinction: Effects of D-cycloserine. *Acta Psychol (Amst).* Mar 2008; 127(3): 601–613.
120. de Quervain DJ, Margraf J. Glucocorticoids for the treatment of post-traumatic stress disorder and phobias: A novel therapeutic approach. *Eur J Pharmacol.* Apr 7 2008; 583(2–3): 365–371.
121. Schelling G. Effects of stress hormones on traumatic memory formation and the development of posttraumatic stress disorder in critically ill patients. *Neurobio l Learn Mem.* Nov 2002; 78(3): 596–609.

7 Traumatic Brain Injury
Improved Management by Micronutrients

INTRODUCTION

Traumatic brain injury (TBI), also called head injury, occurs when a sudden trauma causes damage to the brain. Because of current military conflicts around the world and explosions of bombs by the terrorists, the number of troops and civilians with TBI is increasing. TBI can occur with or without penetrating head injury. TBI without penetrating head injury is also called concussive injury, which may express as a mild, moderate, or severe form. The concussive injury has been discussed in detail in Chapter 8. A concussion occurs when the brain is violently rocked back and forth within the skull, following a blow to the head or neck such as observed in contact sports like football, or when in close proximity to a concussive blast pressure wave, following detonation of the improvised explosion devices (IEDs). Most TBI without penetrating head injury occur as a mild form. This form of TBI also increases the risk of posttraumatic disorder (PTSD), which has been discussed in detail in Chapter 6.

TBI with penetrating head injury could also be mild, moderate, or severe and occur when an object penetrates the skull and damages the brain. This form of TBI is caused by vehicle crashes, gunshot wounds to the head, and exposure to IED explosion and combat-related head injuries. The damage to the brain after severe TBI occurs in three phases. The first phase involves primary injury to the brain tissue that cannot be reversed. The second phase occurs soon after injury and continues for days to weeks and contributes to the development of secondary damage that eventually leads to neurological disorders and neuronal death. During this period, intervention with appropriate agents can slow down the progression of the damage. The third phase of severe TBI appears as late effects, which depend upon the initial areas of the brain damaged. The late effects may include cognitive dysfunction, PTSD, and other behavior abnormalities.

There has been a significant improvement in the management of severe TBI. However, despite measures such as standardized treatment guidelines, several clinical studies aimed at identifying therapeutic agents, and improved understanding of the mechanisms of cellular damage, treatment strategies for patients with severe TBI remain unsatisfactory, and morbidity and mortality continue to be high. In addition, there is no effective strategy to reduce the risk of dementia and other forms of mental disorders associated with severe TBI. In order to develop a rational strategy for reducing the progression of severe TBI, it would be important to identify major biological events that play a crucial role in the progression of this type of injury.

A few studies on animals and humans suggest that increased levels of oxidative stress, inflammation, and the release of glutamate into extracellular spaces of the brain are involved in the progression of damage following acute TBI. Since antioxidants neutralize free radicals and reduce inflammation, and can prevent the release and toxicity of glutamate, they appear to be one of the rational choices for improving the current management of TBI with penetrating head injury as an adjunctive therapy. The clinical studies to evaluate the efficacy of antioxidants in these injuries have not been performed in a satisfactory manner. Most studies with a single antioxidant have been performed in animal models and cell culture models of TBI.

This chapter describes briefly the incidence, cost, causes, symptoms, and major biochemical events that contribute to the progression of severe TBI. In addition, this chapter presents scientific and rational evidence in support of a hypothesis that daily supplementation with multiple micronutrients including dietary and endogenous antioxidants and certain phenolic compounds may reduce oxidative stress indirectly by increasing antioxidant enzymes through a nuclear transcriptional factor (Nrf2)/ antioxidant response element (ARE) pathway and directly by scavenging free radicals and, in combination with standard care, may improve the acute and long-term management of severe TBI more than that produced by the standard care alone.

INCIDENCE AND COST OF TBI

U.S. TROOPS

There is no precise estimate of TBI in injured soldiers returning from Iraq and Afghanistan. About 65% of the soldiers are injured by explosive devices. Because of an excellent trauma care in the battlefield, the number of survivors has increased, resulting in a higher number of soldiers with TBI. In the Editorial section of *The Lancet* (a British clinical medical journal), December 6, 2007, it was mentioned that the proportion of injured soldiers with TBI increased from 14–20% in the previous U.S. wars to 60% in the current wars in Iraq and Afghanistan. About 90% of TBI are of the mild type.

U.S. CIVILIANS

The Center for Disease Control and Prevention (CDC) estimates that about 1.7 million people sustain severe TBI each year. TBI accounts for about 30.5% of all injury-related deaths and for substantial cases of permanent disability. The CDC has estimated that at least 5.3 million Americans who suffered from TBI have a long-term or lifelong need for help performing activities of daily living.

COST

The cost per year per person with mild TBI is about $32,000, with moderate to severe TBI is $268,000 to more than $408,000. In 2010, the direct medical and indirect costs (such as lost productivity) are estimated to be $76.5 billion.

CAUSES OF SEVERE TBI

This type of TBI occurs when an object penetrates the skull and damages the brain, which could be confined to a small or larger area of the brain. Among the U.S. soldiers deployed to the wars in Iraq and Afghanistan, blasts, IEDs, vehicle crashes, and other combat-related injuries are the main causes of the increased incidence of TBI with penetrating head injury. Among civilians, transportation accidents involving automobiles, motorcycles, bicycles and pedestrians, and gunshot wounds to the head are the major causes of TBI with penetrating head injury. This is a serious and life-threatening injury and requires an emergency medical care.

SYMPTOMS

The clinical outcomes depend upon the severity of brain damage and the area of the brain affected. The acute symptoms of severe TBI are the following: (a) heavy bleeding from the head, (b) bleeding from the ears, (c) difficulty in breathing, (d) seizure, (e) loss of bladder and bowel functions, (f) loss of movement and sensation in the limbs, and (g) loss of consciousness. If the damage to the brain is extensive, patients may die within a few days to a few weeks.

The long-term consequences also include impairment of cognitive function (attention and memory), motor (extreme weakness, poor coordination, and balance), and sensation (hearing vision, impaired perception, and touch), emotion (depression, anxiety, aggression, impulse control, and personality changes), and posttraumatic disorders. The survivors of severe TBI may face long-term serious disabilities that can cause very poor quality of life.

NEUROPATHOLOGY

The neuropathology of TBI with penetrating head injury is very complex, depending upon the type and velocity of inducing agents, the area and size of the affected brain tissue, and the loss of brain tissue. Generally, swelling, edema, hematoma, hemorrhage, contusion, focal cerebral vasospasm, increased blood–brain barrier (BBB) disruption, and diffuse axonal injury are observed immediately after injury.[1] It has been reported that penetrating ballistic-like injury and hemorrhagic shock can cause persistent damage of cerebral blood flow and brain tissue oxygen tension. These changes increase the probability of cortical spreading depolarization that may contribute to secondary neuropathology and compromise neurological recovery.[2]

SCORING SYSTEM OF SEVERITY OF TBI

The Glasgow Coma Scale (GCS) is one of the most commonly used severity scoring systems. Individuals with GCS scores of 3–8 are classified with a severe TBI, those with scores of 9–12 are classified with a moderate TBI, and those with scores of 13–15 are classified with a mild TBI. Other classification systems include the Abbreviated Injury Scale (AIS), the Trauma Score, and the Abbreviated Trauma

Scores. These classifications are useful in clinical management of TBI, because the prognosis for mild TBI is better than for moderate or severe TBI.

RISK OF PTSD ASSOCIATED WITH TBI

Epidemiologic studies on TBI and its relationship with PTSD on U.S. soldiers returning from Iraq and Afghanistan have been described.[3] Among 2525 soldiers, 4.9% reported injuries with loss of consciousness, 10.3% reported injuries with altered mental status, and 17.2% reported other injuries during deployment. Among those who reported loss of consciousness, the incidence of PTSD was about 43.9%; among those reporting altered mental status, it was 27.3%; and those who reported other injuries, it was 16.2%. In contrast, those soldiers reporting no injury in combat, the incidence of PTSD was only 9.1%. It was proposed that the strong association between mild TBI and PTSD may be due to life-threatening combat experiences; in some cases, it could reflect neurological deficits as well as traumatic stress. Female soldiers had a higher incidence of PTSD than male soldiers.

BIOCHEMICAL EVENTS THAT CONTRIBUTE TO THE PROGRESSION OF DAMAGE AFTER SEVERE TBI

Both animal and human studies show that TBI causes a significant loss of cortical tissue at the site of injury (primary damage) that is followed by a secondary damage involving abnormal biochemical events, such as increased oxidative damage, mitochondrial dysfunction, release of predominantly proinflammatory cytokines, and glutamate leading to neurological dysfunctions and neuronal death. Therefore, attenuation of these biochemical events in TBI patients may help to reduce the progression of damage, when combined with standard therapy, and may further reduce the risk of developing neurological abnormalities including cognitive impairment.

EVIDENCE FOR INCREASED OXIDATIVE STRESS AFTER SEVERE TBI

Both animal and human studies suggest that increased oxidative stress plays an important role in the progression of injury after severe TBI. A few studies are described here.

STUDIES ON ANIMAL MODELS

Increased oxidative stress due to the production of excessive amounts of free radicals derived from oxygen and nitrogen occur after TBI.[4–7] Increased production of superoxide radicals has been demonstrated in mice.[8] The extent of oxidative damage appeared to be directly proportional to the severity of TBI in rat models of TBI.[9] The levels of antioxidant enzymes Mn-SOD (manganese-dependent superoxide dismutase) and glutathione reductase decreased more in older rats than the younger ones following TBI, whereas the levels of markers of oxidative damage such as products of lipid peroxidation (acrolein and 4-hydroxynonenal) increased more in the older rats than the younger rats.[7] In rats, there appears to be a close relationship between the degree of oxidative stress and the severity of brain damage following TBI as evidenced by the highest values of malondialdehyde (MDA) and lowest value of ascorbate.[10] The total antioxidant reserves of brain homogenates and water-soluble antioxidant reserves as well as tissue concentration of ascorbate, glutathione, and sulfhydryl proteins were reduced after TBI in rats.[11] Peroxynitrite-mediated oxidative damage to mitochondrial function after severe TBI precedes neuronal loss in the brain. The oxidation of nitric oxide forms peroxynitrite. Animal studies have revealed that TBI increased nitric oxide (NO) production that impairs mitochondrial function by inhibiting cytochrome oxidase.[12] Cytochrome oxidase is a key enzyme needed to generate energy. Thus, the energy level in tissue decreased after TBI that may interfere with repair process. TBI also increased inducible nitric oxide synthase (iNOS) activity that contributes to neurological deficits, but not to cerebral edema by generating excessive amounts of NO.[13] In a rat model of traumatic injury (unilateral moderate cortical contusion), increased oxidative damage occurs as early as 3 h following TBI that adversely affects synaptic function and plasticity of hippocampal neurons, and thereby, enhances cognitive dysfunction.[14] In another model of TBI (fluid percussion brain injury in rat), it was observed that protein carbonylation and thiobarbituric acid-reactive substance (TBARS) levels increased in parietal cortex 1 and 3 months following injury. These changes in markers of oxidative damage were associated with the progressive decrease in the activity of Na^+, K^+-ATPase.[15] These results suggest that increase in oxidative stress associated with decrease in Na^+, K^+-ATPase activity may account for cognitive dysfunction observed following TBI.

It has been found that Nrf2 pathway, which activates antioxidant enzyme through ARE, is enhanced during early brain damage after inducing subarachnoid hemorrhage in rats.[16] Since transient increased in oxidative stress is required for the activation of Nrf2 pathway, it can be concluded that increase oxidative stress occurred as an early biochemical event, which may contribute to the progression of the lesion in the brain.

Human Studies

A few human studies also confirm the role of oxidative stress in the progression of brain damage after TBI. F2-isoprostane is a marker of lipid peroxidation, whereas neuron-specific enolase (NSE) is considered a marker of neuronal damage. The levels of F2-isoprostane and NSE increased in the cerebral spinal fluid samples following TBI in children and infants.[17] Both levels of ascorbate and glutathione decreased in the CSF of children and infants following TBI.[18] Metabolic function of the brain in children with severe TBI is impaired. Although cerebral blood flow is variable after severe TBI in children, low-oxygen metabolic index and hypoperfusion were observed.[19] A clinical study showed that the level of 3-nitrotyrosine increased in the CSF of the patients with TBI.[20] Another clinical study reported that increased levels of cytochrome C and activated caspases-9 were detected in the CSF of the adult patients with severe TBI.[21] Increased levels of cytochrome C and activated caspase-9 play a significant role in causing neuronal death. It has been reported that the levels of beta-amyloid fragments (Aβ1–42) increased in the cerebral spinal fluid of patients after severe TBI.[22] This peptide has been implicated in causing neuronal damage in patients with Alzheimer's disease, and one of the mechanisms of injury induced by amyloid beta fragments generated from splicing of amyloid precursor protein (APP) involves increased oxidative stress.[23–26]

In a clinical study on 106 healthy subjects and 106 patients with severe TBI (GCS of 1–3), it was demonstrated that the plasma levels of 8-iso-prostaglandin F2-alpha, a marker of oxidative damage in vivo, were higher in patients with severe TBI than in healthy subjects.[27] Another clinical study has shown a close relationship between oxidative stress and excitotoxicity following severe TBI in humans.[28] A clinical study on 30 severe TBI patients (GCS score of 8 or less), 20 patients with mild TBI, and 36 age- and sex-matched healthy individuals showed that the levels of erythrocyte TBARS were significantly higher and the levels of glutathione lower in severe and mild TBI patients compared to those in healthy individuals.[29] In another clinical study, it was demonstrated that plasma levels of TBARS and protein oxidation (carbonyl) increased significantly in the first 70 h after severe TBI.[30]

Copeptin, a stable glycopeptide, a product of vasopressin, is secreted from the posterior pituitary gland. It is also known as an antidiuretic hormone. Higher plasma levels appear to be associated with poor clinical outcomes of severely ill patients. In a clinical study on 126 healthy children and 126 children with severe TBI (GCS scores of 1–3), it was observed that the plasma levels of copeptin were elevated in patients with severe TBI than in healthy children.[31] Therefore, plasma levels of copeptin may be used as a diagnostic marker for TBI.

MITOCHONDRIAL DYSFUNCTION AFTER SEVERE TBI

Both animal and human studies suggest that mitochondrial dysfunction plays an important role in the progression of injury after severe TBI. A few studies are described here.

ANIMAL STUDIES

Increased oxidative stress contributes to the mitochondrial dysfunction that plays a central role in causing cognitive impairment and eventually neuronal death following TBI.[32,33] Experimental TBI causes a significant loss of cortical tissue at the site of injury (primary damage), which is followed by a secondary injury involving mitochondria that enhances the primary injury leading to neurological dysfunction. In a rat model of TBI, several mitochondrial proteins involved in bioenergetics were oxidized following injury causing mitochondrial dysfunction that eventually led to neuronal death.[34] In a rat model of TBI, it was found that the activity of mitochondrial enzyme pyruvate dehydrogenase decreased, acid–base balance disrupted, and the levels of oxidative stress increased in blood following injury. The decrease in blood levels of pyruvate dehydrogenase (PDH) was associated with an increased gliosis and loss of subunit PDHE1-infinity of PDH in the brain tissue, and these effects can be prevented by pyruvate treatment.[35] These changes contribute to the severity of brain injury. Cytochrome c oxidase is important for oxidative phosphorylation in the mitochondria. The expression of cytochrome c oxidase I, II, and III mRNA in injured cortex was reduced following TBI in rats, whereas the expression of these mRNAs was slightly elevated in contralateral cortex.[36] Generally, oxidative stress-induced mitochondrial dysfunction in rat models of TBI is observed 1–3 h after TBI, suggesting the importance of an early intervention to reduce the oxidative stress.[37] In a mice model of TBI, it was observed that cortical mitochondrial damages include swelling, a disruption of cristae and rupture of outer membranes, a decrease in calcium-buffering capacity, and an increase in oxidation of protein and lipids. The levels of cortical 3-nitrotyrosine were elevated as early as 30 min after injury.[38]

N-methyl-4-isoleucine-cyclosporin (NIM811), a nonimmunosuppressive cyclosporine A analog, inhibits the mitochondrial permeability transition pore. Supplementation with NIM811 improved mitochondrial function, cognitive function, and reduced oxidative damage in a severe unilateral controlled cortical impact rat model of TBI.[39] Mitochondrial dysfunction can cause increased oxidative damage, loss of respiratory functions, and diminished ability to buffer cytosolic calcium, all of which can cause neuronal death. It was demonstrated that supplementation with U-83836E, a potent inhibitor of lipid peroxyl radicals, reduced both oxidative and nitrosylative damage in cortical homogenates and mitochondria after severe TBI in mice model.[40]

HUMAN STUDIES

It has been reported that mitochondrial DNA polymorphism was associated with mitochondrial dysfunction and neurobehavioral abnormalities after severe TBI.[41] There is a direct link between energy metabolism and N-acetylaspartate. In a clinical study on 14 patients (6 patients with diffuse brain injury and 8 with focal brain lesions), it was observed that reduction in the brain levels of N-acetylaspartate in the absence of ischemic insult reflected mitochondrial dysfunction.[42] It has been proposed that reduction in the levels of extracellular N-acetylaspartate can be used as a potential marker for mitochondrial function in humans after TBI.[43] The role of mitochondrial dysfunction in the progression of damage following TBI is further supported by the fact that treatment with mitochondrial uncouplers, 2,4-dinitrophenol (2, 4-DNP), and p-trifluoromethoxyphenylhydrazone (FCCP), significantly reduced the loss of cortical damage and improved behavioral deficits following TBI in rats.[44]

EVIDENCE FOR INCREASED LEVELS OF MARKERS OF INFLAMMATION AFTER SEVERE TBI

Both animal and human studies suggest that increased inflammation plays an important role in the progression of injury after severe TBI. A few studies are described here.

ANIMAL STUDIES

The levels of inflammation markers such as iNOS and cyclooxygenase 2 (COX-2) activities, and markers of oxidative stress (loss of glutathione and oxidized, reduced glutathione ratio, 3-nitrotyrosine, and 4-hydroxynonenal) increased after TBI in an animal model, and treatment with fenofibrate reduced the levels of these markers.[45] The levels of proinflammatory cytokines, tumor necrosis factor-alpha (TNF-alpha) increased after TBI in rats. The delayed elevation of soluble tumor necrosis factor receptors p75 and p55 was observed in cerebral spinal fluid and plasma after TBI.[46] The levels of TNF-alpha and Fas are elevated after TBI. Using TNF-alpha and Fas-deficient transgenic mice (TNF-alpha/Fas–/–), it was demonstrated that the motor performance and spatial memory acquisition were improved in transgenic animal compared to wild type mice after subjecting them to a controlled cortical impact (a model of TBI). The results suggested that TNF-alpha and Fas play an important role in TBI-induced neurological dysfunction. This was further supported by the fact that in immature mice models of TBI, genetic inhibition of TNF-alpha and Fas conferred beneficial effects on histology and spatial memory acquisition in adulthood.[47] In a rat model of TBI, animals received impact acceleration head injuries as a sustained mild head injury or a severe head injury. The levels of NO metabolites decreased in the cortex, cerebellum, hippocampus, and brain stem in both groups after 5 min. The extent of decrease in NO levels depended upon the extent of injury being lowest in the brain regions, where the direct trauma was most severe.[48]

The role of proinflammatory cytokines in the progression of damage after TBI is further supported by the fact that inhibitors of these cytokines improved neuronal loss and cognitive dysfunction in animal models of TBI. For example, IL-1 beta neutralizing antibody (IgG2a/k)[49]; dexanabinol (HU-211), an inhibitor of TNF-alpha at a posttranscriptional stage[50] and antioxidants[51]; Minozac (Mzc), an inhibitor of glial activation and proinflammatory cytokines[52]; and a synthetic analogue of tripeptide Glypromate (NNZ-2566),[53] an inhibitor of activation of astrocytes (simvastatin)[54] provide neuroprotection by reducing neuronal loss and neurological deficits.

It has been reported that the levels of cerebral vascular permeability increased fourfold in TBI mice models compared to that in normal mice. In addition, the expression of aquaporin-4 (AQP-4), a protein which causes blood–brain barrier-mediated edema in brain, was increased twofold in TBI mice compared to that in normal mice. Vagal nerve stimulation after TBI decreased the levels of cerebral vascular permeability as well as the expression of AQP-4.[55] It has been demonstrated that the levels of substance-P, a neuropeptide, increased after severe diffuse TBI in rats. These rats developed edema and functional neurological deficits. Neurokinin-1 (NK-1) antagonist acetyl-L-tryptophan inhibits action of substance P. The administration of NK-1 antagonist after TBI reduced edema and vascular permeability and improved both motor and cognitive functions. These data suggest that the increased levels of substance P contribute to the development of brain edema and increased vascular permeability.[56]

HUMAN STUDIES

A review on the role of inflammation in acute TBI has revealed that a strong inflammatory response occurs immediately after injury. Inflammatory response activates resident glia cells, microglia, and astrocytes, which secrete proinflammatory cytokines (IL-1, IL-6, and tumor necrosis factor-alpha) and anti-inflammatory cytokines (IL-4, IL-10, and TGF-beta)-0 and chemokines.[57] The examination of 21 autopsied brain samples from patients with severe TBI showed that the levels of proinflammatory cytokines were elevated, whereas the levels of anti-inflammatory cytokines did not change.[58] This is in contrast to the acute phase of TBI, when both proinflammatory and anti-inflammatory cytokines are released.[57] It has been demonstrated that activated microglia persists as long as 17 years after injury.[59] This suggests that the toxic products of inflammation continue to be released long after TBI.

Diffuse axonal injury is the leading cause of lasting vegetative state and death of the patients after TBI. A clinical study on 159 patients with severe TBI, who survived the acute phase, showed that about 72% of the patients had diffuse axonal injury.[60] A review has shown that increased levels of proinflammatory cytokines play an important role in the development of diffuse axonal injury.[61]

Following TBI, resident cells in the brain such as microglia generate excessive amounts of proinflammatory cytokines, prostaglandins, reactive oxygen species, complement proteins, and adhesion molecules that are highly toxic to neurons.[62–66] The evidence of inflammation is also found by the infiltration and accumulation of polymorphonuclear leukocytes. Proinflammatory cytokines increased the expression of iNOS, which can produce excessive amounts of NO that may in turn become oxidized to form peroxynitrite, which contribute to the pathogenesis of TBI.[67–69] An inhibitor of iNOS provided neuroprotection against damage produced by peroxynitrite.[70] The proinflammatory cytokine interleukin-6 (IL-6) is elevated in patients with acute TBI, and a significant relationship exists between the severity of TBI and the transcranial IL-6 gradient at admission.[71] In addition, the activation of nuclear factor-kappa B (NF-kappaB) occurs after TBI in both animals and humans.[72,73] Treatment with beta-aescin inhibited the activation of NF-kappaB and the expression of TNF-alpha in rat models of TBI.[72]

The levels of IL-10, an anti-inflammatory cytokine, in 46 adult patients with TBI (N = 18), nontraumatic intracranial hemorrhage (N = 11), and polytrauma with concomitant brain injury (N = 17) were detectable independent of types of lesion,[74] whereas it was barely detectable in control subjects.[75] The significance of this rise in the levels of IL-10 remains uncertain; however, it was associated with the increased rate of infection and mild to moderate to severe damage to blood–brain barrier. A clinical study on 74 patients with severe TBI showed that elevated serum levels of IL-10 were correlated with the severity of GCS score. Elevated levels of IL-10 were also associated with hospital mortality in a subset of patients with severe TBI.[76] These results suggest that the serum levels of IL-10 could be used as a marker for severe TBI prognosis.

A clinical study on 75 patients with moderate to severe TBI on the role of cytokines and lipids in patient outcomes on the criteria of 30-day mortality was evaluated. The results showed that the levels of cytokines (IL-6 and IL-8) increased and lipid decreased in all patients compared to healthy control subjects. In addition, the levels of two cytokines were higher, and the levels of low-density lipoproteins (LDL) were lower in nonsurvivors than in survivors. These results suggested that the level of LDL alone or in combination with IL-6 and IL-8 could be a prognostic value for a 30-day survival outcome.[77]

Severe TBI in infants and children (N = 36) increased the levels of proinflammatory cytokines (IL-1beta, IL-6, and IL-12p70) and anti-inflammatory cytokines (IL-10) and chemokines (IL-8 and MIP-1-alpha) compared to controls. Moderate hypothermia, which is frequently used in the management of TBI, did not decrease the levels of cytokines in children with TBI.[78]

EVIDENCE FOR INCREASED RELEASE OF GLUTAMATE AFTER SEVERE TBI

Both animal and human studies suggest that the increased levels of extracellular glutamate in the brain plays an important role in the progression of injury after severe TBI. A few studies are described here.

ANIMAL STUDIES

The levels of extracellular glutamate and aspartate increased in the brain regions following TBI in animals.[79] In rat model of TBI, it was shown that the levels of two high-affinity sodium-dependent glial transporters, glutamate transporter 1(GLT-1), and glutamate-aspartame transporter (GLAST) decreased following TBI.[80,81] GLT-1 is primarily responsible for clearing extracellular glutamate; therefore, decreased levels of GLT-1 may contribute to the increased levels of extracellular glutamate. Thus, increased levels of GLT-1 appear to be of neuroprotective value by reducing the levels of glutamate. This is supported by the observation in which the administration of ceftriaxone, which increases the expression of GLT-1, reversed the TBI-induced elevation of glia fibrillary acid protein (GFAP) and seizures in rat models of TBI.[82] It has been reported that disruption in calcium-dependent neuronal glutamate release and glia-regulated extracellular glutamate contribute to the progression of damage in the striatum of rats 2 days after the diffuse brain injury.[83] It has been demonstrated that increases in the levels of extracellular glutamate occur due to excessive release of glutamate from neurons.[84] Thus, both neurons and glia contribute to the increased levels of extracellular glutamate after TBI.

In a rat model of TBI, hypothermia treatment reduced the levels of hydroxyl radicals and glutamate release.[85] The administration of N-methyl-D-aspartame, an (NMDA) antagonist, significantly reduced glutamate release,[86,87] and improved motor function and cognitive dysfunction following TBI in animal models. It has been demonstrated that injection of premarin, a conjugated estrogen commonly used as hormone replacement in postmenopausal women, decreased blood glutamate levels in rat models of TBI.[88]

The activation of presynaptic group II metabotropic glutamate (mGlu II) receptor reduces synaptic glutamate release. Indeed, (-)-2-oxa-4-aminobicyclo (3.1.0) hexane-4,6-dicarboxylate (LY379268), a selective agonist ofmGlu II, significantly reduced cell death following TBI in mice.[89] In another animal model of TBI (lateral fluid percussion-induced brain injury), the administration of mGlu II agonist improved behavior deficits compared to control following injury.[90]

The levels of extracellular glutamate and adenosine increase rapidly after TBI; however, the relationship between them in the progression of injury is not well defined. Normally, adenosine A(2A) receptor (A2AR) exerts neuroprotective action, but it can contribute to neurodegeneration depending upon the levels of glutamate. It has been demonstrated that high concentration of glutamate switched the effect of activated A2AR from anti-inflammation to pro-inflammation in microglia cells in culture and in mice TBI models.[91]

HUMAN STUDIES

The excitatory amino acids play a significant role in the progression of injury following TBI. Excessive amounts of glutamate in the extracellular space may lead to uncontrolled shift of sodium, potassium, and calcium, which may cause swelling, edema, and eventually neuronal death. In addition, increased synaptic release of glutamate also occurs at the site of injury.[81,92] In a clinical study on 80 patients with severe head injury, it was observed that the levels of excitatory amino acids increased, which may enhance neuronal damage in these patients.[93] In patients with focal and diffuse brain injury, the levels of glutamate were elevated in both cerebrospinal fluid and extracellular space following TBI.[94] In another clinical study, it was found that patients who died of their head injury had higher levels of dialysate glutamate and aspartame compared to those who recovered from injury. The highest levels of glutamate were present in patients with gunshot wounds, followed by those who had mass lesions. Patients with diffuse brain injury had the lowest levels of glutamate and aspartame.[79] Excessive amounts of glutamate and aspartame are released in 85 severely head injured patients, and patients with contusions had the highest level of glutamate and aspartate.[95] In a clinical study on 28 severely brain injured patients, the levels of glutamate and taurine in ventricular cerebrospinal fluid (CSF) were elevated in patients with subdural or epidural hematomas, contusions, and generalized brain edema. The simultaneous release of taurine, which has inhibitory and antiexcitotoxic functions with glutamate, suggests that the injured brain is attempting to counteract the action of glutamate.[96] Similar results were obtained in rat models of TBI.[97] A clinical study on 165 patients with severe TBI showed that the increased levels of glutamate measured by microdialysis were correlated with higher mortality and poor functional outcomes.[98] The concentrations of glutamate and glycerol in microdialysate from older patients with severe TBI were higher compared to younger patients.[99] This suggested that the increased concentrations of glycerol and glutamate would indicate more extensive damage in older patients. A clinical study on 223 patients with severe TBI showed that higher concentrations of glutamate, glucose, lactate/pyruvate ratio, intracranial pressure, cerebrovascular pressure reactivity index, and age were predictors of increased mortality.[100]

In a clinical study on 27 children with severe TBI and 21 children without TBI or meningitis, it was observed that the levels of adenosine and glutamate were elevated in the ventricular CSF following TBI. The release of adenosine following TBI may reflect an attempt by adenosine to provide neuroprotection against glutamate-induced toxicity.[101]

ROLE OF MATRIX METALLOPROTEINASES AFTER SEVERE TBI

Experimental data in animal models of severe TBI suggested that an increase in the levels of matrix metalloproteinases 3 and 9 that are considered responsible for inflammation in the brain, blood–barrier disruption, hemorrhage, and neuronal death occurred after TBI. Indeed, a clinical study on six patients with TBI showed that the CSF levels of matrix metalloproteinase (MMP)-9 were elevated; however, elevated levels of MMP-3 were observed in the plasma, but not in the CSF.[102] These data suggest that MMPs play an important role in the progression of damage after TBI. In another clinical study on 20 patients with a mild head injury and normal CT scan, 15 patients with moderate polytrauma without TBI and 20 healthy volunteers showed that the levels of MMP-2 and MMP-9 increased in the plasma and microdialysis samples of patients compared to control volunteers. These changes were followed by a significant decrease in the levels of both MMP-2 and MMP-9.[103] It was further demonstrated that the increased levels of MMP-8 and MMP-9 was associated with increases in the levels of proinflammatory cytokines (IL-1 alpha, IL-2, and TNF-alpha) in the microdialysis samples of eight patients with severe TBI. In contrast, the levels of MMP-7 decreased with increases in the levels of IL-1beta, IL-2, and IL-6.[104]

HOW TO REDUCE OXIDATIVE STRESS, CHRONIC INFLAMMATION, AND GLUTAMATE RELEASE

Significant studies discussed in this chapter suggest that increased oxidative stress, chronic inflammation, and the release of glutamate are involved in the initiation and progression of TBI.

How to Reduce Oxidative Stress

Oxidative stress in the body occurs when the antioxidant system fails to provide adequate protection against damage produced by free radicals (reactive oxygen species and reactive nitrogen species). Increased oxidative stress in the body can be most effectively reduced by up-regulating antioxidant enzymes as well as by existing levels of dietary and endogenous antioxidant chemicals, because they work by different mechanisms. For example, antioxidant enzymes reduce free radicals by catalysis, whereas dietary and endogenous antioxidant chemicals reduce free radicals by directly scavenging them. In response to reactive oxygen species (ROS), a nuclear transcriptional factor, Nrf2 (nuclear factor-erythroid 2-related factor 2) translocated from the cytoplasm to the nucleus, where it binds with ARE, which increases the levels of antioxidant enzymes (gamma-glutamylcysteine ligase, glutathione peroxidase, glutathione reductase, and heme oxygenase-1) and phase 2 detoxifying enzymes (NAD(P)H: quinine oxidoreductase 1 and glutathione-S-transferase), in order to reduce oxidative damage.[105–107] In response to increased oxidative stress, existing levels of dietary and endogenous antioxidant chemical levels cannot be elevated without supplementation.

Factors Regulating Response of Nrf2 and Its Action

Several studies suggest that antioxidant enzymes are elevated by Nrf2 activation, which depends upon ROS-dependent[108] and -independent[109–113] mechanisms. In addition, the levels of antioxidant enzymes are also dependent upon the binding ability of Nrf2 with ARE in the nucleus.[114]

DIFFERENTIAL RESPONSE OF Nrf2 TO ROS GENERATED DURING ACUTE AND CHRONIC OXIDATIVE STRESS

It appears that Nrf2 responds to ROS generated during acute and chronic oxidative stress differently. For example, excessive amounts of ROS are generated during acute oxidative stress observed during strenuous exercise. In response to ROS, Nrf2 translocates to the nucleus where it binds with ARE to up-regulate antioxidant genes. Excessive amounts of ROS are also present during chronic oxidative stress commonly observed in older individuals and neurological diseases, such as Parkinson's disease, Alzheimer's disease, and PTSD, suggesting that the Nrf2/ARE regulatory system has become unresponsive to ROS in these diseases. Age-related decline in antioxidant enzymes in the liver of older rats compared to that in younger rats was due to the reduction in the binding ability of Nrf2 with ARE; however, treatment with alpha-lipoic acid restored this defect, increased the levels of antioxidant enzymes, and restored the loss of glutathione from the liver of older rats.[114] The exact reasons for the Nrf2/ARE regulatory system to become unresponsive to ROS during chronic oxidative stress are unknown; however, defects in the binding ability of Nrf2 with ARE may be one of the reasons.

Nrf2 IN TBI

A few studies have been performed to evaluate the role of Nrf2 in TBI. Since increased oxidative stress plays an important role in the initiation and progression of TBI, the following groups of agents in combination may be useful in improved management of TBI:

1. *Agents that can reduce oxidative stress by directly scavenging free radicals without activating Nrf2-regulated antioxidant enzymes*: Some examples are dietary antioxidants, such as vitamin A, beta-carotene, vitamin C, and vitamin E, and endogenous antioxidants, such as glutathione, alpha-lipoic acid, and coenzyme Q_{10}.
2. *Agents that can reduce oxidative stress by activating Nfr2-regulated antioxidant genes without ROS stimulation*: Some examples are organosulfur compound sulforaphane found in cruciferous vegetables, kavalactones found in Kava shrubs, and Puerarin, a major flavonoid from the root of *Pueraria lobata*.[111,112,115] Genistein and vitamin E,[109] and coenzyme Q_{10}[116] also activate Nrf2 without ROS.
3. *Agents that can reduce oxidative stress directly by scavenging free radicals as well as indirectly by activating Nrf2/ARE pathway*: Some examples

are vitamin E,[109] alpha-lipoic acid,[114] curcumin,[117] resveratrol,[118,119] omega-3 fatty acids,[120,121] and NAC.[122]

4. *Agents that can reduce oxidative stress by ROS stimulation*: They include L-carnitine which generates transient ROS.[123]

How to Reduce Chronic Inflammation and Glutamate

Some individual antioxidants from the above groups have been shown to reduce chronic inflammation[124–136] and prevent the release[137] and toxicity[138,139] of glutamate. A combination of selected agents from the above groups may reduce chronic inflammation and release of glutamate and its toxicity optimally, and thereby, may reduce the progression of severe TBI, and in combination with standard therapy, may improve the management of this disease.

Nrf2 IN TBI

Nrf2 is an important transcriptional factor that provides protection against toxic products of inflammation. Using transgenic mice deficient in Nrf2 (–/–), it was demonstrated that the activation of NF-kappaB, the levels of proinflammatory cytokines, TNF-alpha, IL-1beta and IL-6, and the expression of intracellular adhesion molecule 1 (ICAN-1) were higher in the brain compared to the wild-type Nrf2 (+/+) mice following TBI (moderate to severe weight-drop impact head injury).[140,141]

STUDIES ON EFFECTS OF SINGLE ANTIOXIDANTS AFTER SEVERE TBI

Despite great potential of antioxidants in the improved management of severe TBI, very little attention has been paid to test the efficacy of these micronutrients either for primary prevention after secondary prevention of severe TBI in humans. A few studies on the effect of antioxidants on severe TBI in animals and humans are described here.

Animal Studies

Resveratrol, a polyphenolic compound which exhibits antioxidant and anti-inflammation activities, administered immediately after TBI reduced oxidative damage and lesion volume in rats.[142,143] Treatment with alpha-lipoic acid reduced markers of proinflammatory cytokines and oxidative stress, improved histological changes in the brain, preserved BBB permeability, and reduced edema following TBI in animals.[144] The administration of N-acetylcysteine provided neuroprotection (reduction in brain edema and BBB permeability) in animal models following TBI by reducing markers of proinflammatory cytokines and adhesion molecules.[145] The early rise in complex I and complex II proteins of mitochondria that regulate excitatory neurotransmitter release following TBI was blocked by N-acetylcysteine (NAC).[92] In addition, the TBI-induced elevation of heme oxygenase-1 (HO-1) levels in glial cells as well as neurons, and the loss of tissue volume was markedly reduced by N-acetylcysteine treatment in the animal model of TBI (lateral fluid percussion injury).[146]

Melatonin, a pineal hormone exhibiting antioxidant activity, protected against TBI-induced damage by attenuating the activation of NF-kappaB and AP-1.[147] S-nitrosoglutathione (GSNO), a modulator of nitric oxide, plays an important role in maintaining redox balance. The administration of GSNO after severe TBI reduced blood–brain barrier disruption, infiltration/activation of macrophages, and reduced expression of ICAM-1, MMPs, and iNOS. This treatment also reduced neuronal cell and myelin loss in TBI model rats.[148] The administration of an endogenous fatty acid palmitoylethanolamide (PEA), which maintains redox balance, reduced edema, brain infarction, and neuronal loss and improved neurological functions in mice models of severe TBI.[149]

In a rat model of TBI (mild fluid percussion injury), increased oxidation of proteins and reduced levels of SOD and Sir2 (silent information regulator), and poor performance associated with a decline in the levels of brain-derived neurotrophic factor (BDNF) and its downstream effectors on synaptic plasticity, synapsin I, and cAMP-response element-binding protein (CREB), were observed following injury. Dietary supplementation with vitamin E or curcumin protected the brain against mild TBI-induced damage by reducing the above biochemical changes involved in synaptic plasticity and cognitive function.[150,151] Superoxide dismutase improved TBI-induced mitochondrial dysfunction in transgenic mice overexpressing CuZn SOD or Mn SOD.[152] In transgenic mice overexpressing glutathione peroxidase (GPxTg), it was observed that markers of oxidative stress including nitrotyrosine were reduced and spatial memory improved compared to wild-type animals following TBI.[153]

It has been reported that dietary supplementation omega-3 fatty acids in animal models of TBI (mild fluid percussion injury) protected against TBI-induced, reduced synaptic plasticity and cognitive impairment.[154] In contrast, supplementation with saturated fat diet[155] or caffeine[156] aggravated TBI-induced injury in animals.

HUMAN STUDIES

Edaravone, a FDA approved drug, reduced oxidative damage by neutralizing free radicals after TBI in humans.[157] It is well established that antioxidants are scavengers of free radicals; however, their role in reducing inflammation has not drawn significant attention. There are substantial amounts of data that show that dietary and endogenous antioxidants and antioxidants derived from herbs and fruits and vegetables inhibit inflammation.[124–130,132–136,158]

EFFECTS OF PREPARATION OF MULTIPLE MICRONUTRIENTS IN TROOPS WITH TBI

A commercial formulation of multiple micronutrients was tested in a clinical study in troops returning from Iraq with mild to moderate TBI. Thirty-four patients with posttraumatic dizziness were admitted to the Naval Medical Center San Diego Clinic over a 2-month period and agreed to participate in the study under the supervision of Dr. Michael Hoffer and his colleagues.[159] All patients had received their injury 3–20 weeks prior to admission, and they received identical treatment consisting of medical therapy (for any migraines), supportive care, steroids, and vestibular rehabilitation therapy. Fifteen of the 34 patients also received a dose of an antioxidant and micronutrient formula (two capsules by mouth twice a day). At the onset of therapy, all patients were evaluated in outcome measures, which included the Sensory Organization Test (SOT) by Computerized Dynamic Posturography (CDP), the Dynamic Gait Index (DGI), the Activities Balance Confidence (ABC) scale, the Dizziness Handicap Index (DHI), the Vestibular Disorders Activities of Daily Living (VADL) score, and the Balance Scoring System (BESS) test. The study was carried out for 12 weeks. The therapist who graded these outcomes and performed the testing was blinded as to whether the patient was receiving antioxidant therapy or not. The pretrial test scores did not differ significantly between the two groups on any of the tests.

Both groups of patients showed trends toward significant improvement on all the tests after the 12 weeks of therapy, but the combination treatment trend was stronger than that of the standard therapy alone group. After only 4 weeks, the SOT score by CDP was 78 for the antioxidant group as compared to 63 for the nonantioxidant group. This difference was statistically significant at the $P < 0.05$ level. The improvement noted by the antioxidant group on the other tests was also greater than the nonantioxidant group, although these differences did not reach statistical significance because of the short trial period and small sample size.

ANTIOXIDANTS REDUCE GLUTAMATE RELEASE

Glutamate is released following TBI. It has been reported that increased proinflammatory stimuli and oxidative stress cause microglia to release excessive amounts of glutamate, which contribute to the loss of neurons.[137] The release of glutamate was blocked by vitamin E.[137] Both vitamin E[138] and coenzyme Q_{10}[139] also protect against glutamate-induced neurotoxicity in cell culture models.

PREVENTION STRATEGIES FOR SEVERE TBI

Primary Prevention

The purpose of primary prevention is to protect healthy individuals from severe TBI. In case of this form of TBI, it is not feasible to develop a primary prevention strategy, because acute TBI may occur suddenly. However, in some cases such as troops to be deployed in a military conflict, in which the risk of severe TBI is high, it is possible to develop a primary prevention strategy, which can decrease the initial damage during the first phase of TBI. Since severe TBI generates excessive amounts of free radicals and inflammation soon after injury, and since antioxidants and certain phenolic compounds reduce free radicals and inflammation, supplementation with a preparation of micronutrients containing dietary and endogenous antioxidants and certain phenolic compounds may be one of the rational choices for primary prevention of severe TBI. A micronutrient preparation containing dietary and endogenous antioxidants and certain phenolic compounds, which can reduce oxidative stress indirectly by enhancing the levels of antioxidant enzymes through Nrf2/ARE pathway and directly by scavenging free radicals, can be used for primary prevention.

SECONDARY PREVENTION

The purpose of secondary prevention is to delay the progression of severe TBI in order to reduce the risk of developing edema, increased cerebral vascular permeability, and neuronal death during acute phase of injury. The purpose of secondary prevention is also to reduce the risk of developing late adverse health effects, such as cognitive dysfunction, PTSD, and behavior abnormalities, among those who survive severe TBI. During acute phase of severe TBI, excessive amounts of free radicals, inflammation, and glutamate, which play an important role in the progression of acute injury, are produced, and since antioxidants and certain polyphenolic compounds reduce oxidative damage and inflammation, and glutamate release and toxicity, supplementation with a preparation of micronutrients containing dietary and endogenous antioxidants and certain polyphenolic compounds may be one of the rational choices for secondary prevention of severe TBI. Since individuals exposed to severe TBI require emergency care, secondary prevention cannot be performed in the absence of standard care. Therefore, this form of prevention cannot be distinguish from treatment.

PROBLEMS OF USING SINGLE MICRONUTRIENTS AFTER SEVERE TBI

The use of single agents, such as NAC, melatonin, vitamin E, curcumin, omega-3 fatty acids and flavonoids, produced some benefits in a few animal models of severe TBI. These studies are not sufficient to draw any conclusion regarding the value of multiple micronutrients in reducing the progression of TBI in humans. Previous studies on the effect of single antioxidants in chronic diseases have produced inconsistent results. For example, the study on beta-carotene in male heavy smokers for reducing the risk of lung cancer, vitamin E in Alzheimer's disease (AD) for improving cognitive function, and vitamin E in Parkinson disease (PD) for improving the symptoms and as expected, produced inconsistent results varying from no effect[160] to modest beneficial[161] as in PD, no effect affects as in AD,[162] or harmful effects as in heavy male smokers.[163] This is due to the fact that patients with the above diseases have a high internal oxidative environment, in which an individual antioxidant is oxidized, and then acts as a pro-oxidant rather than as an antioxidant. An oxidized antioxidant is likely to increase the risk of chronic diseases after long-term consumption. Because of the failure to obtain consistent results with individual antioxidants in other neurodegenerative diseases, I recommend a preparation of micronutrients containing dietary and endogenous antioxidants, vitamin D, B vitamins, certain minerals and polyphenolic compounds (resveratrol and curcumin), and omega-3 fatty acids for reducing the progression of TBI.

RATIONALE FOR USING MULTIPLE MICRONUTRIENTS FOR REDUCING THE PROGRESSION OF TBI

The references for this section are described in a review.[164] The mechanisms of action of micronutrients and polyphenolic compounds in the proposed formulation are in part different; their distribution in various organs and cells, their affinity to various types of free radicals, and their biological half-lives are also different. Beta-carotene (BC) is more effective in quenching oxygen radicals than most other antioxidants. BC can perform certain biological functions that cannot be produced by its metabolite vitamin A, and vice versa. It has been reported that BC treatment enhances the expression of the connexin gene, which codes for a gap junction protein in mammalian fibroblasts in culture, whereas vitamin A treatment does not produce such an effect. Vitamin A can induce differentiation in certain normal and cancer cells, whereas BC and other carotenoids do not. Thus, BC and vitamin A have, in part, different biological functions in the body. The gradient of oxygen pressure varies within cells. Some antioxidants, such as vitamin E, are more effective as quenchers of free radicals in reduced oxygen pressure, whereas BC and vitamin A are more effective in higher atmospheric pressures. Vitamin C is necessary to protect cellular components in aqueous environments, whereas carotenoids and vitamins A and E protect cellular components in lipid environments. Vitamin C also plays an important role in maintaining the cellular levels of vitamin E by recycling vitamin E radical (oxidized) to the reduced (antioxidant) form.

The form of vitamin E used in a preparation of micronutrients is also important. It has been established that D-alpha-tocopheryl succinate (vitamin E succinate) is the most effective form of vitamin in both in vitro and in vivo. This form of vitamin E is more soluble than alpha-tocopherol and enters cells more readily, and therefore, it is expected that vitamin E succinate would cross the blood–brain barrier in greater amounts than alpha-tocopherol. However, this idea has not yet been tested in animals or humans. We have reported that an oral ingestion of vitamin E succinate (800 IU/day) in humans increased plasma levels of not only alpha-tocopherol but also of vitamin E succinate, suggesting that a portion of this form of vitamin E can be absorbed from the intestinal tract before hydrolysis to alpha-tocopherol, provided that the plasma pool of alpha-tocopherol is saturated. This observation is important, because the conventional assumption based on the studies in rodents has indicated that esterified forms of vitamin E, such as alpha-tocopheryl succinate, alpha-tocopheryl nicotinate, and alpha-tocopheryl acetate, can be absorbed from the intestinal tract only after they are hydrolyzed to alpha-tocopherol. Our preliminary data showed that this assumption may not be true for the absorption of vitamin E succinate in humans, provided that the plasma pool of alpha-tocopherol is saturated.

An endogenous antioxidant, glutathione, is effective in catabolizing H_2O_2 and anions. However, oral supplementation with glutathione failed to significantly increase plasma levels of glutathione in human subjects, suggesting that this tripeptide is completely hydrolyzed in the GI tract.Therefore, I propose to add N-acetylcysteine and alpha-lipoic acid, which increase the cellular levels of glutathione by different mechanisms in a multiple micronutrient preparation.

Another endogenous antioxidant, coenzyme Q_{10}, may have some potential value in reducing the progression of TBI. Since coenzyme Q_{10} is needed for the generation of ATP by mitochondria, it is essential to add this antioxidant in a multiple micronutrient preparation. A study has shown that coenzyme Q_{10} scavenges peroxy radicals faster than alpha-tocopherol and, like vitamin C, can regenerate vitamin E in a redox cycle. However, it is a weaker antioxidant than alpha-tocopherol. Coenzyme Q_{10} administration has been shown to improve clinical symptoms in patients with mitochondrial encephalomyopathies.[165]

Since memory loss occurs among survivors of TBI as a late effect, nicotinamide, a precursor of NAD^+, attenuated glutamate-induced toxicity and preserved cellular levels of NAD^+ to support the activity of SIRT1. It is also a competitive inhibitor of histone deacetylase activity, and restored memory deficits in AD transgenic mice. These preclinical data suggest that oral supplementation with nicotinamide may be safe and useful in preventing memory deficits.

Selenium is a cofactor of glutathione peroxidase, and Se-glutathione peroxidase acts as an antioxidant by increasing the level of intracellular glutathione. Therefore, selenium should be added to a multiple micronutrient preparation for reducing the progression of TBI.

In addition to dietary and endogenous antioxidants, all B vitamins with high doses of vitamin B_3 (nicotinamide) and vitamin D should be added to a multiple micronutrient preparation for maintaining normal health. Curcumin and omega-3 fatty acids were also added, because they appear to produce some benefits in reducing the progression of TBI. Resveratrol is also added, because it has produced some beneficial effects in animal models of TBI.

Two recent studies on supplementation with multiple vitamin preparations reduced cancer incidence by 10% in men[166] and improved clinical outcomes in patients with HIV/AIDS, who were not taking medication.[167]

Dietary and endogenous antioxidants and polyphenolic compounds derived from herbs, fruits, and vegetables inhibit chronic inflammation.[124–136]

Animal studies have suggested that increased proinflammatory stimuli and oxidative stress cause microglia to release excessive amounts of glutamate, which not only maintains anxiety disorders through NMDA receptors but which also contribute to neurodegeneration.[137] The release of glutamate was blocked by vitamin E,[137] and this could help in improving anxiety disorders. Indeed, an inhibitor of the NMDA receptor reduces anxiety,[168] but is toxic. Both vitamin E[138] and coenzyme Q_{10}[139] also protect against glutamate-induced neurotoxicity in cell culture models.

PROPOSED MICRONUTRIENTS FOR PRIMARY PREVENTION OF TBI

Studies on primary prevention can be performed on individuals, such as combat troops who are to be deployed in a military conflict, where they are likely to sustain TBI. A preparation of multiple micronutrients may include vitamin A (retinyl palmitate); vitamin E (both D-alpha-tocopherol and D-alpha-TS); natural mixed carotenoids; vitamin C (calcium ascorbate); coenzyme Q_{10}, R-alpha-lipoic acid; N-acetylcysteine; L-carnitine; vitamin D, all B vitamins, selenium, zinc, chromium, and omega-3 fatty acids; and certain polyphenolic compounds (curcumin and resveratrol) for reducing the initial damage to the brain.

No iron, copper, or manganese would be included, because these trace minerals are known to interact with vitamin C to produce free radicals. These trace minerals are absorbed from the intestinal tract more in the presence of antioxidants than in their absence that could result in increased body stores of free forms of these minerals. Increased iron stores have been linked to increased risk of some neurodegenerative diseases.[169] No heavy metals such as zirconium and molybdenum were added because of their potential neurotoxicity after long-term consumption.

The recommended micronutrient supplements should be taken daily, orally, divided into two doses, one half in the morning and the other half in the evening with meal. This is because the biological half-lives of micronutrients are highly viable, which can create high levels of fluctuations in the tissue levels of micronutrients if they are consumed once-a-day. A twofold difference in the levels of certain micronutrients such as alpha-tocopheryl succinate can cause a marked difference in the expression of gene profiles.[170] In order to maintain relatively consistent levels of micronutrients in the brain, the proposed micronutrients should be taken twice a day.

The efficacy of proposed micronutrient formulation in troops to be deployed in military conflicts should be tested by well-designed clinical studies. Meanwhile, the proposed micronutrient recommendations may be adopted by the individuals who are in combat theater but have not sustained TBI with their physicians or health professionals. It is expected that the proposed recommendations would reduce the level of initial damage to brain following TBI.

TOXICITY OF INGREDIENTS IN PROPOSED MICRONUTRIENT PREPARATION

Antioxidants and B vitamins used in a proposed micronutrient preparation are considered safe. Antioxidants at doses higher than those that are recommended for the proposed micronutrient preparation have been consumed by the U.S. population for decades without a significant toxicity. However, a few of them could produce harmful effects at certain high doses in some individuals when consumed daily for a long period of time. For example, vitamin A at doses of 10,000 IU or more per day can cause birth defects in pregnant women, and beta-carotene at a 50 mg dose or more can produce bronzing of the skin, which is reversible on discontinuation. Vitamin C as ascorbic acid at high doses (10 g or more per day) can cause diarrhea in some individuals. Vitamin E at high doses (2000 IU or more per day) can induce clotting defects after long-term consumption. Vitamin B_6 at high doses (50 mg or more per day) may produce peripheral neuropathy, and selenium at a 400 mcg dose or more per day can cause skin and liver toxicity after long-term consumption. Coenzyme Q_{10} has no known toxicity, and recommended daily doses are 30–400 mg. N-acetylcysteine doses of 250–1500 mg and alpha-lipoic acid doses of 600 mg are used in humans without toxicity at these doses. All ingredients present in the proposed micronutrient preparations are safe and come under category of "Food Supplement" and therefore do not require FDA approval for their use.

PROPOSED MICRONUTRIENTS FOR SECONDARY PREVENTION IN COMBINATION WITH STANDARD THERAPY

Individuals who sustain severe TBI provide an excellent opportunity to study the efficacy of a multiple micronutrients preparation, in combination with standard therapy, in reducing the secondary damage during the acute and chronic phases of injury. These patients require immediate emergency care in the hospital to receive standard therapy in order to stabilize their conditions.

Standard Therapy

The severe TBI is extremely difficult to treat, because of the inherent complexity of the brain structures and functions as well as extreme variations in the pattern of injury. Approximately half of severely brain-injured patients will need surgery to remove or repair hematomas (rupture of blood vessels) or contusions (bruised brain tissue) (National Institute of Neurological Disorders and Stroke, 2009). Initial treatment focuses on preventing secondary injury following TBI. This includes proper oxygen supply to the brain and the rest of the body, maintaining adequate blood flow, and controlling blood pressure.

Hypothermia (32–33°C) has been used in the management of TBI. In a clinical study, it was demonstrated that hypothermia attenuated the levels of markers of oxidative stress in infants and children after severe TBI.[171] The effect of hypothermia was analyzed in 12 studies with 1327 patients, in which 8 studies cooled according to long-term or goal-directed strategy, and 4 studies cooled according to short-term strategy. The results revealed that when only short-term strategy cooling was performed, neither mortality nor neurological outcomes were improved; however, when long-term cooling was used, mortality was reduced and neurological outcomes were improved.[172] The optimal results were obtained when cooling was continued for at least 72 h and/or until intracranial pressure is normalized for at least 24 h. In children with severe TBI, the CSF levels of alpha-synuclein were elevated in patients with TBI than in control subjects; however, the CSF levels of alpha-synuclein decreased after hypothermia treatment.[173]

Medications to reduce the secondary damage to the brain immediately after injury may include diuretics (to reduce pressure from the brain by eliminating fluid through urine), antiseizure drugs during the first week (to avoid additional damage to the brain that might be caused by seizures, and coma-inducing drugs (the brain at this state uses less oxygen for survival and function; this procedure is particularly helpful if the blood vessels are unable to supply sufficient nutrients and oxygen to the brain). In addition, emergency surgery may be needed to remove blood clots, repair skull fractures, and open a window in the skull to relieve pressure inside the brain by draining accumulated fluid. Patients with severe TBI receive rehabilitation therapy that includes an individually tailored treatment program in the area of physical therapy, occupational therapy, speech/language therapy, medications, psychology/psychiatry therapy, and social support. The standard therapy has markedly improved the management of severe TBI and has improved the survival rate of patients.

Based on the studies on animal models of TBI, several potential therapeutic agents have been identified. They include erythropoietin[174,175]; antibodies of serotonin receptors[176]; histone deacetylase inhibitors[177,178]; protease inhibitors[179]; fenofibrate, a peroxisome proliferator-activated receptor alpha agonist[45]; meloxicam, a COX-2 inhibitor[180]; and interferon-gamma.[181] These drugs will require FDA approval.

At present, increased oxidative stress, inflammation, and glutamate release contribute to the development of secondary injury to the brain during acute phase, and to the development of late adverse effects during chronic phase of injury are not being adequately addressed. This is essential in order to improve current management of severe TBI. Antioxidants and certain polyphenolic compounds reduce oxidative stress, inflammation, and the release and toxicity of glutamate, in combination with standard therapy, may further improve the acute and chronic management of TBI. A separate preparation of micronutrients, in combination with standard therapy, is recommended during the acute phase of injury. This preparation of micronutrients contains doses of ingredients higher than those recommended for primary prevention. It should be pointed out that oral supplementation with a preparation of micronutrients can be started 24 h after injury, and not immediately after injury. This is due to the fact that both anti-inflammatory and proinflammatory cytokines are released immediately after injury. Anti-inflammatory cytokines help to repair cellular damage. Supplementation with a preparation of micronutrients immediately after injury may reduce both proinflammatory and anti-inflammatory cytokines. Inhibition of anti-inflammatory cytokine release may interfere with the repair processes in the brain. The above treatment with a preparation of micronutrients should be continued for 4–6 weeks after which the micronutrient preparation used for primary prevention should be adopted for the entire lifespan in order to reduce late adverse health effects of severe TBI.

The efficacy of the proposed micronutrient formulations, in combination with standard therapy, on individuals who have sustained severe TBI should be tested by well-designed clinical studies. Meanwhile, the proposed micronutrient recommendations may be adopted by the individuals who have sustained severe traumatic injury in consultation with their physicians. It is expected that the proposed recommendations, in combination with standard therapy, would improve the current management of severe TBI during the acute and chronic phases of injury.

DIET AND LIFESTYLE RECOMMENDATIONS FOR SEVERE TBI

A balanced diet, in addition to supplementation with multiple micronutrients, is necessary for reducing the risk of long-term adverse effects on brain functions, as well as for improving the efficacy of standard therapy in the management of acute and long-term consequences of TBI with penetrating head injury. Lifestyle recommendations include daily moderate exercise, reduced stress, no tobacco smoking, and reduced intake of caffeine. A high saturated fat diet[155] and caffeine[156] appear to increase the progression of damage following TBI in animal models. Therefore high-fat diet and excessive use of caffeine should be avoided. I recommend a balanced diet containing a low-fat and high-fiber diet with plenty of fruits and vegetables.

CONCLUSIONS

Severe TBI occurs when an object penetrates the skull and damages the brain. This form of TBI is caused by vehicle crashes, gunshot wounds to the head, and exposure to improvised explosive devices and combat-related injuries. The damage to the brain after severe TBI occurs in three phases. The first phase involves injury to the brain tissue that cannot be reversed; however, standard therapy together with micronutrient supplements may reduce the progression of damage. The second phase of TBI occurs soon after injury and continues for days to weeks and contributes to the progression of injury leading to neurological disorders and neuronal death. During this period, intervention with standard therapy and micronutrient supplements can slow down the progression of the damage. The third phase of severe TBI appears as late effects to the extent of which TBI depends upon the size of initial areas of the brain damaged. The late effects may include cognitive dysfunction, PTSD, and other behavior abnormalities.

Recent advances in surgical techniques and improved management by hypothermia and medications have improved survival and clinical outcomes of patients with severe TBI. Most survivors need long-term rehabilitation and physical therapy and suffer from poor quality of life, such as cognitive dysfunction and abnormal behavior. Therefore, additional approaches during acute and late phases of injury are needed in order to reduce the incidence of cognitive dysfunction and abnormal behavior.

Both animal and human studies reveal that increased oxidative stress, inflammation, and release of glutamate play an important role in progression of the damage, leading to cognitive dysfunction and abnormal behavior. Antioxidants which reduce oxidative stress, chronic inflammation, and glutamate release and its toxicity appear to be one of the rational choices for reducing the progression of damage during acute and late phases of injury. Despite these observations, only a few studies with individual antioxidants primarily in animal models of TBI have been performed. No studies have been performed with multiple antioxidants either on animal models of TBI or humans with TBI.

I have proposed a micronutrient preparation containing multiple dietary and endogenous antioxidants, vitamin D, L-carnitine, all B vitamins with high doses of vitamin B_3, selenium, curcumin, resveratrol, omega-3 fatty acids, and selenium for primary prevention. This preparation of micronutrients would reduce oxidative stress, chronic inflammation, and glutamate release and its toxicity by enhancing the levels of antioxidant enzymes through the Nrf2/ARE pathway as well as the levels of dietary and endogenous antioxidants. A micronutrient preparation similar to that proposed for primary prevention except for higher doses of certain ingredients, in combination with standard therapy, has been proposed for secondary prevention or treatment.

The efficacy of these formulations can be tested by clinical studies in the following groups: (1) troops to be employed in combat and, (2) in combination with standard therapy, in individuals who have sustained and/or survive severe TBI. Meanwhile, the proposed micronutrient recommendations may be adopted by the individuals who belong to one of the above groups in consultation with their physicians. It is expected that the proposed recommendations would reduce the progression of damage and enhance the efficacy of standard therapy in the management of severe TBI during acute and late phases of injury.

REFERENCES

1. Hicks RR, Fertig SJ, Desrocher RE, Koroshetz WJ, Pancrazio JJ. Neurological effects of blast injury. *J Trauma*. May 2010; 68(5): 1257–1263.
2. Leung LY, Wei G, Shear DA, Tortella FC. The acute effects of hemorrhagic shock on cerebral blood flow, brain tissue oxygen tension, and spreading depolarization following penetrating ballistic-like brain injury. *J Neurotrauma*. Jul 15 2013; 30(14): 1288–1298.

3. Schneiderman AI, Braver ER, Kang HK. Understanding the sequelae of injury mechanisms and mild traumatic brain injury incurred during the conflicts in Iraq and Afghanistan: Persistent postconcussive symptoms and posttraumatic stress disorder. *Am J Epidemiol.* Apr 17 2008.

4. Graham DI, McIntosh TK, Maxwell WL, Nicoll JA. Recent advances in neurotrauma. *J Neuropathol Exp Neurol.* Aug 2000; 59(8): 641–651.

5. Bayir H, Kochanek PM, Kagan VE. Oxidative stress in immature brain after traumatic brain injury. *Dev Neurosci.* 2006; 28(4–5): 420–431.

6. Rael LT, Bar-Or R, Mains CW, Slone DS, Levy AS, Bar-Or D. Plasma oxidation-reduction potential and protein oxidation in traumatic brain injury. *J Neurotrauma.* Mar 24 2009.

7. Shao C, Roberts KN, Markesbery WR, Scheff SW, Lovell MA. Oxidative stress in head trauma in aging. *Free Radic Biol Med.* Jul 1 2006; 41(1): 77–85.

8. Mikawa S, Kinouchi H, Kamii H et al. Attenuation of acute and chronic damage following traumatic brain injury in copper, zinc-superoxide dismutase transgenic mice. *J Neurosurg.* Nov 1996; 85(5): 885–891.

9. Petronilho F, Feier G, de Souza B et al. Oxidative stress in brain according to traumatic brain injury intensity. *J Surg Res.* May 19 2009.

10. Tavazzi B, Signoretti S, Lazzarino G et al. Cerebral oxidative stress and depression of energy metabolism correlate with severity of diffuse brain injury in rats. *Neurosurgery.* Mar 2005; 56(3): 582–589; discussion 582–589.

11. Singh IN, Sullivan PG, Hall ED. Peroxynitrite-mediated oxidative damage to brain mitochondria: Protective effects of peroxynitrite scavengers. *J Neurosci Res.* Aug 1 2007; 85(10): 2216–2223.

12. Huttemann M, Lee I, Kreipke CW, Petrov T. Suppression of the inducible form of nitric oxide synthase prior to traumatic brain injury improves cytochrome c oxidase activity and normalizes cellular energy levels. *Neuroscience.* Jan 2 2008; 151(1): 148–154.

13. Louin G, Marchand-Verrecchia C, Palmier B, Plotkine M, Jafarian-Tehrani M. Selective inhibition of inducible nitric oxide synthase reduces neurological deficit but not cerebral edema following traumatic brain injury. *Neuropharmacology.* Feb 2006; 50(2): 182–190.

14. Ansari MA, Roberts KN, Scheff SW. Oxidative stress and modification of synaptic proteins in hippocampus after traumatic brain injury. *Free Radic Biol Med.* Aug 15 2008; 45(4): 443–452.

15. Lima FD, Souza MA, Furian AF et al. Na$^+$, K$^+$-ATPase activity impairment after experimental traumatic brain injury: Relationship to spatial learning deficits and oxidative stress. *Behav Brain Res.* Nov 21 2008; 193(2): 306–310.

16. Chen G, Fang Q, Zhang J, Zhou D, Wang Z. Role of the Nrf2-ARE pathway in early brain injury after experimental subarachnoid hemorrhage. *J Neurosci Res.* Apr 2011; 89(4): 515–523.

17. Varma S, Janesko KL, Wisniewski SR et al. F2-isoprostane and neuron-specific enolase in cerebrospinal fluid after severe traumatic brain injury in infants and children. *J Neurotrauma.* Aug 2003; 20(8): 781–786.

18. Bayir H, Kagan VE, Tyurina YY et al. Assessment of antioxidant reserves and oxidative stress in cerebrospinal fluid after severe traumatic brain injury in infants and children. *Pediatr Res.* May 2002; 51(5): 571–578.

19. Ragan DK, McKinstry R, Benzinger T, Leonard JR, Pineda JA. Alterations in cerebral oxygen metabolism after traumatic brain injury in children. *J Cereb Blood Flow Metab.* Jan 2013; 33(1): 48–52.

20. Darwish RS, Amiridze N, Aarabi B. Nitrotyrosine as an oxidative stress marker: Evidence for involvement in neurologic outcome in human traumatic brain injury. *J Trauma.* Aug 2007; 63(2): 439–442.

21. Darwish RS, Amiridze NS. Detectable levels of cytochrome C and activated caspase-9 in cerebrospinal fluid after human traumatic brain injury. *Neurocrit Care.* Jun 2010; 12(3): 337–341.

22. Emmerling MR, Morganti-Kossmann MC, Kossmann T et al. Traumatic brain injury elevates the Alzheimer's amyloid peptide A beta 42 in human CSF: A possible role for nerve cell injury. *Ann N Y Acad Sci.* Apr 2000; 903: 118–122.

23. Pappolla MA, Chyan YJ, Omar RA et al. Evidence of oxidative stress and in vivo neurotoxicity of beta-amyloid in a transgenic mouse model of Alzheimer's disease: A chronic oxidative paradigm for testing antioxidant therapies in vivo. *Am J Pathol.* Apr 1998; 152(4): 871–877.

24. Butterfield DA. Amyloid beta-peptide (1–42)-induced oxidative stress and neurotoxicity: Implications for neurodegeneration in Alzheimer's disease brain. A review. *Free Radic Res.* Dec 2002; 36(12): 1307–1313.

25. Butterfield DA, Castegna A, Lauderback CM, Drake J. Evidence that amyloid beta-peptide-induced lipid peroxidation and its sequelae in Alzheimer's disease brain contribute to neuronal death. *Neurobiol Aging.* Sep–Oct 2002; 23(5): 655–664.

26. Qi XL, Xiu J, Shan KR et al. Oxidative stress induced by beta-amyloid peptide(1–42) is involved in the altered composition of cellular membrane lipids and the decreased expression of nicotinic receptors in human SH-SY5Y neuroblastoma cells. *Neurochem Int.* Jun 2005; 46(8): 613–621.

27. Yu GF, Jie YQ, Wu A, Huang Q, Dai WM, Fan XF. Increased plasma 8-iso-prostaglandin F2alpha concentration in severe human traumatic brain injury. *Clin Chim Acta.* Jun 5 2013; 421: 7–11.

28. Clausen F, Marklund N, Lewen A, Enblad P, Basu S, Hillered L. Interstitial F(2)-isoprostane 8-iso-PGF(2alpha) as a biomarker of oxidative stress after severe human traumatic brain injury. *J Neurotrauma.* Mar 20 2012; 29(5): 766–775.

29. Nayak CD, Nayak DM, Raja A, Rao A. Erythrocyte indicators of oxidative changes in patients with graded traumatic head injury. *Neurol India.* Jan–Mar 2008; 56(1): 31–35.

30. Hohl A, Gullo Jda S, Silva CC et al. Plasma levels of oxidative stress biomarkers and hospital mortality in severe head injury: A multivariate analysis. *J Crit Care.* Oct 2012; 27(5): 523 e511–e529.

31. Lin C, Wang N, Shen ZP, Zhao ZY. Plasma copeptin concentration and outcome after pediatric traumatic brain injury. *Peptides.* Apr 2013; 42: 43–47.

32. Robertson CL, Scafidi S, McKenna MC, Fiskum G. Mitochondrial mechanisms of cell death and neuroprotection in pediatric ischemic and traumatic brain injury. *Exp Neurol.* Aug 2009; 218(2): 371–380.

33. Mazzeo AT, Beat A, Singh A, Bullock MR. The role of mitochondrial transition pore, and its modulation, in traumatic brain injury and delayed neurodegeneration after TBI. *Exp Neurol.* Aug 2009; 218(2): 363–370.

34. Opii WO, Nukala VN, Sultana R et al. Proteomic identification of oxidized mitochondrial proteins following experimental traumatic brain injury. *J Neurotrauma.* May 2007; 24(5): 772–789.

35. Sharma P, Benford B, Li ZZ, Ling GS. Role of pyruvate dehydrogenase complex in traumatic brain injury and measurement of pyruvate dehydrogenase enzyme by dipstick test. *J Emerg Trauma Shock.* May 2009; 2(2): 67–72.

36. Dai W, Cheng HL, Huang RQ, Zhuang Z, Shi JX. Quantitative detection of the expression of mitochondrial cytochrome c oxidase subunits mRNA in the cerebral cortex after experimental traumatic brain injury. *Brain Res.* Jan 28 2009; 1251: 287–295.

37. Gilmer LK, Roberts KN, Joy K, Sullivan PG, Scheff SW. Early mitochondrial dysfunction after cortical contusion injury. *J Neurotrauma.* Aug 2009; 26(8): 1271–1280.

38. Singh IN, Sullivan PG, Deng Y, Mbye LH, Hall ED. Time course of post-traumatic mitochondrial oxidative damage and dysfunction in a mouse model of focal traumatic brain injury: Implications for neuroprotective therapy. *J Cereb Blood Flow Metab.* Nov 2006; 26(11): 1407–1418.

39. Readnower RD, Pandya JD, McEwen ML, Pauly JR, Springer JE, Sullivan PG. Post-injury administration of the mitochondrial permeability transition pore inhibitor, NIM811, is neuroprotective and improves cognition after traumatic brain injury in rats. *J Neurotrauma.* Sep 2011; 28(9): 1845–1853.

40. Mustafa AG, Singh IN, Wang J, Carrico KM, Hall ED. Mitochondrial protection after traumatic brain injury by scavenging lipid peroxyl radicals. *J Neurochem.* Jul 2010; 114(1): 271–280.

41. Conley YP, Okonkwo DO, Deslouches S, Alexander SA, Beers SR, Ren D. Mitochondrial polymorphisms impact outcomes after severe traumatic brain injfsury. *J Neurotrauma.* Jul 24 2013.

42. Aygok GA, Marmarou A, Fatouros P, Kettenmann B, Bullock RM. Assessment of mitochondrial impairment and cerebral blood flow in severe brain injured patients. *Acta Neurochir Suppl.* 2008; 102: 57–61.

43. Belli A, Sen J, Petzold A et al. Extracellular N-acetylaspartate depletion in traumatic brain injury. *J Neurochem.* Feb 2006; 96(3): 861–869.

44. Pandya JD, Pauly JR, Nukala VN et al. Post-injury administration of mitochondrial uncouplers increases tissue sparing and improves behavioral outcome following traumatic brain injury in rodents. *J Neurotrauma.* May 2007; 24(5): 798–811.

45. Chen XR, Besson VC, Palmier B, Garcia Y, Plotkine M, Marchand-Leroux C. Neurological recovery-promoting, anti-inflammatory, and anti-oxidative effects afforded by fenofibrate, a PPAR alpha agonist, in traumatic brain injury. *J Neurotrauma.* Jul 2007; 24(7): 1119–1131.

46. Maier B, Lehnert M, Laurer HL, Mautes AE, Steudel WI, Marzi I. Delayed elevation of soluble tumor necrosis factor receptors p75 and p55 in cerebrospinal fluid and plasma after traumatic brain injury. *Shock.* Aug 2006; 26(2): 122–127.

47. Bermpohl D, You Z, Lo EH, Kim HH, Whalen MJ. TNF alpha and Fas mediate tissue damage and functional outcome after traumatic brain injury in mice. *J Cereb Blood Flow Metab.* Nov 2007; 27(11): 1806–1818.

48. Tuzgen S, Tanriover N, Uzan M et al. Nitric oxide levels in rat cortex, hippocampus, cerebellum, and brainstem after impact acceleration head injury. *Neurol Res.* Jan 2003; 25(1): 31–34.

49. Clausen F, Hanell A, Bjork M et al. Neutralization of interleukin-1beta modifies the inflammatory response and improves histological and cognitive outcome following traumatic brain injury in mice. *Eur J Neurosci.* Aug 2009; 30(3): 385–396.

50. Shohami E, Gallily R, Mechoulam R, Bass R, Ben-Hur T. Cytokine production in the brain following closed head injury: Dexanabinol (HU-211) is a novel TNF-alpha inhibitor and an effective neuroprotectant. *J Neuroimmunol.* Feb 1997; 72(2): 169–177.

51. Trembovler V, Beit-Yannai E, Younis F, Gallily R, Horowitz M, Shohami E. Antioxidants attenuate acute toxicity of tumor necrosis factor-alpha induced by brain injury in rat. *J Interferon Cytokine Res.* Jul 1999; 19(7): 791–795.

52. Lloyd E, Somera-Molina K, Van Eldik LJ, Watterson DM, Wainwright MS. Suppression of acute proinflammatory cytokine and chemokine upregulation by post-injury administration of a novel small molecule improves long-term neurologic outcome in a mouse model of traumatic brain injury. *J Neuroinflammation.* 2008; 5: 28.

53. Wei HH, Lu XC, Shear DA et al. NNZ-2566 treatment inhibits neuroinflammation and pro-inflammatory cytokine expression induced by experimental penetrating ballistic-like brain injury in rats. *J Neuroinflammation.* 2009; 6: 19.

54. Wu H, Mahmood A, Lu D et al. Attenuation of astrogliosis and modulation of endothelial growth factor receptor in lipid rafts by simvastatin after traumatic brain injury. *J Neurosurg.* Nov 6 2009.

55. Lopez NE, Krzyzaniak MJ, Costantini TW et al. Vagal nerve stimulation decreases blood-brain barrier disruption after traumatic brain injury. *J Trauma Acute Care Surg.* Jun 2012; 72(6): 1562–1566.

56. Donkin JJ, Nimmo AJ, Cernak I, Blumbergs PC, Vink R. Substance P is associated with the development of brain edema and functional deficits after traumatic brain injury. *J Cereb Blood Flow Metab.* Aug 2009; 29(8): 1388–1398.

57. Woodcock T, Morganti-Kossmann MC. The role of markers of inflammation in traumatic brain injury. *Front Neurol.* 2013; 4: 18.

58. Frugier T, Morganti-Kossmann MC, O'Reilly D, McLean CA. In situ detection of inflammatory mediators in post mortem human brain tissue after traumatic injury. *J Neurotrauma.* Mar 2010; 27(3): 497–507.

59. Ramlackhansingh AF, Brooks DJ, Greenwood RJ et al. Inflammation after trauma: Microglial activation and traumatic brain injury. *Ann Neurol.* Sep 2011; 70(3): 374–383.

60. Skandsen T, Kvistad KA, Solheim O, Strand IH, Folvik M, Vik A. Prevalence and impact of diffuse axonal injury in patients with moderate and severe head injury: A cohort study of early magnetic resonance imaging findings and 1-year outcome. *J Neurosurg.* Sep 2010; 113(3): 556–563.

61. Lin Y, Wen L. Inflammatory response following diffuse axonal injury. *Int J Med Sci.* 2013; 10(5): 515–521.

62. Lucas SM, Rothwell NJ, Gibson RM. The role of inflammation in CNS injury and disease. *Br J Pharmacol.* Jan 2006; 147 Suppl 1: S232–S240.

63. Goodman JC, Van M, Gopinath SP, Robertson CS. Pro-inflammatory and pro-apoptotic elements of the neuroinflammatory response are activated in traumatic brain injury. *Acta Neurochir Suppl.* 2008; 102: 437–439.

64. Hutchinson PJ, O'Connell MT, Rothwell NJ et al. Inflammation in human brain injury: Intracerebral concentrations of IL-1alpha, IL-1beta, and their endogenous inhibitor IL-1ra. *J Neurotrauma.* Oct 2007; 24(10): 1545–1557.

65. You Z, Yang J, Takahashi K et al. Reduced tissue damage and improved recovery of motor function after traumatic brain injury in mice deficient in complement component C4. *J Cereb Blood Flow Metab.* Dec 2007; 27(12): 1954–1964.

66. Hein AM, O'Banion MK. Neuroinflammation and memory: The role of prostaglandins. *Mol Neurobiol.* Aug 2009; 40(1): 15–32.

67. Dietrich WD, Chatzipanteli K, Vitarbo E, Wada K, Kinoshita K. The role of inflammatory processes in the pathophysiology and treatment of brain and spinal cord trauma. *Acta Neurochir Suppl.* 2004; 89: 69–74.

68. Potts MB, Koh SE, Whetstone WD et al. Traumatic injury to the immature brain: Inflammation, oxidative injury, and iron-mediated damage as potential therapeutic targets. *NeuroRx.* Apr 2006; 3(2): 143–153.

69. Hall ED, Detloff MR, Johnson K, Kupina NC. Peroxynitrite-mediated protein nitration and lipid peroxidation in a mouse model of traumatic brain injury. *J Neurotrauma.* Jan 2004; 21(1): 9–20.

70. Gahm C, Holmin S, Wiklund PN, Brundin L, Mathiesen T. Neuroprotection by selective inhibition of inducible nitric oxide synthase after experimental brain contusion. *J Neurotrauma.* Sep 2006; 23(9): 1343–1354.

71. Minambres EC, Sanchez-Velasco, P et al. Correlation between transcranial interleukin-6 gradient and outcome in patients with acute brain injury. *Crit Care Med.* 2003; 31: 33–38.

72. Xiao GM, Wei J. Effects of beta-Aescin on the expression of nuclear factor-kappaB and tumor necrosis factor-alpha after traumatic brain injury in rats. *J Zhejiang Univ Sci B.* Jan 2005; 6(1): 28–32.

73. Hang CH, Chen G, Shi JX, Zhang X, Li JS. Cortical expression of nuclear factor kappaB after human brain contusion. *Brain Res.* Sep 13 2006; 1109(1): 14–21.

74. Dziurdzik P, Krawczyk L, Jalowiecki P, Kondera-Anasz Z, Menon L. Serum interleukin-10 in ICU patients with severe acute central nervous system injuries. *Inflamm Res.* Aug 2004; 53(8): 338–343.

75. Kirchhoff C, Buhmann S, Bogner V et al. Cerebrospinal IL-10 concentration is elevated in non-survivors as compared to survivors after severe traumatic brain injury. *Eur J Med Res.* Oct 27 2008; 13(10): 464–468.

76. Schneider Soares FM, Menezes de Souza N, Liborio Schwarzbold M et al. Interleukin-10 is an independent biomarker of severe traumatic brain injury prognosis. *Neuroimmunomodulation.* 2012; 19(6): 377–385.

77. Venetsanou K, Vlachos K, Moles A, Fragakis G, Fildissis G, Baltopoulos G. Hypolipoproteinemia and hyperinflammatory cytokines in serum of severe and moderate traumatic brain injury (TBI) patients. *Eur Cytokine Netw.* Dec 2007; 18(4): 206–209.

78. Buttram SD, Wisniewski SR, Jackson EK et al. Multiplex assessment of cytokine and chemokine levels in cerebrospinal fluid following severe pediatric traumatic brain injury: Effects of moderate hypothermia. *J Neurotrauma.* Nov 2007; 24(11): 1707–1717.

79. Gopinath SP, Valadka AB, Goodman JC, Robertson CS. Extracellular glutamate and aspartate in head injured patients. *Acta Neurochir Suppl.* 2000; 76: 437–438.

80. Rao VL, Baskaya MK, Dogan A, Rothstein JD, Dempsey RJ. Traumatic brain injury down-regulates glial glutamate transporter (GLT-1 and GLAST) proteins in rat brain. *J Neurochem.* May 1998; 70(5): 2020–2027.

81. Yi JH, Hazell AS. Excitotoxic mechanisms and the role of astrocytic glutamate transporters in traumatic brain injury. *Neurochem Int.* Apr 2006; 48(5): 394–403.

82. Goodrich GS, Kabakov AY, Hameed MQ, Dhamne SC, Rosenberg PA, Rotenberg A. Ceftriaxone treatment after traumatic brain injury restores expression of the glutamate transporter, GLT-1, reduces regional gliosis, and reduces post-traumatic seizures in the rat. *J Neurotrauma.* Aug 15 2013; 30(16): 1434–1441.

83. Hinzman JM, Thomas TC, Quintero JE, Gerhardt GA, Lifshitz J. Disruptions in the regulation of extracellular glutamate by neurons and glia in the rat striatum two days after diffuse brain injury. *J Neurotrauma.* Apr 10 2012; 29(6): 1197–1208.

84. Hascup ER, Hascup KN, Stephens M et al. Rapid microelectrode measurements and the origin and regulation of extracellular glutamate in rat prefrontal cortex. *J Neurochem.* Dec 2010; 115(6): 1608–1620.

85. Globus MY, Alonso O, Dietrich WD, Busto R, Ginsberg MD. Glutamate release and free radical production following brain injury: Effects of posttraumatic hypothermia. *J Neurochem.* Oct 1995; 65(4): 1704–1711.

86. Panter SS, Faden AI. Pretreatment with NMDA antagonists limits release of excitatory amino acids following traumatic brain injury. *Neurosci Lett.* Mar 2 1992; 136(2): 165–168.

87. Obrenovitch TP, Urenjak J. Is high extracellular glutamate the key to excitotoxicity in traumatic brain injury? *J Neurotrauma.* Oct 1997; 14(10): 677–698.

88. Zlotnik A, Leibowitz A, Gurevich B et al. Effect of estrogens on blood glutamate levels in relation to neurological outcome after TBI in male rats. *Intensive Care Med.* Jan 2012; 38(1): 137–144.

89. Movsesyan VA, Faden AI. Neuroprotective effects of selective group II mGluR activation in brain trauma and traumatic neuronal injury. *J Neurotrauma.* Feb 2006; 23(2): 117–127.

90. Allen JW, Ivanova SA, Fan L, Espey MG, Basile AS, Faden AI. Group II metabotropic glutamate receptor activation attenuates traumatic neuronal injury and improves neurological recovery after traumatic brain injury. *J Pharmacol Exp Ther.* Jul 1999; 290(1): 112–120.

91. Dai SS, Zhou YG, Li W et al. Local glutamate level dictates adenosine A2A receptor regulation of neuroinflammation and traumatic brain injury. *J Neurosci.* Apr 21 2010; 30(16): 5802–5810.

92. Yi JH, Hoover R, McIntosh TK, Hazell AS. Early, transient increase in complexin I and complexin II in the cerebral cortex following traumatic brain injury is attenuated by N-acetylcysteine. *J Neurotrauma.* Jan 2006; 23(1): 86–96.

93. Bullock R, Zauner A, Woodward JJ et al. Factors affecting excitatory amino acid release following severe human head injury. *J Neurosurg.* Oct 1998; 89(4): 507–518.

94. Yamamoto T, Rossi S, Stiefel M et al. CSF and ECF glutamate concentrations in head injured patients. *Acta Neurochir Suppl.* 1999; 75: 17–19.

95. Koura SS, Doppenberg EM, Marmarou A, Choi S, Young HF, Bullock R. Relationship between excitatory amino acid release and outcome after severe human head injury. *Acta Neurochir Suppl.* 1998; 71: 244–246.

96. Stover JF, Morganti-Kosmann MC, Lenzlinger PM, Stocker R, Kempski OS, Kossmann T. Glutamate and taurine are increased in ventricular cerebrospinal fluid of severely brain-injured patients. *J Neurotrauma.* Feb 1999; 16(2): 135–142.

97. Stover JF, Unterberg AW. Increased cerebrospinal fluid glutamate and taurine concentrations are associated with traumatic brain edema formation in rats. *Brain Res.* Sep 1 2000; 875(1–2): 51–55.

98. Chamoun R, Suki D, Gopinath SP, Goodman JC, Robertson C. Role of extracellular glutamate measured by cerebral microdialysis in severe traumatic brain injury. *J Neurosurg.* Sep 2010; 113(3): 564–570.

99. Mellergard P, Sjogren F, Hillman J. The cerebral extracellular release of glycerol, glutamate, and FGF2 is increased in older patients following severe traumatic brain injury. *J Neurotrauma.* Jan 1 2012; 29(1): 112–118.

100. Timofeev I, Carpenter KL, Nortje J et al. Cerebral extracellular chemistry and outcome following traumatic brain injury: A microdialysis study of 223 patients. *Brain.* Feb 2011; 134(Pt 2): 484–494.

101. Robertson CL, Bell MJ, Kochanek PM et al. Increased adenosine in cerebrospinal fluid after severe traumatic brain injury in infants and children: Association with severity of injury and excitotoxicity. *Crit Care Med.* Dec 2001; 29(12): 2287–2293.

102. Grossetete M, Phelps J, Arko L, Yonas H, Rosenberg GA. Elevation of matrix metalloproteinases 3 and 9 in cerebrospinal fluid and blood in patients with severe traumatic brain injury. *Neurosurgery.* Oct 2009; 65(4): 702–708.

103. Vilalta A, Sahuquillo J, Rosell A, Poca MA, Riveiro M, Montaner J. Moderate and severe traumatic brain injury induce early overexpression of systemic and brain gelatinases. *Intensive Care Med.* Aug 2008; 34(8): 1384–1392.

104. Roberts DJ, Jenne CN, Leger C et al. Association between the cerebral inflammatory and matrix metalloproteinase responses after severe traumatic brain injury in humans. *J Neurotrauma.* Oct 15 2013; 30(20): 1727–1736.

105. Itoh K, Chiba T, Takahashi S et al. An Nrf2/small Maf heterodimer mediates the induction of phase II detoxifying enzyme genes through antioxidant response elements. *Biochem Biophys Res Commun.* Jul 18 1997; 236(2): 313–322.

106. Hayes JD, Chanas SA, Henderson CJ et al. The Nrf2 transcription factor contributes both to the basal expression of glutathione S-transferases in mouse liver and to their induction by the chemopreventive synthetic antioxidants, butylated hydroxyanisole and ethoxyquin. *Biochem Soc Trans.* Feb 2000; 28(2): 33–41.

107. Chan K, Han XD, Kan YW. An important function of Nrf2 in combating oxidative stress: Detoxification of acetaminophen. *Proc Natl Acad Sci U S A*. Apr 10 2001; 98(8): 4611–4616.

108. Niture SK, Kaspar JW, Shen J, Jaiswal AK. Nrf2 signaling and cell survival. *Toxicol Appl Pharmacol*. Apr 1 2010; 244(1): 37–42.

109. Xi YD, Yu HL, Ding J et al. Flavonoids protect cerebrovascular endothelial cells through Nrf2 and PI3K from beta-amyloid peptide-induced oxidative damage. *Curr Neurovasc Res*. Feb 2012; 9(1): 32–41.

110. Li XH, Li CY, Lu JM, Tian RB, Wei J. Allicin ameliorates cognitive deficits ageing-induced learning and memory deficits through enhancing of Nrf2 antioxidant signaling pathways. *Neurosci Lett*. Apr 11 2012; 514(1): 46–50.

111. Bergstrom P, Andersson HC, Gao Y et al. Repeated transient sulforaphane stimulation in astrocytes leads to prolonged Nrf2-mediated gene expression and protection from superoxide-induced damage. *Neuropharmacology*. Feb–Mar 2011; 60(2–3): 343–353.

112. Wruck CJ, Gotz ME, Herdegen T, Varoga D, Brandenburg LO, Pufe T. Kavalactones protect neural cells against amyloid beta peptide-induced neurotoxicity via extracellular signal-regulated kinase 1/2-dependent nuclear factor erythroid 2-related factor 2 activation. *Mol Pharmacol*. Jun 2008; 73(6): 1785–1795.

113. Hine CM, Mitchell JR. NRF2 and the phase II response in acute stress resistance induced by dietary restriction. *J Clin Exp Pathol*. Jun 19 2012; S4(4).

114. Suh JH, Shenvi SV, Dixon BM et al. Decline in transcriptional activity of Nrf2 causes age-related loss of glutathione synthesis, which is reversible with lipoic acid. *Proc Natl Acad Sci U S A*. Mar 9 2004; 101(10): 3381–3386.

115. Zou Y, Hong B, Fan L et al. Protective effect of puerarin against beta-amyloid-induced oxidative stress in neuronal cultures from rat hippocampus: Involvement of the GSK-3beta/Nrf2 signaling pathway. *Free Radic Res*. Jan 2013; 47(1): 55–63.

116. Choi HK, Pokharel YR, Lim SC et al. Inhibition of liver fibrosis by solubilized coenzyme Q_{10}: Role of Nrf2 activation in inhibiting transforming growth factor-beta1 expression. *Toxicol Appl Pharmacol*. Nov 1 2009; 240(3): 377–384.

117. Trujillo J, Chirino YI, Molina-Jijon E, Anderica-Romero AC, Tapia E, Pedraza-Chaverri J. Renoprotective effect of the antioxidant curcumin: Recent findings. *Redox Biol*. 2013; 1(1): 448–456.

118. Steele ML, Fuller S, Patel M, Kersaitis C, Ooi L, Munch G. Effect of Nrf2 activators on release of glutathione, cysteinylglycine and homocysteine by human U373 astroglial cells. *Redox Biol*. 2013; 1(1): 441–445.

119. Kode A, Rajendrasozhan S, Caito S, Yang SR, Megson IL, Rahman I. Resveratrol induces glutathione synthesis by activation of Nrf2 and protects against cigarette smoke-mediated oxidative stress in human lung epithelial cells. *Am J Physiol Lung Cell Mol Physiol*. Mar 2008; 294(3): L478–L488.

120. Gao L, Wang J, Sekhar KR et al. Novel n-3 fatty acid oxidation products activate Nrf2 by destabilizing the association between Keap1 and Cullin3. *J Biol Chem*. Jan 26 2007; 282(4): 2529–2537.

121. Saw CL, Yang AY, Guo Y, Kong AN. Astaxanthin and omega-3 fatty acids individually and in combination protect against oxidative stress via the Nrf2-ARE pathway. *Food Chem Toxicol*. Dec 2013; 62: 869–875.

122. Ji L, Liu R, Zhang XD et al. N-acetylcysteine attenuates phosgene-induced acute lung injury via up-regulation of Nrf2 expression. *Inhal Toxicol*. Jun 2010; 22(7): 535–542.

123. Zambrano S, Blanca AJ, Ruiz-Armenta MV et al. The renoprotective effect of L-carnitine in hypertensive rats is mediated by modulation of oxidative stress-related gene expression. *Eur J Nutr*. Sep 2013; 52(6): 1649–1659.

124. Abate A, Yang G, Dennery PA, Oberle S, Schroder H. Synergistic inhibition of cyclo-oxygenase-2 expression by vitamin E and aspirin. *Free Radic Biol Med*. Dec 2000; 29(11): 1135–1142.

125. Devaraj S, Tang R, Adams-Huet B et al. Effect of high-dose alpha-tocopherol supplementation on biomarkers of oxidative stress and inflammation and carotid atherosclerosis in patients with coronary artery disease. *Am J Clin Nutr.* Nov 2007; 86(5): 1392–1398.

126. Fu Y, Zheng S, Lin J, Ryerse J, Chen A. Curcumin protects the rat liver from CCl4-caused injury and fibrogenesis by attenuating oxidative stress and suppressing inflammation. *Mol Pharmacol.* Feb 2008; 73(2): 399–409.

127. Hori K, Hatfield D, Maldarelli F, Lee BJ, Clouse KA. Selenium supplementation suppresses tumor necrosis factor alpha-induced human immunodeficiency virus type 1 replication in vitro. *AIDS Res Hum Retroviruses.* Oct 10 1997; 13(15): 1325–1332.

128. Jesudason EP, Masilamoni JG, Ashok BS et al. Inhibitory effects of short-term administration of DL-alpha-lipoic acid on oxidative vulnerability induced by Abeta amyloid fibrils (25–35) in mice. *Mol Cell Biochem.* Apr 2008; 311(1–2): 145–156.

129. Kuhlmann MK, Levin NW. Potential interplay between nutrition and inflammation in dialysis patients. *Contrib Nephrol.* 2008; 161: 76–82.

130. Lee HS, Jung KK, Cho JY et al. Neuroprotective effect of curcumin is mainly mediated by blockade of microglial cell activation. *Pharmazie.* Dec 2007; 62(12): 937–942.

131. Brinjikji W, Rabinstein AA, Cloft HJ. Hospitalization costs for acute ischemic stroke patients treated with intravenous thrombolysis in the United States are substantially higher than medicare payments. *Stroke.* Apr 2012; 43(4): 1131–1133.

132. Peairs AT, Rankin JW. Inflammatory response to a high-fat, low-carbohydrate weight loss diet: Effect of antioxidants. *Obesity (Silver Spring).* May 1 2008.

133. Rahman S, Bhatia K, Khan AQ et al. Topically applied vitamin E prevents massive cutaneous inflammatory and oxidative stress responses induced by double application of 12-O-tetradecanoylphorbol-13-acetate (TPA) in mice. *Chem Biol Interact.* Apr 15 2008; 172(3): 195–205.

134. Suzuki YJ, Aggarwal BB, Packer L. Alpha-lipoic acid is a potent inhibitor of NF-kappa B activation in human T cells. *Biochem Biophys Res Commun.* Dec 30 1992; 189(3): 1709–1715.

135. Wood LG, Garg ML, Powell H, Gibson PG. Lycopene-rich treatments modify noneosinophilic airway inflammation in asthma: Proof of concept. *Free Radic Res.* Jan 2008; 42(1): 94–102.

136. Zhu J, Yong W, Wu X et al. Anti-inflammatory effect of resveratrol on TNF-alpha-induced MCP-1 expression in adipocytes. *Biochem Biophys Res Commun.* May 2 2008; 369(2): 471–477.

137. Barger SW, Goodwin ME, Porter MM, Beggs ML. Glutamate release from activated microglia requires the oxidative burst and lipid peroxidation. *J Neurochem.* Jun 2007; 101(5): 1205–1213.

138. Schubert D, Kimura H, Maher P. Growth factors and vitamin E modify neuronal glutamate toxicity. *Proc Natl Acad Sci U S A.* Sep 1 1992; 89(17): 8264–8267.

139. Sandhu JK, Pandey S, Ribecco-Lutkiewicz M et al. Molecular mechanisms of glutamate neurotoxicity in mixed cultures of NT2-derived neurons and astrocytes: Protective effects of coenzyme Q_{10}. *J Neurosci Res.* Jun 15 2003; 72(6): 691–703.

140. Jin W, Wang H, Yan W et al. Disruption of Nrf2 enhances upregulation of nuclear factor-kappaB activity, proinflammatory cytokines, and intercellular adhesion molecule-1 in the brain after traumatic brain injury. *Mediators Inflamm.* 2008; 2008: 725174.

141. Jin W, Wang H, Yan W et al. Role of Nrf2 in protection against traumatic brain injury in mice. *J Neurotrauma.* Jan 2009; 26(1): 131–139.

142. Ates O, Cayli S, Altinoz E et al. Neuroprotection by resveratrol against traumatic brain injury in rats. *Mol Cell Biochem.* Jan 2007; 294(1–2): 137–144.

143. Sonmez U, Sonmez A, Erbil G, Tekmen I, Baykara B. Neuroprotective effects of resveratrol against traumatic brain injury in immature rats. *Neurosci Lett.* Jun 13 2007; 420(2): 133–137.

144. Toklu HZ, Hakan T, Biber N, Solakoglu S, Ogunc AV, Sener G. The protective effect of alpha lipoic acid against traumatic brain injury in rats. *Free Radic Res.* Jul 2009; 43(7): 658–667.
145. Chen G, Shi J, Hu Z, Hang C. Inhibitory effect on cerebral inflammatory response following traumatic brain injury in rats: A potential neuroprotective mechanism of N-acetylcysteine. *Mediators Inflamm.* 2008; 2008: 716458.
146. Yi JH, Hazell AS. N-acetylcysteine attenuates early induction of heme oxygenase-1 following traumatic brain injury. *Brain Res.* Feb 1 2005; 1033(1): 13–19.
147. Beni SM, Kohen R, Reiter RJ, Tan DX, Shohami E. Melatonin-induced neuroprotection after closed head injury is associated with increased brain antioxidants and attenuated late-phase activation of NF-kappaB and AP-1. *FASEB J.* Jan 2004; 18(1): 149–151.
148. Khan M, Im YB, Shunmugavel A et al. Administration of S-nitrosoglutathione after traumatic brain injury protects the neurovascular unit and reduces secondary injury in a rat model of controlled cortical impact. *J Neuroinflamm.* 2009; 6: 32.
149. Ahmad A, Crupi R, Impellizzeri D et al. Administration of palmitoylethanolamide (PEA) protects the neurovascular unit and reduces secondary injury after traumatic brain injury in mice. *Brain Behav Immun.* Nov 2012; 26(8): 1310–1321.
150. Wu A, Ying Z, Gomez-Pinilla F. Vitamin E protects against oxidative damage and learning disability after mild traumatic brain injury in rats. *Neurorehabil Neural Repair.* Oct 19 2009.
151. Wu A, Ying Z, Gomez-Pinilla F. Dietary curcumin counteracts the outcome of traumatic brain injury on oxidative stress, synaptic plasticity, and cognition. *Exp Neurol.* Feb 2006; 197(2): 309–317.
152. Xiong Y, Shie FS, Zhang J, Lee CP, Ho YS. Prevention of mitochondrial dysfunction in post-traumatic mouse brain by superoxide dismutase. *J Neurochem.* Nov 2005; 95(3): 732–744.
153. Tsuru-Aoyagi K, Potts MB, Trivedi A et al. Glutathione peroxidase activity modulates recovery in the injured immature brain. *Ann Neurol.* May 2009; 65(5): 540–549.
154. Wu A, Ying Z, Gomez-Pinilla F. Dietary omega-3 fatty acids normalize BDNF levels, reduce oxidative damage, and counteract learning disability after traumatic brain injury in rats. *J Neurotrauma.* Oct 2004; 21(10): 1457–1467.
155. Wu A, Molteni R, Ying Z, Gomez-Pinilla F. A saturated-fat diet aggravates the outcome of traumatic brain injury on hippocampal plasticity and cognitive function by reducing brain-derived neurotrophic factor. *Neuroscience.* 2003; 119(2): 365–375.
156. Al Moutaery K, Al Deeb S, Ahmad Khan H, Tariq M. Caffeine impairs short-term neurological outcome after concussive head injury in rats. *Neurosurgery.* Sep 2003; 53(3): 704–711; discussion 711–702.
157. Dohi K, Satoh K, Mihara Y et al. Alkoxyl radical-scavenging activity of edaravone in patients with traumatic brain injury. *J Neurotrauma.* Nov 2006; 23(11): 1591–1599.
158. Albini A, Morini M, D'Agostini F et al. Inhibition of angiogenesis-driven Kaposi's sarcoma tumor growth in nude mice by oral N-acetylcysteine. *Cancer Res.* Nov 15 2001; 61(22): 8171–8178.
159. Gottshall K, Hoffer, ME, Balough, BJ. Use of antioxidants micronutrient compounds in vestibular rehabilitation after operational head trauma or blast injury. Paper presented at *Barany International Balance Meeting, June, 2006, Stockholm, Sweden.*
160. Shoulson I. DATATOP: A decade of neuroprotective inquiry. Parkinson Study Group. Deprenyl and tocopherol antioxidative therapy of parkinsonism. *Ann Neurol.* Sep 1998; 44(3 Suppl 1): S160–S166.
161. Sano M, Ernesto C, Thomas RG et al. A controlled trial of selegiline, alpha-tocopherol, or both as treatment for Alzheimer's disease. The Alzheimer's Disease Cooperative Study. *N Engl J Med.* Apr 24 1997; 336(17): 1216–1222.
162. Farina N, Isaac MG, Clark AR, Rusted J, Tabet N. Vitamin E for Alzheimer's dementia and mild cognitive impairment. *Cochrane Database Syst Rev.* 2012; 11: CD002854.

163. Albanes D, Heinonen OP, Huttunen JK et al. Effects of alpha-tocopherol and beta-carotene supplements on cancer incidence in the Alpha-Tocopherol Beta-Carotene Cancer Prevention Study. *Am J Clin Nutr.* Dec 1995; 62(6 Suppl): 1427S–1430S.

164. Prasad KN, Cole WC, Prasad KC. Risk factors for Alzheimer's disease: Role of multiple antioxidants, non-steroidal anti-inflammatory and cholinergic agents alone or in combination in prevention and treatment. *J Am Coll Nutr.* Dec 2002; 21(6): 506–522.

165. Chen RS, Huang CC, Chu NS. Coenzyme Q_{10} treatment in mitochondrial encephalomyopathies. Short-term double-blind, crossover study. *Eur Neurol.* 1997; 37(4): 212–218.

166. Gaziano JM, Sesso HD, Christen WG et al. Multivitamins in the prevention of cancer in men: The Physicians' Health Study II randomized controlled trial. *JAMA.* Nov 14 2012; 308(18): 1871–1880.

167. Baum MK, Campa A, Lai S et al. Effect of micronutrient supplementation on disease progression in asymptomatic, antiretroviral-naive, HIV-infected adults in Botswana: A randomized clinical trial. *JAMA.* Nov 27 2013; 310(20): 2154–2163.

168. Davis M, Ressler K, Rothbaum BO, Richardson R. Effects of D-cycloserine on extinction: Translation from preclinical to clinical work. *Biol Psychiatry.* Aug 15 2006; 60(4): 369–375.

169. Olanow CW, Arendash GW. Metals and free radicals in neurodegeneration. *Curr Opin Neurol.* Dec 1994; 7(6): 548–558.

170. Prasad KN, Kumar B, Yan XD, Hanson AJ, Cole WC. Alpha-tocopheryl succinate, the most effective form of vitamin E for adjuvant cancer treatment: A review. *J Am Coll Nutr.* Apr 2003; 22(2): 108–117.

171. Bayir H, Adelson PD, Wisniewski SR et al. Therapeutic hypothermia preserves antioxidant defenses after severe traumatic brain injury in infants and children. *Crit Care Med.* Feb 2009; 37(2): 689–695.

172. Fox JL, Vu EN, Doyle-Waters M, Brubacher JR, Abu-Laban R, Hu Z. Prophylactic hypothermia for traumatic brain injury: A quantitative systematic review. *CJEM.* Jul 2010; 12(4): 355–364.

173. Su E, Bell MJ, Wisniewski SR et al. alpha-Synuclein levels are elevated in cerebrospinal fluid following traumatic brain injury in infants and children: The effect of therapeutic hypothermia. *Dev Neurosci.* 2010; 32(5–6): 385–395.

174. Grasso G, Sfacteria A, Meli F, Fodale V, Buemi M, Iacopino DG. Neuroprotection by erythropoietin administration after experimental traumatic brain injury. *Brain Res.* Nov 28 2007; 1182: 99–105.

175. Xiong Y, Chopp M, Lee CP. Erythropoietin improves brain mitochondrial function in rats after traumatic brain injury. *Neurol Res.* Jun 2009; 31(5): 496–502.

176. Sharma HS, Patnaik R, Patnaik S, Mohanty S, Sharma A, Vannemreddy P. Antibodies to serotonin attenuate closed head injury induced blood brain barrier disruption and brain pathology. *Ann N Y Acad Sci.* Dec 2007; 1122: 295–312.

177. Zhang B, West EJ, Van KC et al. HDAC inhibitor increases histone H3 acetylation and reduces microglia inflammatory response following traumatic brain injury in rats. *Brain Res.* Aug 21 2008; 1226: 181–191.

178. Dash PK, Orsi SA, Zhang M et al. Valproate administered after traumatic brain injury provides neuroprotection and improves cognitive function in rats. *PloS One.* 2010; 5(6): e11383.

179. Foley K, Kast RE, Altschuler EL. Ritonavir and disulfiram have potential to inhibit caspase-1 mediated inflammation and reduce neurological sequelae after minor blast exposure. *Med Hypotheses.* Feb 2009; 72(2): 150–152.

180. Hakan T, Toklu HZ, Biber N et al. Effect of COX-2 inhibitor meloxicam against traumatic brain injury-induced biochemical, histopathological changes and blood-brain barrier permeability. *Neurol Res.* Aug 5 2009.

181. Chen X, Choi IY, Chang TS et al. Pretreatment with interferon-gamma protects microglia from oxidative stress via up-regulation of Mn-SOD. *Free Radic Biol Med.* Apr 15 2009; 46(8): 1204–1210.

8 Concussive Brain Injuries
Prevention and Improved Management by Micronutrients

INTRODUCTION

Concussive brain injury is also referred to as mild traumatic brain injury (TBI). It can express as a mild, moderate, or severe form. Concussive injury occurs when the brain is violently rocked back and forth within the skull following a blow to the head or neck such as that observed in contact sports like football and soccer. Concussive injury also can occur during the rapid displacement and rotation of the cranium after peak head acceleration and momentum transfer in helmet impacts.[1] Concussive damage occurs in troops when exposed to blast pressure waves, such as following detonation of an explosive device (IED). This injury is characterized by the immediate and transient changes in brain function which include temporary loss of memory, confusion, poor balance, and reflexes and hearing loss. Although concussive injury has occurred in players of contact sports and in troops returning from previous wars, only recently it has drawn scientific, public, and administrative interest. This is due to the recognition of serious mental disorders including cognitive dysfunction and abnormal behavior (fear, anxiety, anger, and suicidal tendency) that are being observed at increased rates in professional football players and veterans of foreign wars.

Current efforts on reducing the adverse impacts of concussion on brain function have focused on the development of physical protection of the outer skull. Introduction of newer football helmets appears to lower the risk of concussion by about 10–20%.[2] Despite evolutionary changes in protective equipment, concussive injuries in the brain remain a major health risk for professional football players.[3,4] Despite state of the art physical protection, U.S. troops continue to suffer from the adverse consequences of mild TBI. Currently available physical protective devices are not sufficient to reduce the acute and long-term adverse consequences of concussions on brain function. At present, treatments involving medications and psychotherapy are not satisfactory. A novel concept of PAMARA (protection as much as reasonably achievable) is proposed. This concept includes protection of the skull by physical devices and protection of the brain by antioxidant supplementation before and after concussions.

Most studies on concussions in humans have focused on the incidence, cost and physical, cognitive, and behavioral symptoms following injury to the brain. A few studies have investigated changes in brain structures, and markers of oxidative damage and chronic inflammation and glutamate release following concussive injury primarily in animal models of TBI (fluid percussion injury model, cortical model of closed head injury, and blunt head injury model). From these studies, it appears that an increase in oxidative stress, chronic inflammation, and glutamate release may contribute to the development of cognitive dysfunction and behavioral changes following concussive injuries. Free radical-scavenging role of antioxidants is well established. Some studies have revealed that antioxidants attenuate chronic inflammation and release of glutamate.[5–17] Therefore, antioxidants appear to be one of the rational choices for biological protection of the brain before and after concussions. However, only a few studies on the effects of antioxidants on concussive injury in animal models are available. No such studies have been performed in humans.

This review briefly describes incidence, cost, causes, and major biochemical pathways that contribute to the development and progression of concussive injury. This review provides scientific rationale and data in support of the concept of PAMARA that may reduce the acute and long-term adverse health consequences of concussive injury. The concept of PAMARA includes physical protection of skull and biological protection of brain tissue by multiple antioxidants.

INCIDENCE

The Center for Disease Control and Prevention (CDC, 2012) estimates that 1.7 million people in the USA sustain a TBI annually from all causes, out of which about 75% represent concussive injury. Concussive injury primarily occurs in contact sports such as football and soccer, in civilians such as during accidental falls involving the head, and in combat zones such as during exposures to blast waves.

NATIONAL FOOTBALL LEAGUE

In 2002–2007, 152 players had repeat concussions.[18] The defensive secondary, kick unit, running back, and linebacker have the highest incidence of repeat concussion. About 7.6% of all repeat concussions occurred within 2 weeks of the prior concussion. More than half of players with repeat concussion were removed from play.

HIGH SCHOOL AND COLLEGE SPORTS

A prospective 11-year study revealed that annual increase in concussive injury was 14% in boys and 21% in girls.[19] Football accounted for more than half of all concussions. Among girls' sports, soccer accounted for the highest proportion of concussive injury. It was found that concussive injury increased fourfold between the years 1998 and 2008. Another study has estimated that about 300,000 sports related TBI, primarily concussive injury occur among high school and college athletes. It has been determined that concussive injury represented 8.9% of all high school athletic injuries and 5.8% of all collegiate athletic injuries.[20] The rates of concussions were highest among athletes playing football and soccer. The rate of concussive injury was higher in girls than in boys. Among young people ages 15–24 years, sports are second to motor vehicle crashes as the leading cause of TBI. The number of students participating in high school and college sports is increasing. In 2005–2006, more than seven million high school students and in 2004–2005, about 385,000 college students participated in sports. According to the National Federation of State High School Association, in 2008–2009, about 7.5 million high school students participated in sports.

VETERANS

Among U.S. veterans returning from the military conflicts in Iraq and Afghanistan, TBI represents one of the major injuries. The prevalence of TBI ranges from 15 to 20%, and 85% of the TBI are mild concussions.[21] The majority of these concussions were due to exposure to blasts. Most of them experienced exposure to multiple blasts. About 20% of them were exposed to a second blast within 2 weeks of the first and 87% within 3 months.

CIVILIANS

In civilians, falls, motor vehicle accidents, being struck by/against moving or stationary objects, and assaults involving the head contribute to concussive injury or mild to severe TBI (CDC, Traumatic Brain Injury and Causes, 2012). Falls contribute to 35.2% of TBI, motor vehicle accidents to 17.3%, being struck by/against moving or stationary objects to 16.5%, assaults to 10%, and other unknown factors to 21%. Falls are the major cause of concussive injury among children ages up to 14 years and among adults ages 65 years or older.

COST

Direct medical costs and indirect costs such as lost productivity of TBI is estimated to be $56 billion in the USA each year. The cost of mild TBI or concussive injury each year is estimated to be $17 billion (CDC, Traumatic Brain Injury and Causes, 2012).

CAUSES AND SYMPTOMS OF CONCUSSIVE INJURY

Concussive injury occurs when the brain is violently rocked back and forth within the skull following a blow to the head or neck such as that observed in contact sports like football and soccer. Concussive damage occurs in troops when exposed to a blast pressure wave, such as following detonation of an explosive device. Among civilian, falls, and crashes involving automobile, motorcycle, and bicycles can cause concussive injury.

The major acute physical symptoms include transient confusion, disorientation, and loss of consciousness, headache, dizziness, nausea, blurred vision, uneven gait, insomnia, blurred vision, and fatigue. The cognitive symptoms include memory loss, attention deficits, and lack of concentration. The behavioral changes include irritability, depression, fear and anxiety, emotional control, and problems with relationships.

LONG-TERM HEALTH CONSEQUENCES OF CONCUSSIONS

Brain deformation may occur after the primary head acceleration.[1] Damage to the midbrain correlated with memory and cognitive problems after concussions. The major changes after concussions included impairment of memory, processing speed, verbal memory, and executive function.[22–24] An early onset of dementia may be initiated by repetitive concussions in professional football players.[25,26] Balance disorders are also considered one of the major health problems with mild TBI.[2,26]

In a clinical study involving 1044 members of the National Football League Retired Players Association, the effect of one or more concussions on the incidence of depression 9 years after the incident was evaluated, using General Health Survey Questionnaires.[27] The results showed that 10.2% of participating players had depression which increased with an increasing number of concussions compared to those retired players who reported no concussions. An increase in concussion-induced depression was independent of depression induced by other agents. In another study involving 2552 retired professional football players with an average age of 45.8 ± 13.4 years and an average professional football playing career of 6.6 ± 3.6 years, the effect of concussions on the risk of developing mild cognitive dysfunction and Alzheimer's disease was evaluated.[25] The results showed that retired players with three or more concussions had a fivefold prevalence of mild cognitive dysfunction and a threefold increase in significant memory loss compared to those retired players who did not suffer concussions. There was no association between recurrent concussions and Alzheimer's disease; however, the onset of this disease in the retired players was earlier than in the general American population.

In study involving college football players, it was found that players with a history of previous concussions are more likely to have future concussions than those with no history of concussion. About 85.2% of retired players reported headache that lasted up to 82 h. Previous concussions were associated with slower recovery.[28]

Increased risk of chronic traumatic encephalopathy (CTE) remains one of the measurable health concerns of repeated concussions. In studies with high school football players, it was found that repetitive blows to the head are cumulative and that repeated subconcussive blows can cause CTE and neurophysiological abnormalities.[29]

Concussions can cause decline in motor and cognitive function and increased risk of Alzheimer's disease in young athletes. Animal models of TBI have shown that impaired learning ability was related to synaptic plasticity suppression. In humans, single or repeated concussions can cause lifelong or cumulative enhancement of gamma-aminobutyric acid (GABA)-mediated suppression of synaptic plasticity. It has been reported that repeated concussions induced persistent elevation of GABA-mediated inhibition in the primary motor cortex which caused suppressed synaptic plasticity.[30] These changes accounted for impaired learning ability.

In a study involving 79 concussed college athletes, a computerized neuropsychological test was given during the preseason and on 2 and 8 days after concussions. The results showed that concussed female athletes performed significantly worse than concussed male athletes on visual memory tasks.[31] Male athletes were more likely to report symptoms of vomiting and sadness than female athletes. The analysis of performance data further revealed that at 2 days after injury, 58% of concussed athletes exhibited a decline in performance and increase in other symptoms whereas at 8 days after concussions, 30% continue to show one or more changes in neuropsychological tests.

In a study involving 1502 U.S. Army soldiers, an anonymous mental health survey was performed at 4 to 6 months after returning from deployment to Iraq or Afghanistan.[32] The results showed that 17% of soldiers reported a mild TBI during their previous deployment, and 59% of these soldiers suffered more than one mild TBI. After adjusting for post-traumatic syndrome (PTSD), depression, and other factors, multiple mild TBI with loss of consciousness increased the risk of headache compared to those who had only one mild TBI. Mild TBI is also associated with an increased incidence of PTSD. The similarity in some of the symptoms makes it difficult to distinguish them while evaluating the treatment of these brain dysfunctions. A review of three large studies evaluating the frequency of mild TBI and PTSD in veterans of Iraq and Afghanistan showed that frequencies of probable mild TBI/ PTSD were from 5% to 7%; among those with probable mild TBI, frequencies of probable PTSD were from 33% to 39%.[33]

Recent evidence from functional and metabolic imaging suggest that abnormalities in the electric responses, metabolic balance, and oxygen consumption in neurons persist several months after concussions.[34]

INCREASED OXIDATIVE STRESS AND INFLAMMATION

OXIDATIVE STRESS IN ANIMAL MODELS OF MILD TBI (CONCUSSION)

Evidence for increased oxidative stress comes from the levels of markers of oxidative damage and from the use of antioxidants that reduce their levels. It has been reported that elevated levels of protein carbonyls (a marker of oxidative damage), reduced levels of superoxide dismutase (SOS), and silent information regulator-2 (Sir2) in the hippocampus was observed after a mild TBI in rats.[35] In addition, poor performance by the animals were associated with reduced levels of brain-derived neurotrophic factor (BDNF). BDNF facilitates synaptic function and support learning by modulating the CaMKII system (Ca^{2+}- and calmodulin-dependent protein kinase II), synapsin 1, and cAMP response element-binding protein (CREB). Feeding diet supplemented with vitamin E for 4 weeks before a mild TBI prevented impairment in learning ability and the above biochemical changes in these rats. These results suggest the involvement of increased oxidative stress in causing impaired learning ability in animals with a mild TBI. In transgenic mouse models of Alzheimer amyloidosis (Tg2576 mice), repetitive concussive brain injury induced by a modified cortical impact model of closed head injury, increased the levels of brain lipid peroxidation, accelerated beta amyloid deposition, and caused learning deficits. Feeding a diet supplemented with vitamin E for 4 weeks before mild TBI prevented lipid peroxidation, impairment in learning ability, and reduction in the levels of BDNF in these transgenic mice.[36] It has been reported that feeding a high-fat diet decreased hippocampal plasticity and cognitive function by reducing BDNF in rats with a mild TBI.[37] Feeding a diet supplemented with curcumin, which exhibit antioxidant and anti-inflammation activities, prevented oxidative stress, restored BDNF, and improved synaptic plasticity and cognitive function in rats with a mild TBI.[38] Similar results were obtained by feeding a diet supplemented with omega-3 fatty acid doco-sahexaenoic acid (DHA) prior to inducing a mild TBI in rats.[39] Repetitive concussive injuries increased the levels of markers of oxidative damage (malondialdehyde [MDA]), reduced/oxidized glutathione ratio, nitrite, nitrate, and decreased ascorbic acid and glutathione in rats. These biochemical changes were observed in rats in which mild TBI was delivered 1, 2, or 3 days after the first one. However, if the time interval between the first one and the second one was 5 days, biochemical markers of oxidative and nitrosylative stress were nearly at control levels.[40]

OXIDATIVE STRESS IN HUMANS WITH MILD TBI (CONCUSSION)

No human studies have been performed on changes in markers of oxidative damage or the levels of antioxidants following concussive injury in active or retired football players. However, it should be pointed out that during the active season football players are exposed to excessive amounts of oxygen during the game. Normally, about 20% of respired oxygen is used by the brain. Mitochondria utilize oxygen to generate energy, and free radicals are produced during this process. About 2% of unused oxygen leaks out of mitochondria that makes about 20 billion molecules of superoxide anions and hydrogen peroxide per cell per day. Thus, it is likely that during the game when excessive amounts of oxygen are used, the brain may be exposed to higher levels of oxidative stress that may overwhelm endogenous defense systems. Such an event may enhance the effects of concussions on acute and long-term adverse effects on brain functions.

INFLAMMATION IN ANIMAL MODELS OF MILD TBI (CONCUSSION)

Rats exposed to repetitive concussions (one, three, or five times) spaced 5 days apart displayed increased anxiety- and depression-like behaviors, short- and long-term cognitive dysfunction, neuroinflammation, and cortical damage.[41]

INFLAMMATION IN HUMANS WITH MILD TBI (CONCUSSION)

Time-dependent changes in inflammatory cellular response in human cortical contusions were investigated during the first 30 weeks after blunt head injury, by immunohistochemistry.[42] The results showed that CD-15 (3-fucosyl-N-acertyl-lactosamine)-labeled granulocytes were detected as early as 10 minutes after brain injury. In addition, increased numbers of mononuclear leukocytes labeled with LCA (leukocyte common antigen), CD-3, and UCHL-1, a clone of CD45RO that is an isoform of LCA, were detected at 1.1 days, 2 days, and 3.7 days after injury in cortical contusions. In another study, time-dependent alterations in inflammatory responses in 12 consecutive patients undergoing surgery for brain contusions 3 h to 5 days after trauma were determined by immunohistochemistry.[43] If the inflammatory responses were determined in less than 24 h after injury, they were limited to vascular margination of polymorphonuclear cells. In patients undergoing surgery 3–5 days after injury, an extensive inflammatory reaction consisting of monocyte/macrophages, reactive microglia, polymorphonuclear cells, and CD-4- and CD-8-labeled T lymphocytes was observed. Human lymphocyte antigen-DQ was expressed on reactive microglia and infiltrating leukocytes later on.

These inflammatory reactions following contusions may produce several potentially harmful effects, including acute and long-term degeneration of nerve cells. Expression of pro- and anti-inflammatory cytokines on the above brain tissues was determined.[44] The results showed that in patients undergoing surgery in less than 24 h after injury, elevated levels of pro-inflammatory cytokines Interleukin-1 beta (IL-1 beta), IL-6, and interferon-gamma (INF-gamma) and the anti-inflammatory cytokine IL-4 were present. However, in patients undergoing surgery 3–5 days after injury, expression of IL-4 was lower compared to those who were operated on earlier. However, expression of IL-1 beta and IFN-gamma remained high compared to IL-6. The persistence of pro-inflammatory cytokines causes neurodegeneration in the brain.

In a study involving brain tissue obtained at autopsy from 24 patients who had TBI and five control brains, changes in CD-14, a pattern recognition receptor of the immune system, were investigated.[45] In control brains, CD-14 expressed constitutively in perivascular cells but not in parenchymal cells. However, after TBI, expression of CD-14 in perivascular cells and parenchymal cells reached maximal levels within 4–8 days and remained elevated until weeks after injury. These results suggest that increased expression of CD-14 is one of the major responses of acute inflammatory reaction in the brain following TBI.

INCREASED GLUTAMATE RELEASE

Mild traumatic injury (brain concussive injury) can cause cognitive and emotional dysfunction and increases the risk for the development of anxiety disorders, including PTSD commonly observed in veterans of foreign wars. Glutamate receptor N-methy-D-aspartate (NMDA) in the amygdala appears to regulate fear and anxiety. In a rat model of mild TBI, the levels of NMDA receptors in the amydala increased. In addition, GABA-related inhibition decreased in amygdala and hippocampus.[46] These results suggest excitatory events created by an elevation of NMDA receptor levels and a decrease in GABA activity may increase the risk for developing fear and anxiety. It appears that following concussive brain injury, excessive amounts of glutamate are released that can cause a massive efflux of K^+ ions and increased accumulation of lactate. This was confirmed by the fact that administration of ouabain, an inhibitor of Na^+/K^+-ATPase, before injury reduced lactate accumulation.

MOLECULAR CHANGES IN BRAIN AFTER CONCUSSIONS

The expression of oncogene proteins, c-myc, and c-fos was elevated in rat brains after brain concussions.[47,48] In addition, cortical expression of nuclear factor kappaB (NF-kappaB) was elevated in human contused brain.[49] The fact that antioxidants reduced expression of c-myc oncogene[50] and activation of NF-kappaB[51] further suggested that supplementation with antioxidants may reduce acute and long-term health consequences of concussive injury in the brain. The levels of inducible nitric oxide synthase (iNOS) in human neurons, macrophages, neutrophils, astrocytes, and oligodendrocytes increased within 6 h after trauma and peaked at about 8–23 h.[52] Increased levels of iNOS can generate excessive amounts of NO that can form peroxynitrite that is very toxic to nerve cells.

HOW TO REDUCE OXIDATIVE STRESS, CHRONIC INFLAMMATION, AND GLUTAMATE RELEASE

Significant studies discussed in this chapter suggest that increased oxidative stress, chronic inflammation, and release of glutamate are involved in the initiation and progression of TBI.

HOW TO REDUCE OXIDATIVE STRESS

Oxidative stress in the body occurs when the antioxidant system fails to provide adequate protection against damage produced by free radicals (reactive oxygen species and reactive nitrogen species). Increased oxidative stress in the body can be most effectively reduced by upregulating antioxidant enzymes as well as by existing levels of dietary and endogenous antioxidant chemicals, because they work by different mechanisms. For example, antioxidant enzymes reduce free radicals by catalysis, whereas dietary and endogenous antioxidant chemicals reduce free radicals by directly scavenging them. In response to reactive oxygen species (ROS), a nuclear transcriptional factor, Nrf2 (nuclear factor-erythroid 2-related factor 2) translocated from the cytoplasm to the nucleus where it binds with ARE (antioxidant response element) which increases the levels of antioxidant enzymes (gamma-glutamylcysteine ligase, glutathione peroxidase, glutathione reductase, and heme oxygenase-1) and phase 2 detoxifying enzymes (NAD(P)H): quinine oxidoreductase 1 and glutathione-S-transferase) in order to reduce oxidative damage.[53-55] In response to increased oxidative stress, existing levels of dietary and endogenous antioxidant chemicals levels cannot be elevated without supplementation.

FACTORS REGULATING RESPONSE OF NRF2 AND ITS ACTION

Several studies suggest that antioxidant enzymes are elevated by Nrf2 activation which depends upon ROS-dependent[56] and ROS-independent[57-61] mechanisms. In addition, the levels of antioxidant enzymes are also dependent upon the binding ability of Nrf2 with ARE in the nucleus.[62]

DIFFERENTIAL RESPONSE OF Nrf2 TO ROS GENERATED DURING ACUTE AND CHRONIC OXIDATIVE STRESS

It appears that Nrf2 responds to ROS generated during acute and chronic oxidative stress differently. For example, excessive amounts of ROS are generated during acute oxidative stress observed during strenuous exercise. In response to ROS, Nrf2 translocates to the nucleus where it binds with ARE to upregulate antioxidant genes. Excessive amounts of ROS are also present during chronic oxidative stress commonly observed in older individuals and neurological diseases, such as Parkinson disease, Alzheimer's disease, and PTSD, suggesting that the Nrf2/ARE regulatory system has become unresponsive to ROS in these diseases. Age-related decline in antioxidant enzymes in the liver of older rats compared to that in younger rats was due to reduction in the binding ability of Nrf2 with ARE; however, treatment with alpha-lipoic acid restored this defect, increased the levels of antioxidant enzymes and restored the loss of glutathione from the liver of older rats.[62] The exact reasons for the Nrf2/ARE regulatory system to become unresponsive to ROS during chronic oxidative stress are unknown; however, defects in the binding ability of Nrf2 with ARE may be one of the reasons.

Nrf2 IN CONCUSSIVE BRAIN INJURY

No studies have been performed to evaluate the role of Nrf2 in the brain following concussion. Since increased oxidative stress plays an important role in the initiation and progression of concussive injury, the following groups of agents in combination may be useful in reducing the development and progression of brain injury following concussions:

1. *Agents that can reduce oxidative stress by directly scavenging free radicals without activating Nrf2-regulated antioxidant enzymes*: Some examples are dietary antioxidants, such as vitamin A, beta-carotene, vitamin C, and vitamin E, and endogenous antioxidants, such as glutathione, alpha-lipoic acid, and coenzyme Q_{10}.
2. *Agents that can reduce oxidative stress by activating Nfr2-regulated antioxidant genes without ROS stimulation*: Some examples are organosulfur compound sulforaphane found in cruciferous vegetables, kavalactones found in Kava shrubs, and Puerarin, a major flavonoid from the root of *Pueraria lobata*.[59,60,63] Genistein and vitamin E[57] and coenzyme Q_{10}[64] also activate Nrf2 without ROS.
3. *Agents that reduce oxidative stress directly by scavenging free radicals as well as indirectly by activating Nrf2/ARE pathway*: Some examples are vitamin E,[57] alpha-lipoic acid,[62] curcumin,[65] resveratrol,[66,67] omega-3 fatty acids,[68,69] and NAC.[70]
4. *Agents that can reduce oxidative stress by ROS stimulation*: They include L-carnitine which generates transient ROS.[71]

How to Reduce Chronic Inflammation and Glutamate

Some individual antioxidants from the above groups have been shown to reduce chronic inflammation[5-11,13-17,72] and prevent the release[73] and toxicity[74,75] of glutamate. A combination of selected agents from the above groups may reduce chronic inflammation and release of glutamate and its toxicity optimally, and thereby, may reduce the progression of concussive injury, and in combination with standard therapy, may improve the management of this disease.

PREVENTION STRATEGIES FOR CONCUSSIVE INJURY

Primary Prevention

The purpose of primary prevention is to protect healthy individuals from brain damage following concussion. Football and soccer players before the start of training and

U.S. troops to be deployed in combat are the suitable populations for primary prevention studies. Since concussion generates excessive amounts of free radicals and inflammation soon after injury, and since antioxidants and certain phenolic compounds reduce free radicals and inflammation, supplementation with a preparation of micronutrients containing dietary and endogenous antioxidants and certain phenolic compounds may be one of the rational choices for primary prevention of concussive injury. A micronutrient preparation containing dietary and endogenous antioxidants and certain phenolic compounds, which can reduce oxidative stress indirectly by enhancing the levels of antioxidant enzymes through the Nrf2/ARE pathway and directly by scavenging free radicals by antioxidants, can be used for primary prevention.

SECONDARY PREVENTION

The purpose of secondary prevention is to slow the progression of brain injury following concussions in order to reduce the risk of developing late adverse health effects, such as cognitive dysfunction and behavior abnormalities. During the period of progression of injury following concussions, excessive amounts of free radicals, products of chronic inflammation, and glutamate are produced. Antioxidants and certain polyphenolic compounds reduce oxidative damage, chronic inflammation, and glutamate release and toxicity. Therefore, supplementation with a preparation of micronutrients containing dietary and endogenous antioxidants and certain polyphenolic compounds may be one of the rational choices for secondary prevention of brain injury following concussions.

PROBLEMS OF USING SINGLE MICRONUTRIENTS IN CONCUSSIVE INJURY

Although no well-designed clinical studies have been performed with one antioxidant following concussive brain injury, previous clinical studies with a single antioxidant in high-risk populations of other diseases, such as cancer, heart disease, and certain neurological diseases, have produced inconsistent results. The oxidative environment of the brain following concussions may be high. It is also known that individual antioxidants when oxidized act as a pro-oxidant. Therefore, administration of a single antioxidant under the above conditions may produce pro-oxidant effects rather than antioxidant effects on the risk of developing chronic diseases. The effects of oxidized antioxidant may have contributed to the inconsistent results varying from beneficial effects, no effect, to harmful effects in the previous studies on other chronic diseases. For example, the study on beta-carotene in male heavy smokers for reducing the risk of lung cancer, vitamin E in Alzheimer's disease (AD) for improving cognitive function, and vitamin E in Parkinson's disease (PD) for improving the symptoms, and as expected, produced inconsistent results varying from no effect in PD,[76] to modest beneficial effects in AD,[77] and to harmful effects in heavy male smokers.[78] Because of the failure to obtain consistent results with individual antioxidants in other neurodegenerative diseases, I recommend a preparation of micronutrients containing dietary and endogenous antioxidants, vitamin D, B vitamins, certain minerals, polyphenolic compounds (resveratrol and curcumin), and omega-3 fatty acids before and after concussions for reducing the development and progression of concussive injury. The implementation of this micronutrient strategy would increase the efficacy of physical devices that are used to protect the brain from concussive injury as well as from drugs and other complementary approaches that are provided after concussive injury. Additional rationales are described here.

RATIONALE FOR USING MULTIPLE MICRONUTRIENTS FOR REDUCING DEVELOPMENT AND PROGRESSION OF CONCUSSIVE INJURY

The references for this section are described in a review.[79] The mechanisms of action of micronutrients and polyphenolic compounds in the proposed formulation are in part different; their distribution in various organs and cells, their affinity to various types of free radicals, and their biological half lives are also different. Beta-carotene (BC) is more effective in quenching oxygen radicals than most other antioxidants. BC can perform certain biological functions that cannot be produced by its metabolite vitamin A and vice versa. It has been reported that BC treatment enhances the expression of the connexin gene which codes for a gap junction protein in mammalian fibroblasts in culture, whereas vitamin A treatment does not produce such an effect. Vitamin A can induce differentiation in certain normal and cancer cells, whereas BC and other carotenoids do not. Thus, BC and vitamin A have, in part, different biological functions in the body. The gradient of oxygen pressure varies within cells. Some antioxidants, such as vitamin E, are more effective as quenchers of free radicals in reduced oxygen pressure, whereas BC and vitamin A are more effective in higher atmospheric pressures. Vitamin C is necessary to protect cellular components in aqueous environments, whereas carotenoids and vitamins A and E protect cellular components in lipid environments. Vitamin C also plays an important role in maintaining cellular levels of vitamin E by recycling vitamin E radical (oxidized) to the reduced (antioxidant) form.

The form of vitamin E used in a preparation of micronutrients is also important. It has been established that D-alpha-tocopheryl succinate (vitamin E succinate) is the most effective form of vitamin both *in vitro* and *in vivo*. This form of vitamin E is more soluble than alpha-tocopherol and enters cells more readily, and therefore, it is expected that vitamin E succinate would cross the blood–brain barrier in greater amounts than alpha-tocopherol. However, this idea has not yet been tested in animals or humans. We have reported that an oral ingestion of vitamin E succinate (800 IU/day) in humans increased plasma levels of not only alpha-tocopherol but also of vitamin E succinate, suggesting that a portion of this form of vitamin E can be absorbed from the intestinal tract before hydrolysis to alpha-tocopherol, provided that the plasma pool of alpha-tocopherol is saturated. This observation is important because the conventional assumption based on the studies in rodents has been that esterified forms of vitamin E, such as alpha-tocopheryl succinate, alpha-tocopheryl nicotinate, and alpha-tocopheryl acetate, can be absorbed from the intestinal tract only after they are hydrolyzed to alpha-tocopherol. Our preliminary data showed that this assumption may not be true for the absorption of vitamin E succinate in humans provided that the plasma pool of alpha-tocopherol is saturated.

An endogenous antioxidant, glutathione, is effective in catabolizing H_2O_2 and anions. However, oral supplementation with glutathione failed to significantly increase plasma levels of glutathione in human subjects, suggesting that this tripeptide is completely hydrolyzed in the GI tract. Therefore, I propose to add N-acetylcysteine and alpha-lipoic acid which increase the cellular levels of glutathione by different mechanisms in a multiple micronutrient preparation.

Another endogenous antioxidant, coenzyme Q_{10}, may have some potential value in reducing the progression of TBI. Since coenzyme Q_{10} is needed for the generation of ATP by mitochondria, it is essential to add this antioxidant in a multiple micronutrient preparation. A study has shown that coenzyme Q_{10} scavenges peroxy radicals faster than alpha-tocopherol, and like vitamin C, can regenerate vitamin E in a redox cycle. However, it is a weaker antioxidant than alpha-tocopherol. Coenzyme Q_{10} administration has been shown to improve clinical symptoms in patients with mitochondrial encephalomyopathies.[80]

Since memory loss occurs after concussions, nicotinamide, a precursor of NAD^+, attenuated glutamate-induced toxicity and preserved cellular levels of NAD^+ to support the activity of SIRT-1. It is also a competitive inhibitor of histone deacetylase activity and restored memory deficits in AD transgenic mice. These preclinical data suggest that oral supplementation with nicotinamide may be safe and useful in the prevention of memory deficits.

Selenium is a cofactor of glutathione peroxidase, and Se-glutathione peroxidase acts as an antioxidant by increasing the intracellular level of glutathione. Therefore, selenium should be added to a multiple micronutrient preparation for reducing the progression of TBI.

In addition to dietary and endogenous antioxidants, all B vitamins with high doses of vitamin B_3 (nicotinamide) and vitamin D should be added to a multiple micronutrient preparation for maintaining normal health. Curcumin and omega-3 fatty acids were also added because they appear to produce some benefits in reducing the progression of TBI. Resveratrol is also added because it has produced some beneficial effects in animal models of TBI.

Two recent studies supplemented with multiple vitamin preparations reduced cancer incidence by 10 percent in men[81] and improved clinical outcomes in patients with HIV/AIDS who were not taking medication.[82]

EVIDENCE SUPPORTING EFFECTIVENESS OF MICRONUTRIENT PREPARATION

VETERANS EXPOSED TO CONCUSSIVE INJURY FROM BLAST EXPOSURE

A commercial preparation of micronutrients containing multiple dietary and endogenous antioxidants was tested in a clinical study in troops returning from Iraq with mild to moderate TBI. Thirty-four patients with post-traumatic dizziness were admitted to the Naval Medical Center San Diego Clinic over a 2-month period and agreed to participate in the study under the supervision of Dr. Michael Hoffer and his colleagues.[83] All patients had received their injury 3–20 weeks prior to admission, and they received identical treatment consisting of medical therapy (for any migraines), supportive care, steroids, and vestibular rehabilitation therapy. Fifteen of the thirty-four patients also received a dose of an antioxidant and micronutrient formula (two capsules by mouth twice a day). At the onset of therapy, all patients were evaluated in outcome measures which included the Sensory Organization Test (SOT) by Computerized Dynamic Posturography (CDP), the Dynamic Gait Index (DGI), the Activities Balance Confidence (ABC) scale, the Dizziness Handicap Index (DHI), the Vestibular Disorders Activities of Daily Living (VADL) score, and the Balance Scoring System (BESS) test. The study was carried out for 12 weeks. The therapist who graded these outcomes and performed the testing was blinded as to whether the patient was receiving antioxidant therapy or not. The pretrial test scores did not differ significantly between the two groups on any of the tests.

Both groups of patients showed trends toward significant improvement on all tests after the 12 weeks of therapy, but the combination treatment trend was stronger than that of the standard therapy alone group. After only 4 weeks, the SOT score by CDP was 78 for the antioxidant group as compared to 63 for the nonantioxidant group. This difference was statistically significant at the $p < 0.05$ level. The improvement noted by the antioxidant group on the other tests was also greater than the nonantioxidant group, although these differences did not reach statistical significance because of the short trial period and small sample size.

PROPOSED MICRONUTRIENTS FOR PRIMARY PREVENTION OF CONCUSSIVE INJURY

Studies on primary prevention can be performed on football players, soccer players or combat troops who are going to be deployed in a military conflict where they are likely to sustain concussive injury. A preparation of multiple micronutrients may include vitamin A (retinyl palmitate), vitamin E (both D-alpha-tocopherol and D-alpha-TS), natural mixed carotenoids, vitamin C (calcium ascorbate), coenzyme Q_{10}, R-alpha-lipoic acid, n-acetylcysteine, L-carnitine, vitamin D, all B vitamins, selenium, zinc, chromium, and omega-3 fatty acids, certain polyphenolic compounds (curcumin and resveratrol) for reducing the initial damage to the brain following concussive injury.

No iron, copper, or manganese would be included, because these trace minerals are known to interact with vitamin C to produce free radicals. These trace minerals are absorbed from the intestinal tract more in the presence of antioxidants than in their absence that could result in increased body stores of free forms of these minerals. Increased iron stores have been linked to increased risk of some neurodegenerative diseases.[84] No heavy metals such as zirconium and molybdenum were added because of their potential neurotoxicity after long-term consumption.

The recommended micronutrient supplements should be taken daily orally divided into two doses: one half in the morning and the other half in the evening with meal. This is because the biological half lives of micronutrients are highly variable which can create high levels of fluctuations in the tissue levels of micronutrients if they are consumed once-a-day. A twofold difference in the levels of certain micronutrients such as alpha-tocopheryl succinate can cause a marked difference in the expression of gene profiles.[85] In order to maintain relatively consistent levels of micronutrients in the brain, the proposed micronutrients should be taken twice a day.

The efficacy of proposed micronutrient formulation in troops to be deployed in military conflicts or in football players should be tested by well-designed clinical studies. In the meantime, the proposed micronutrient recommendations may be adopted by the individuals who are at risk of receiving concussions with their physicians or health professionals. It is expected that the proposed recommendations would reduce the level of initial damage to the brain following concussions.

TOXICITY OF INGREDIENTS IN PROPOSED MICRONUTRIENT PREPARATION

Antioxidants and B vitamins used in proposed micronutrient preparation are considered safe. Antioxidants at doses higher than those that are recommended for the proposed micronutrient preparation have been consumed by the U.S. population for decades without significant toxicity. However, a few of them could produce harmful effects at certain high doses in some individuals when consumed daily for a long period of time. For example, vitamin A at doses of 10,000 IU or more per day can cause birth defects in pregnant women, and beta-carotene at doses of 50 mg or more can produce bronzing of the skin that is reversible on discontinuation. Vitamin C as ascorbic acid at high doses (10 g or more per day) can cause diarrhea in some individuals. Vitamin E at high doses (2000 IU or more per day) can induce clotting defects after long-term consumption. Vitamin B_6 at high doses (50 mg or more per day) may produce peripheral neuropathy, and selenium at doses of 400 mcg or more per day can cause skin and liver toxicity after long-term consumption. Coenzyme Q_{10} has no known toxicity, and recommended daily doses are 30–400 mg. N-acetylcysteine doses of 250–1500 mg and alpha-lipoic acid doses of 600 mg are used in humans without toxicity at these doses. All ingredients present in the proposed micronutrient preparations are safe and come under the category of "Food Supplement" and therefore do not require FDA approval for their use.

PROPOSED MICRONUTRIENTS FOR SECONDARY PREVENTION IN COMBINATION WITH STANDARD THERAPY AFTER CONCUSSIONS

Antioxidants and certain polyphenolic compounds reduce oxidative stress, inflammation, and release and toxicity of glutamate, in combination with standard therapy, and may further improve the acute and chronic management of concussive injury. A separate preparation of micronutrients, in combination with standard therapy, is recommended after concussive injury. This preparation of micronutrients contains doses of ingredients higher than those recommended for primary prevention. The above treatment with a preparation of micronutrients should be continued for 4–6 weeks after which the micronutrient preparation used for primary prevention should be adopted for the entire lifespan in order to reduce late adverse health effects of concussions.

The efficacy of proposed micronutrient formulations, in combination with standard therapy, on individuals who have sustained concussive injury should be tested by well-designed clinical studies. In the meantime, the proposed micronutrient recommendations may be adopted by the individuals who have received repeated concussions in consultation with their physicians. It is expected that the proposed recommendations, in combination with standard therapy, would decrease the progression and improve the current management of concussive injury.

RECOMMENDED MICRONUTRIENT PREPARATION BEFORE AND AFTER CONCUSSIVE INJURY FOR HIGH SCHOOL ATHLETES

INGREDIENTS

A preparation of multiple micronutrients may include vitamin A (retinyl palmitate), vitamin E (both D-alpha-tocopherol and D-TS), natural mixed carotenoids, vitamin C (calcium ascorbate), coenzyme Q_{10}, R-alpha-lipoic acid, n-acetylcysteine, L-carnitine, vitamin D, all B vitamins with high doses of vitamin B_3, selenium, zinc, curcumin, resveratrol, and omega-3 fatty acids.

DOSE SCHEDULE

Most clinical studies have utilized a once-a-day dose schedule. Taking vitamins and antioxidants once-a-day can create large fluctuations in their levels in the body. This is due to the fact that the biological half lives of vitamins and antioxidants markedly vary, depending upon their lipid or water solubility. A twofold difference in the levels of vitamin E succinate can produce marked alterations in the expression profiles of several genes in neuroblastoma cells in culture. Therefore, taking a multiple vitamin preparation once-a-day may produce large fluctuation in the levels of micronutrients in the body which could potentially cause genetic stress in cells that may compromise the effectiveness of the vitamin supplementation after long-term consumption. I recommend taking a preparation of micronutrients containing multiple dietary and endogenous antioxidants twice-a-day (half in the morning and another half in the evening preferably with meal) in order to reduce fluctuations in the levels of gene expressions in the brain. Such a dose schedule may improve the effectiveness of a multiple vitamin preparation in reducing the risk of developing acute and long-term adverse health consequences of concussion.

RECOMMENDED MICRONUTRIENT PREPARATION BEFORE AND AFTER CONCUSSIVE INJURY FOR PROFESSIONAL/COLLEGE SPORTS

Except for higher doses of certain ingredients, the micronutrient preparation and dose schedule are similar to those of high school sports.

UNIQUENESS OF THIS FORMULATION

No iron, copper, or manganese is included because these trace minerals are known to interact with vitamin C to produce free radicals. These trace minerals are absorbed from the intestinal tract more in the presence of antioxidants than in their absence that could result in increased body stores of free forms of these minerals after long-term consumption. Increased free iron stores have been linked to increased risk of several chronic diseases.[84] This preparation also does not contain heavy metals, such as zirconium or molybdenum. The excretion of these heavy metals is very little; therefore, daily supplementation even with small amounts of these metals may accumulate in the brain after long-term consumption. Heavy metals are known to be neurotoxic. Antioxidants from herbs, fruits, and vegetables are not included because they do not produce any unique biological effects that cannot be produced by antioxidants present in the proposed micronutrient preparation.

CONCEPT OF PAMARA

The validity of the concept of PAMARA, which includes protecting the skull by physical devices and protecting the brain tissue by supplementation with a preparation of micronutrients before and after concussions, should be tested by clinical studies. Some studies have investigated the efficacy of physical devices in reducing the risk of concussion; however, the efficacy of proposed micronutrient preparation for prevention and mitigation of brain concussive injuries has not been tested in players of high school, college, or professional athletes by well-designed clinical studies. It is expected that the implementation of the concept of PAMARA before sustaining concussive injury may reduce the risk of developing abnormal brain functions including cognitive dysfunction and aberrant behavior.

CONCLUSIONS

Concussive injury also referred to as mild TBI occurs when the brain is violently rocked back and forth within the skull following a blow to the head or neck such as that observed in contact sports like football and soccer. Concussive injury occurs in troops when exposed to blast pressure waves, such as following detonation of an IED. This injury is characterized by the immediate and transient changes in brain function which include temporary loss of memory, confusion, poor balance, and reflexes and hearing loss. The long-term health risks of concussive injury include serious mental disorders, such as cognitive dysfunction and abnormal behavior (fear, anxiety, anger, and suicidal tendency) that are being observed at increased rates among retired professional football players and veterans of foreign wars.

The major biochemical abnormalities that contribute to neurodegeneration leading to cognitive dysfunction and aberrant behaviors include increased oxidative stress, chronic inflammation, and glutamate release. Antioxidants, which reduce oxidative stress, chronic inflammation, and release and toxicity of glutamate, appear to be one of the rational choices for prevention and improved management of concussive injury.

Despite evolutionary improvements in protective equipment, concussive injuries in the brain remain a major health risk for professional football players. Despite the use of state of the art physical protection during combat, U.S. troops continue to suffer from the adverse consequences of concussive injury. Currently available physical protective devices are not sufficient to reduce the acute and long-term adverse consequences of concussions on brain function. At present, treatments involving medications and other complementary approaches are not satisfactory.

A novel concept of PAMARA is proposed. This concept includes protection of the skull by physical protective devices and protection of the brain tissue by micronutrient supplementation before and after concussions. The validity of the proposed concept of PAMARA should be tested by well-designed clinical studies. A separate preparation of micronutrients including dietary and endogenous antioxidants and certain polyphenolic compounds (curcumin and resveratrol) and omega-3 fatty acids for professionals and high school/college athletes is proposed. This preparation of micronutrients would reduce oxidative stress, chronic inflammation, and release and toxicity of glutamate indirectly by increasing the levels of antioxidant enzyme through the Nrf2/ARE pathway as well as directly by scavenging free radicals. In a preliminary clinical study, a commercial preparation of micronutrients containing multiple dietary and endogenous antioxidants in combination with standard care improved some of the symptoms of concussive injury in troops returning from wars in Iraq and Afghanistan with mild to moderate TBI. The efficacy of proposed micronutrient preparation should be tested before and after concussive injury by well-designed clinical studies.

REFERENCES

1. Viano DC, Casson IR, Pellman EJ et al. Concussion in professional football: Comparison with boxing head impacts—Part 10. *Neurosurgery.* Dec 2005; 57(6): 1154–1172; discussion 1154–1172.
2. Viano DC, Pellman EJ, Withnall C, Shewchenko N. Concussion in professional football: Performance of newer helmets in reconstructed game impacts—Part 13. *Neurosurgery.* Sep 2006; 59(3): 591–606; discussion 591–606.
3. Guskiewicz KM, Weaver NL, Padua DA, Garrett WE, Jr. Epidemiology of concussion in collegiate and high school football players. *Am J Sports Med.* Sep–Oct 2000; 28(5): 643–650.
4. Levy ML, Ozgur BM, Berry C, Aryan HE, Apuzzo ML. Analysis and evolution of head injury in football. *Neurosurgery.* Sep 2004; 55(3): 649–655.
5. Abate A, Yang G, Dennery PA, Oberle S, Schroder H. Synergistic inhibition of cyclooxygenase-2 expression by vitamin E and aspirin. *Free Radic Biol Med.* Dec 2000; 29(11): 1135–1142.
6. Devaraj S, Tang R, Adams-Huet B et al. Effect of high-dose alpha-tocopherol supplementation on biomarkers of oxidative stress and inflammation and carotid atherosclerosis in patients with coronary artery disease. *Am J Clin Nutr.* Nov 2007; 86(5): 1392–1398.
7. Fu Y, Zheng S, Lin J, Ryerse J, Chen A. Curcumin protects the rat liver from CCl4-caused injury and fibrogenesis by attenuating oxidative stress and suppressing inflammation. *Mol Pharmacol.* Feb 2008; 73(2): 399–409.
8. Hori K, Hatfield D, Maldarelli F, Lee BJ, Clouse KA. Selenium supplementation suppresses tumor necrosis factor alpha-induced human immunodeficiency virus type 1 replication *in vitro*. *AIDS Res Hum Retroviruses.* Oct 10 1997; 13(15): 1325–1332.
9. Jesudason EP, Masilamoni JG, Ashok BS et al. Inhibitory effects of short-term administration of DL-alpha-lipoic acid on oxidative vulnerability induced by Abeta amyloid fibrils (25–35) in mice. *Mol Cell Biochem.* Apr 2008; 311(1–2): 145–156.

10. Kuhlmann MK, Levin NW. Potential interplay between nutrition and inflammation in dialysis patients. *Contrib Nephrol.* 2008; 161: 76–82.

11. Lee HS, Jung KK, Cho JY et al. Neuroprotective effect of curcumin is mainly mediated by blockade of microglial cell activation. *Pharmazie.* Dec 2007; 62(12): 937–942.

12. Albini A, Morini M, D'Agostini F et al. Inhibition of angiogenesis-driven Kaposi's sarcoma tumor growth in nude mice by oral N-acetylcysteine. *Cancer Res.* Nov 15 2001; 61(22): 8171–8178.

13. Peairs AT, Rankin JW. Inflammatory response to a high-fat, low-carbohydrate weight loss diet: Effect of antioxidants. *Obesity (Silver Spring).* May 1 2008.

14. Rahman S, Bhatia K, Khan AQ et al. Topically applied vitamin E prevents massive cutaneous inflammatory and oxidative stress responses induced by double application of 12-O-tetradecanoylphorbol-13-acetate (TPA) in mice. *Chem Biol Interact.* Apr 15 2008; 172(3): 195–205.

15. Suzuki YJ, Aggarwal BB, Packer L. Alpha-lipoic acid is a potent inhibitor of NF-kappaB activation in human T cells. *Biochem Biophys Res Commun.* Dec 30 1992; 189(3): 1709–1715.

16. Wood LG, Garg ML, Powell H, Gibson PG. Lycopene-rich treatments modify noneosinophilic airway inflammation in asthma: Proof of concept. *Free Radic Res.* Jan 2008; 42(1): 94–102.

17. Zhu J, Yong W, Wu X et al. Anti-inflammatory effect of resveratrol on TNF-alpha-induced MCP-1 expression in adipocytes. *Biochem Biophys Res Commun.* May 2 2008; 369(2): 471–477.

18. Casson IR, Viano DC, Powell JW, Pellman EJ. Repeat concussions in the national football league. *Sports health.* Jan 2011; 3(1): 11–24.

19. Lincoln AE, Caswell SV, Almquist JL, Dunn RE, Norris JB, Hinton RY. Trends in concussion incidence in high school sports: A prospective 11-year study. *Am J Sport Med.* May 2011; 39(5): 958–963.

20. Gessel LM, Fields SK, Collins CL, Dick RW, Comstock RD. Concussions among United States high school and collegiate athletes. *J aAthl Train.* Oct–Dec 2007; 42(4): 495–503.

21. MacGregor AJ, Dougherty AL, Morrison RH, Quinn KH, Galarneau MR. Repeated concussion among U.S. military personnel during Operation Iraqi Freedom. *J Rehabil Res Dev.* 2011; 48(10): 1269–1278.

22. Rapoport MJ, McCullagh S, Shammi P, Feinstein A. Cognitive impairment associated with major depression following mild and moderate traumatic brain injury. *J Neuropsychiatry Clin Neurosci.* Winter 2005; 17(1): 61–65.

23. van Donkelaar P, Langan J, Rodriguez E et al. Attentional deficits in concussion. *Brain Inj.* Nov 2005; 19(12): 1031–1039.

24. Halterman CI, Langan J, Drew A et al. Tracking the recovery of visuospatial attention deficits in mild traumatic brain injury. *Brain.* Mar 2006; 129(Pt 3): 747–753.

25. Guskiewicz KM, Marshall SW, Bailes J et al. Association between recurrent concussion and late-life cognitive impairment in retired professional football players. *Neurosurgery.* Oct 2005; 57(4): 719–726; discussion 719–726.

26. Gottshall K, Drake A, Gray N, McDonald E, Hoffer ME. Objective vestibular tests as outcome measures in head injury patients. *Laryngoscope.* Oct 2003; 113(10): 1746–1750.

27. Kerr ZY, Marshall SW, Harding HP, Jr., Guskiewicz KM. Nine year risk of depression diagnosis increases with increasing self-reported concussions in retired professional football players. *Am J Sports Med.* Oct 2012; 40(10): 2206–2212.

28. Guskiewicz KM, McCrea M, Marshall SW et al. Cumulative effects associated with recurrent concussion in collegiate football players: The NCAA Concussion Study. *JAMA.* Nov 19 2003; 290(19): 2549–2555.

29. Breedlove EL, Robinson M, Talavage TM et al. Biomechanical correlates of symptomatic and asymptomatic neurophysiological impairment in high school football. *J Biomech.* Apr 30 2012; 45(7): 1265–1272.

30. De Beaumont L, Tremblay S, Poirier J, Lassonde M, Theoret H. Altered bidirectional plasticity and reduced implicit motor learning in concussed athletes. *Cereb Cortex.* Jan 2012; 22(1): 112–121.

31. Covassin T, Schatz P, Swanik CB. Sex differences in neuropsychological function and postconcussion symptoms of concussed collegiate athletes. *Neurosurgery.* Aug 2007; 61(2): 345–350; discussion 350–341.

32. Wilk JE, Herrell RK, Wynn GH, Riviere LA, Hoge CW. Mild traumatic brain injury (concussion), posttraumatic stress disorder, and depression in U.S. soldiers involved in combat deployments: Association with postdeployment symptoms. *Psychosom Med.* Apr 2012; 74(3): 249–257.

33. Carlson KF, Kehle SM, Meis LA et al. Prevalence, assessment, and treatment of mild traumatic brain injury and posttraumatic stress disorder: A systematic review of the evidence. *J Head Trauma Rehabil.* Mar–Apr 2011; 26(2): 103–115.

34. Ellemberg D, Henry LC, Macciocchi SN, Guskiewicz KM, Broglio SP. Advances in sport concussion assessment: From behavioral to brain imaging measures. *J Neurotrauma.* Dec 2009; 26(12): 2365–2382.

35. Aiguo W, Zhe Y, Gomez-Pinilla F. Vitamin E protects against oxidative damage and learning disability after mild traumatic brain injury in rats. *Neurorehabil Neural Repair.* Mar–Apr 2010; 24(3): 290–298.

36. Conte V, Uryu K, Fujimoto S et al. Vitamin E reduces amyloidosis and improves cognitive function in Tg2576 mice following repetitive concussive brain injury. *J Neurochem.* Aug 2004; 90(3): 758–764.

37. Wu A, Molteni R, Ying Z, Gomez-Pinilla F. A saturated-fat diet aggravates the outcome of traumatic brain injury on hippocampal plasticity and cognitive function by reducing brain-derived neurotrophic factor. *Neuroscience.* 2003; 119(2): 365–375.

38. Wu A, Ying Z, Gomez-Pinilla F. Dietary curcumin counteracts the outcome of traumatic brain injury on oxidative stress, synaptic plasticity, and cognition. *Exp Neurol.* Feb 2006; 197(2): 309–317.

39. Wu A, Ying Z, Gomez-Pinilla F. The salutary effects of DHA dietary supplementation on cognition, neuroplasticity, and membrane homeostasis after brain trauma. *J Neurotrauma.* Oct 2011; 28(10): 2113–2122.

40. Tavazzi B, Vagnozzi R, Signoretti S et al. Temporal window of metabolic brain vulnerability to concussions: Oxidative and nitrosative stresses—Part II. *Neurosurgery.* Aug 2007; 61(2): 390–395; discussion 395–396.

41. Shultz SR, Bao F, Omana V, Chiu C, Brown A, Cain DP. Repeated mild lateral fluid percussion brain injury in the rat causes cumulative long-term behavioral impairments, neuroinflammation, and cortical loss in an animal model of repeated concussion. *J Neurotrauma.* Jan 20 2012; 29(2): 281–294.

42. Hausmann R, Kaiser A, Lang C, Bohnert M, Betz P. A quantitative immunohistochemical study on the time-dependent course of acute inflammatory cellular response to human brain injury. *Int J Legal Med.* 1999;112(4): 227–232.

43. Holmin S, Soderlund J, Biberfeld P, Mathiesen T. Intracerebral inflammation after human brain contusion. *Neurosurgery.* Feb 1998; 42(2): 291–298; discussion 298–299.

44. Holmin S, Hojeberg B. In situ detection of intracerebral cytokine expression after human brain contusion. *Neurosci Lett.* Oct 14 2004; 369(2): 108–114.

45. Beschorner R, Nguyen TD, Gozalan F et al. CD14 expression by activated parenchymal microglia/macrophages and infiltrating monocytes following human traumatic brain injury. *Acta Neuropathol.* Jun 2002; 103(6): 541–549.

46. Reger ML, Poulos AM, Buen F, Giza CC, Hovda DA, Fanselow MS. Concussive brain injury enhances fear learning and excitatory processes in the amygdala. *Biol Psychiatry.* Feb 15 2012; 71(4): 335–343.

47. Fang WH, Wang DL, Wang F. [Expression of c-myc protein on rats' brains after brain concussion]. *Fa Yi Xue Za Zhi.* Oct 15 2006; 22(5): 333–334.

48. Wang F, Li YH, Hu YL. [A study on the expression of C-FOS protein after experimental rat brain concussion]. *Fa Yi Xue Za Zhi.* 2003; 19(1): 8–9.

49. Hang CH, Chen G, Shi JX, Zhang X, Li JS. Cortical expression of nuclear factor kappaB after human brain contusion. *Brain Res.* Sep 13 2006; 1109(1): 14–21.

50. Prasad KN, Cohrs RJ, Sharma OK. Decreased expressions of c-myc and H-ras oncogenes in vitamin E succinate induced morphologically differentiated murine B-16 melanoma cells in culture. *Biochem Cell Biol.* Nov 1990; 68(11): 1250–1255.

51. Shen WH, Zhang CY, Zhang GY. Antioxidants attenuate reperfusion injury after global brain ischemia through inhibiting nuclear factor-kappaB activity in rats. *Acta Pharmacol Sin.* Nov 2003; 24(11): 1125–1130.

52. Gahm C, Holmin S, Mathiesen T. Nitric oxide synthase expression after human brain contusion. *Neurosurgery.* Jun 2002; 50(6): 1319–1326.

53. Itoh K, Chiba T, Takahashi S et al. An Nrf2/small Maf heterodimer mediates the induction of phase II detoxifying enzyme genes through antioxidant response elements. *Biochem Biophys Res Commun.* Jul 18 1997; 236(2): 313–322.

54. Hayes JD, Chanas SA, Henderson CJ et al. The Nrf2 transcription factor contributes both to the basal expression of glutathione S-transferases in mouse liver and to their induction by the chemopreventive synthetic antioxidants, butylated hydroxyanisole, and ethoxyquin. *Biochem Soc Trans.* Feb 2000; 28(2): 33–41.

55. Chan K, Han XD, Kan YW. An important function of Nrf2 in combating oxidative stress: Detoxification of acetaminophen. *Proc Natl Acad Sci U S A.* Apr 10 2001; 98(8): 4611–4616.

56. Niture SK, Kaspar JW, Shen J, Jaiswal AK. Nrf2 signaling and cell survival. *Toxicol Appl Pharmacol.* Apr 1 2010; 244(1): 37–42.

57. Xi YD, Yu HL, Ding J et al. Flavonoids protect cerebrovascular endothelial cells through Nrf2 and PI3K from beta-amyloid peptide-induced oxidative damage. *Curr Neurovasc Res.* Feb 2012; 9(1): 32–41.

58. Li XH, Li CY, Lu JM, Tian RB, Wei J. Allicin ameliorates cognitive deficits ageing-induced learning and memory deficits through enhancing of Nrf2 antioxidant signaling pathways. *Neurosci Lett.* Apr 11 2012; 514(1): 46–50.

59. Bergstrom P, Andersson HC, Gao Y et al. Repeated transient sulforaphane stimulation in astrocytes leads to prolonged Nrf2-mediated gene expression and protection from superoxide-induced damage. *Neuropharmacology.* Feb–Mar 2011; 60(2–3): 343–353.

60. Wruck CJ, Gotz ME, Herdegen T, Varoga D, Brandenburg LO, Pufe T. Kavalactones protect neural cells against amyloid beta peptide-induced neurotoxicity via extracellular signal-regulated kinase 1/2-dependent nuclear factor erythroid 2-related factor 2 activation. *Mol Pharmacol.* Jun 2008; 73(6): 1785–1795.

61. Hine CM, Mitchell JR. NRF2 and the phase II response in acute stress resistance induced by dietary restriction. *J Clin Exp Pathol.* Jun 19 2012; S4(4).

62. Suh JH, Shenvi SV, Dixon BM et al. Decline in transcriptional activity of Nrf2 causes age-related loss of glutathione synthesis, which is reversible with lipoic acid. *Proc Natl Acad Sci U S A.* Mar 9 2004; 101(10): 3381–3386.

63. Zou Y, Hong B, Fan L et al. Protective effect of puerarin against beta-amyloid-induced oxidative stress in neuronal cultures from rat hippocampus: Involvement of the GSK-3beta/Nrf2 signaling pathway. *Free Radic Res.* Jan 2013; 47(1): 55–63.

64. Choi HK, Pokharel YR, Lim SC et al. Inhibition of liver fibrosis by solubilized coenzyme Q_{10}: Role of Nrf2 activation in inhibiting transforming growth factor-beta1 expression. *Toxicol Appl Pharmacol.* Nov 1 2009; 240(3): 377–384.
65. Trujillo J, Chirino YI, Molina-Jijon E, Anderica-Romero AC, Tapia E, Pedraza-Chaverri J. Renoprotective effect of the antioxidant curcumin: Recent findings. *Redox Biol.* 2013; 1(1): 448–456.
66. Steele ML, Fuller S, Patel M, Kersaitis C, Ooi L, Munch G. Effect of Nrf2 activators on release of glutathione, cysteinylglycine, and homocysteine by human U373 astroglial cells. *Redox Biol.* 2013; 1(1): 441–445.
67. Kode A, Rajendrasozhan S, Caito S, Yang SR, Megson IL, Rahman I. Resveratrol induces glutathione synthesis by activation of Nrf2 and protects against cigarette smoke-mediated oxidative stress in human lung epithelial cells. *Am J Physiol Lung Cell Mol Physiol.* Mar 2008; 294(3): L478–L488.
68. Gao L, Wang J, Sekhar KR et al. Novel n-3 fatty acid oxidation products activate Nrf2 by destabilizing the association between Keap1 and Cullin3. *J Biol Chem.* Jan 26 2007; 282(4): 2529–2537.
69. Saw CL, Yang AY, Guo Y, Kong AN. Astaxanthin and omega-3 fatty acids individually and in combination protect against oxidative stress via the Nrf2-ARE pathway. *Food Chem Toxicol.* Dec 2013; 62: 869–875.
70. Ji L, Liu R, Zhang XD et al. N-acetylcysteine attenuates phosgene-induced acute lung injury via upregulation of Nrf2 expression. *Inhal Toxicol.* Jun 2010; 22(7): 535–542.
71. Zambrano S, Blanca AJ, Ruiz-Armenta MV et al. The renoprotective effect of L-carnitine in hypertensive rats is mediated by modulation of oxidative stress-related gene expression. *Eur J Nutr.* Sep 2013; 52(6): 1649–1659.
72. Brinjikji W, Rabinstein AA, Cloft HJ. Hospitalization costs for acute ischemic stroke patients treated with intravenous thrombolysis in the United States are substantially higher than medicare payments. *Stroke.* Apr 2012; 43(4): 1131–1133.
73. Barger SW, Goodwin ME, Porter MM, Beggs ML. Glutamate release from activated microglia requires the oxidative burst and lipid peroxidation. *J Neurochem.* Jun 2007; 101(5): 1205–1213
74. Schubert D, Kimura H, Maher P. Growth factors and vitamin E modify neuronal glutamate toxicity. *Proc Natl Acad Sci U S A.* Sep 1 1992; 89(17): 8264–8267.
75. Sandhu JK, Pandey S, Ribecco-Lutkiewicz M et al. Molecular mechanisms of glutamate neurotoxicity in mixed cultures of NT2-derived neurons and astrocytes: Protective effects of coenzyme Q_{10}. *J Neurosci Res.* Jun 15 2003; 72(6): 691–703.
76. Shoulson I. DATATOP: A decade of neuroprotective inquiry. Parkinson Study Group. Deprenyl and tocopherol antioxidative therapy of Parkinsonism. *Ann Neurol.* Sep 1998; 44(3 Suppl 1): S160–166.
77. Sano M, Ernesto C, Thomas RG et al. A controlled trial of selegiline, alpha-tocopherol, or both as treatment for Alzheimer's disease. The Alzheimer's Disease Cooperative Study. *N Engl J Med.* Apr 24 1997; 336(17): 1216–1222.
78. Albanes D, Heinonen OP, Huttunen JK et al. Effects of alpha-tocopherol and beta-carotene supplements on cancer incidence in the Alpha-Tocopherol Beta-Carotene Cancer Prevention Study. *Am J Clin Nutr.* Dec 1995; 62(6 Suppl): 1427S–1430S.
79. Prasad KN, Cole WC, Prasad KC. Risk factors for Alzheimer's disease: Role of multiple antioxidants, nonsteroidal anti-inflammatory, and cholinergic agents alone or in combination in prevention and treatment. *J Am Coll Nutr.* Dec 2002; 21(6): 506–522.
80. Chen RS, Huang CC, Chu NS. Coenzyme Q_{10} treatment in mitochondrial encephalomyopathies. Short-term double-blind, crossover study. *Eur Neurol.* 1997; 37(4): 212–218.

81. Gaziano JM, Sesso HD, Christen WG et al. Multivitamins in the prevention of cancer in men: The Physicians' Health Study II randomized controlled trial. *JAMA*. Nov 14 2012; 308(18): 1871–1880.

82. Baum MK, Campa A, Lai S et al. Effect of micronutrient supplementation on disease progression in asymptomatic, antiretroviral-naive, HIV-infected adults in Botswana: A randomized clinical trial. *JAMA*. Nov 27 2013; 310(20): 2154–2163.

83. Gottshall K, Hoffer, ME, Balough, BJ. Use of antioxidants micronutrient compounds in vestibular rehabilitation after operational head trauma or blast injury. Paper presented at *Barany International Balance Meeting, June 2006; Stockholm, Sweden.*

84. Olanow CW, Arendash GW. Metals and free radicals in neurodegeneration. *Curr Opin Neurol.* Dec 1994; 7(6): 548–558.

85. Prasad KN, Kumar B, Yan XD, Hanson AJ, Cole WC. Alpha-tocopheryl succinate, the most effective form of vitamin E for adjuvant cancer treatment: A review. *J Am Coll Nutr.* Apr 2003; 22(2): 108–117.

9 Cerebrovascular Insufficiency

Improved Management by Micronutrients

INTRODUCTION

The brain requires a constant supply of oxygen and nutrients through blood vessels for survival and normal function. It consumes about 20% of the total body oxygen consumption. Cerebrovascular insufficiency, a form of cerebrovascular disease, caused by poor blood supply to the brain can lead to transient ischemic stroke (min-stroke) or stroke. Stroke is the third leading cause of death in the USA, causing more than 150,000 deaths annually. Insufficient blood supply to the brain can occur by formation of clot (thrombosis) in the carotid artery that supplies blood to the brain, release of clot from another part of the body and lodged in the carotid artery, or by stenosis of the carotid artery. There are two major zones of ischemic injury referred to as core ischemic zones (necrosis of neurons and glia cells) and ischemic penumbra (surrounding ischemic area containing potentially viable neurons). The damage in the core ischemic zone is irreversible, whereas cells in the ischemic penumbra can regain function if blood circulation to the brain is restored before they become dead. When blood circulation to the brain is restored, reperfusion injury occurs that can aggravate damage caused by ischemia. The existence of ischemic penumbra provides an opportunity to rescue neurons and glia cells and thereby reduce the impact of ischemic/reperfusion injury on the brain functions. However, the window of time for rescuing neurons is very short.

Laboratory and clinical studies have revealed that increased oxidative stress occurs in the brain following ischemic/reperfusion injury. In addition to increased oxidative stress, acute and chronic inflammation which is characterized by the rapid activation of brain resident inflammatory cells (primarily microglia), increased production of pro-inflammatory cytokines, and infiltration of various types of blood-derived inflammatory cells, such as neutrophils, different subtypes of T-lymphocytes, monocytes, and macrophages, into the ischemic brain tissue, occur after ischemia/reperfusion. In addition, glutamate is also released during this form of brain injury. Thus, increased oxidative stress, inflammation, and glutamate play an important role in the progression of brain damage after ischemic/reperfusion. Therefore, reducing these biochemical defects may be one of the rational choices for attenuating the progression of brain damage during the acute phase of ischemic/reperfusion injury and decreasing the risk of developing neurological deficits including cognitive dysfunction during the chronic phase of injury.

This chapter describes incidence, cost, classification, symptoms, and involvement of oxidative stress, inflammation, and glutamate in the progression of brain damage after ischemic/reperfusion. In addition, this chapter provides data and scientific rationale for using a preparation of micronutrients, in combination with standard therapy, to reduce the progression of brain damage after ischemic/reperfusion injury, as well as the risk of developing neurological deficits.

INCIDENCE AND COST

The incidence of ischemic stroke increased by about 50% among individuals who are 85 years or older compared to those who are 75–84 years; however, the incidence of neuroendovascular procedures for acute ischemic stroke among individuals aged 75–84 years was 22.8 per 100,000 persons, and it was only 13.2% among individuals aged 85 years or older.[1] Cerebrovascular diseases remain the fourth leading cause of death in the USA.[2] During 1998–2007, about 4.4 million ischemic stroke patients were hospitalized in the USA. The age-adjusted rate of ischemic stroke hospitalization decreased from 184 to 128 per 100,000 persons.[3]

The cost of hospitalization may differ, depending upon the status of patients with ischemic stroke. Average hospitalization cost of ischemic stroke increased from $9273 to $10,524 per patient.[3] In 2008, the average cost after intravenous thrombolysis for acute ischemic stroke is $14,102 for patients with good outcome, $18,856 for patients with severe disability, and $19,129 for patients with in-hospital mortality.[4]

CLASSIFICATIONS

A report by the *Ad Hoc* Committee established by the Council of the National Institute of Neurological and Communicative Disorders and Stroke, National Institute of Health, Bethesda, MD, will publish a revised classification of cerebrovascular diseases in 2014. The revised classification has been divided into six parts and outlines in broad terms:

Part 1. Clinical Stage
Part 2. Pathophysiological Mechanisms
Part 3. Anatomy (blood vessels, brain)
Part 4. Pathology (blood vessels, brain)
Part 5. Clinical Phenomenon
Part 6. Status of Patients (Performance and Placement)

Part I. Clinical Stage
    A. *Asymptomatic*: Asymptomatic individuals may show risk factors that increase the risk of developing cerebrovascular insufficiency in the future.
    B. *Focal Cerebral Dysfunction*: This form of cerebral dysfunction may include focal ischemia, intracranial hemorrhage, and arteritis. It also

includes transient attacks (transient ischemic attacks) and generally lasts for 2–15 min, but occasionally it can last as long as 24 h. No persistent neurological deficits are observed after the episode. The aura of migraine is commonly attributed to focal cerebral ischemia owing to vasoconstriction. Rarely the symptoms persist long enough to produce a cerebral infarct.

C. *General Cerebral Dysfunction*: This type of cerebral dysfunction refers to general cerebral ischemia in which there is a generalized reduction of cerebral perfusion due to cardiac arrest, shock, or severe hypotension. The transient symptoms may include simple fainting and loss of consciousness.

Part II. Pathophysiological Mechanisms

Primary abnormalities of cerebral circulation include thrombosis, embolism, hemorrhage, compression, and expanding mass.

Part III. Anatomy

The major arteries involved in inducing cerebral ischemia include ascending aorta and aortic arch.

Part IV. Pathology

The pathological changes in blood vessels as well as in neural parenchymal cells are observed.

Part V. Clinical Phenomena

This includes history, physical examination, laboratory examination, x-ray examination, and others.

Part VI. Status of Patient (Performance and Placement)

It includes measurements of performance ability in physical and living environments. Performance may be divided into the following categories: no significant impairment, mildly impaired, modestly impaired, and severely impaired.

Placement may be divided into the following categories: no limitation (require no supervision), mild limitation (require occasional supervision and/or occasional medical care), modest limitation (require much supervision and/or regular available medical care), and severe limitation (require constant supervision and/or immediate available medical-nursing care).

REPERFUSION INJURY

When the blood circulation is restored in patients with cerebral ischemia, reperfusion injury occurs due to formation of reactive oxygen species (ROS) and reactive nitrogen species (RNS), and pro-inflammatory cytokines.

SENSITIVITY OF BRAIN CELLS TO ISCHEMIC/REPERFUSION INJURY

Neurons are much more sensitive to damage than glia cells following ischemic/reperfusion injury. Neurons from different parts of the brain show differential sensitivity due to variations in blood flow and cellular metabolic requirements. Depending upon the severity of ischemia, the patients may live or die. The survivors may suffer from severe neurological deficits including cognitive dysfunctions. The pathological changes and symptoms are very complex because of marked variations in the area of the brain most immediately damaged by ischemia and the total area of the brain involved in the damage.

INCREASED OXIDATIVE STRESS

Extensive studies have revealed that increased generation oxygen-derived and nitrogen-derived free radicals (increased oxidative stress) play an important role in the development of infarct brain swelling and blood–brain barrier disruption after cerebral ischemia/reperfusion.[5–8] Arbitrarily selected studies and reviews are presented in support of the role of increased oxidative stress in the progression of damage during acute and chronic phases of injury. The sources of increased oxidative stress following cerebrovascular insufficiency include mitochondrial dysfunction and activation of cerebral oxidases. Increased oxidative stress contributes to necrosis and apoptosis through a number of pathways in ischemic tissue.[9] A clinical study on the levels of markers of oxidative damage was measured in 70 patients within the first 48 h after stroke and compared with 70 patients with similar stroke risk factors. The results showed that serum levels of malondialdehyde (MDA), nitric oxide (NO), and glutathione were significantly elevated within 24 h after stroke compared to those who did not have stroke. The Canadian Neurological Scale (CNS) was negatively correlated with the levels of NO and MDA; however, there was a significant correlation between plasma levels of glutathione and CNS scores.[10] Elevated plasma levels of glutathione following stroke may reflect adaptive response to increased oxidative stress. It has been reported that the plasma levels of antioxidants, such as ascorbic acid, alpha-tocopherol, and protein thiols were associated with the degree of neurological impairment assessed by scores of NIH Stroke Scale, Barthel index, and Hand Motor Score tests.[11] It has been reported that multiple markers of oxidative damage were increased immediately after ischemic stroke and remained elevated for several days.[12] A clinical study on 93 neonates with perinatal hypoxic-ischemic encephalopathy showed that increased oxidative stress may contribute to brain damage, especially in preterm neonates.[13]

Nicotinamide adenine dinucleotide phosphate (NADPH) oxidases (NOXs) are one of the major sources of ROS in the brain. Among NOXs, NOX4 is a major source of oxidative stress that contributes to degeneration of neurons after ischemic stroke.[14] Therefore, the authors have suggested that the development of an inhibitor of isoform-specific NOX inhibitors may be useful in the management of ischemic stroke. Indeed, several studies have shown that glucose, one of the substrates of NOX, may participate in the progression of damage following reperfusion injury. This was substantiated by the fact that inhibitors of NOX reduced the adverse effects of hyperglycemia on stroke. It was also reported that inhibitors of NOX reduced the complications of thrombolytic therapy by decreasing blood–brain barrier disruption, brain edema, and hemorrhage.[15] It was also reported that NOX produced from circulating inflammatory cells contributes to the brain damage more than that produced from endogenous brain residential cells.

In a clinical study on 160 patients with strokes involving the middle cerebral artery who were treated with tissue plasminogen activators (dissolves clot) and 60 healthy controls, plasma levels of markers of oxidative damage were determined and correlated with arterial recanalization. The results showed that the levels of markers of oxidative damage were elevated at the baseline in patients who had stroke compared to the healthy control; however, there was no association between the levels of markers of oxidative damage and reperfusion injury after arterial recanalization.[16]

The development of infarction after cerebral ischemia is considered due to the death of neurons. Cytosolic superoxide dismutase (Cu/Zn SOD) protects the brain from ischemic injury. The effectiveness of Cu/Zn SOD in protecting the brain after focal cerebral ischemia was tested in mutant mice lacking Cu/Zn SOD (SOD1). The results showed that homozygous mutant (SOD–/–) had no detectable Cu/Zn SOD activity, whereas heterozygous mutant (SOD+/–) had 50% less Cu/Zn SOD activity compared to wild type mice. Homozygous mutant mice showed increased levels of disruption of blood–brain barrier 1 h after occlusion of middle cerebral artery, and all mutant mice died 24 h after onset of ischemia. On the other hand, heterozygous mutant mice revealed increased infarct volume and brain swelling and neuronal death.[17] These results suggest that oxygen-derived free radicals, especially superoxide anions, play an important role in the development of infarction and edema after focal cerebral ischemia. This was further confirmed by experiments in which overexpression of Cu/Zn SOD in transgenic mice reduced damage to the brain (infarct size and edema) after focal cerebral ischemia.[18] The transcriptional factor Nrf2 (nuclear factor erythroid 2-related factor 2) which regulates the levels of antioxidant enzymes through ARE (antioxidant response element) plays an important role in neuroprotection after ischemia/reperfusion injury. This was confirmed using Nrf2 knockout mice in which neurological deficits and infarct volume were greater than in wild type mice after ischemia/reperfusion injury.[19] Furthermore, increased oxidative stress caused translocation of Nrf2 from the cytoplasm to the nucleus which is necessary for the upregulation of antioxidant genes; whereas, glutamate treatment failed to do so.

Global ischemia activates mixed lineage kinase3 (MLK3) via free radicals. It has been reported that overexpressed MLK3 in primary hippocampal neurons in culture (HEK293 cell) is S-nitrosylated by NO. This is supported by the fact that administration of 7-nitroindazole, an inhibitor of neuronal NO synthase (nNOS), reduced the S-nitrosylation of MLK3 and inhibited its activation after cerebral ischemia/reperfusion.[20] It has been reported that endogenous NO induced S-nitrosylation and phosphorylation of P38MAPK-alpha (P38), and the activation of P38 was dependent on its S-nitrosylation after ischemia, whereas sodium nitroprusside, a NO donor, and 7-nitroindazole, an inhibitor of (nNOS), inhibited the activation of P38 signaling pathway induced by cerebral ischemia/reperfusion and reduced damage to the hippocampus. It has been proposed that the N-methyl-D-aspartate receptor may be involved in the S-nitrosylation and phosphorylation of P38.[21] Apoptosis signal-regulating kinase 1 (ASK1) is activated after cerebral ischemia. Overexpressed ASK1 in hippocampal neurons in culture can be S-nitrosylated by both endogenous and exogenous NO. S-Nitrosylated ASK1 enhanced its phosphorylation and thus became activated. Administration of exogenous NO reversed the effects of endogenous NO by inhibiting S-nitrosylation of ASK1 and thereby reduced damage to the brain after ischemia/reperfusion.[22] Thrombolysis and endovascular recanalization cause cerebral reperfusion injury due to increased oxidative/nitrosylative stress. The activities of brain matrix metalloproteinases (MMPs) increase during reperfusion injury which is correlated with increased oxidative/nitrosylative stress. MMPs are Zn-containing proteolytic enzymes which degrade extracellular matrix around cerebral blood vessels and neurons. Free radicals after ischemic/reperfusion activate MMPs which cause blood–brain barrier disruption. Caveiolin-1, a member of integral proteins, protected blood–brain barrier disruption by inhibiting production of RNS and activities of MMPs.[23]

Serum concentration of uric acid increases rapidly after acute ischemic stroke. A low serum concentration of uric acid was modestly associated with improved short-term clinical outcomes in patients with acute ischemic stroke. It has been suggested that serum levels of uric acid is more a marker of severity of cerebral infarction than an independent predictor of clinical outcomes of stroke.[24] Among 724 patients with ischemic stroke, 226 patients (31.2%) had cerebral micro bleeds (CMBs). Elevated uric acid levels were associated with the presence of CMBs. This association was most pronounced in patients with hypertension.[25]

Transglutaminases (TGs) are calcium-dependent multifunctional enzymes which play a role in pathophysiology of brain after stroke. It appears that TG2 isoform in response to increased oxidative stress translocate to the nucleus where it suppresses genes responsible for increasing antioxidant enzymes. Therefore, inhibitors of TGs may be useful in reducing damage to the brain after stroke by restoring the antioxidant ability of neurons.[26]

The sequential cleavage of amyloid precursor protein (APP) by beta- and gamma-secretases produces beta-amyloid fragments (Aβ-142) which are toxic to nerve cells and are considered the primary cause of Alzheimer's disease. It has been reported that the brain ischemia increases the expression and activity of beta- and gamma-secretases and thereby produces excessive amounts of Aβ1–42.[27]

INCREASED INFLAMMATION

Inflammation plays an important role in the repair and progression of damage after ischemic/reperfusion injury. Inflammatory cells release excessive amounts of cytokines, ROS, adhesion molecules, prostaglandins, and complement proteins all of which are toxic to nerve cells. During the period of acute inflammation, both pro- and anti-inflammatory cytokines are released. Pro-inflammatory cytokines include interleukin-6 (IL-6), IL-17, IL-18, IL-23, and tumor necrosis factor-alpha (TNF-alpha) that are toxic to the neurons, whereas anti-inflammatory cytokines include IL-1, IL-4, IL-10, IL-11, and IL-13 that help in the repair at the site of injury. If the tissue damage after ischemic/reperfusion injury is severe, the pro-inflammatory cytokines may overcome the repair function of anti-inflammatory cytokines and participate in the progression of damage. Some pro-inflammatory cytokines such as IL-6 can also act as a neurotrophic factor. It acts as a pro-inflammatory cytokine during the acute phase of injury and as a neurotrophic factor between sub-acute and chronic-phase of injury. Administration of IL-6 directly into the brain after ischemia can reduce the brain damage.[28]

It has been reported that IL-23 released from the infiltrating macrophages induced IL-17 producing T lymphocytes in a mouse stroke model.[29] IL-17 promoted delayed ischemic damage in the brain. In addition, necrotic brain tissue released peroxiredoxin family proteins which induce pro-inflammatory cytokines including IL-23 in macrophages through activation of Toll-like receptors (TLR2 and TLR4). These released cytokines participate in neuronal death after stroke in mice. Some endogenous TLR ligands, such as high-mobility group box 1 and peroxiredoxin family proteins, are released from injured brain cells. These ligands activate the infiltrating macrophages which released pro-inflammatory cytokines which participate in the progression of damage in ischemic brain.[30] It has been shown that extracellular peroxiredoxin family proteins are released from the necrotic brain cells 12 h after the onset of stroke in a mouse models. These proteins participate in neuronal death. This is substantiated by the observation that administration of antibodies of peroxiredoxin family proteins inhibited expression of pro-inflammatory cytokines and reduced infarct volume.[31] The levels of endogenous ligand of TLR, high-mobility group protein box-1 (HMGB1) increased in the acute cerebral infarct (ACI) group compared to that in the control group; and this rise in the levels of HMGB1 correlated with the severity of neurological abnormalities in patients with ACI.[32] In addition, it was found that TLR4 was involved in the development of brain injury following ischemia. IL-17A positive lymphocytes have been found in the brain tissue of patients with stroke, suggesting the role of pro-inflammatory cytokines in the progression of damage after ischemia.[33] This was supported by the fact that administration of IL-17A-blocking antibody 3 h after stroke decreased infarct size and improved neurological functions in a mouse model of stroke.

Using a rat model of cerebral ischemia and reperfusion, it was demonstrated that oxidative activity of neutrophils and the levels of pro-inflammatory cytokines (IL-1beta and TNF-alpha) increased after acute focal cerebral ischemia, prolonged ischemia, and reperfusion. In addition, increased levels of endothelin-1 (ET-1) were also observed after acute and prolonged ischemia.[34] Mast cells of cerebral microvasculature act as potent inflammatory cells which release cytoplasmic granules containing a number of vasoactive mediators, such as TNF-alpha, histamine, heparin, and proteases which play an important role in the progression of damage after cerebral ischemia. These mast cells promote blood–brain barrier disruption, brain edema, prolonged extravasation, and hemorrhage after cerebral ischemia.[35] Using a mouse model of cerebral ischemia-reperfusion, it was shown that CD38 deficiency reduced chemokine production, immune cell infiltration, and brain damage after transient ischemia and reperfusion.[36]

In a clinical study on 75 patients with acute stroke with or without insulin resistance, it was found that serum levels of marker of pro-inflammatory cytokines (IL-6) and oxidative stress (nitric oxide and malondialdehyde) were elevated in all patients; however, in patients with insulin resistance, elevation of these markers of inflammation and oxidative stress correlated with the severity of stroke.[37] On the other hand, the levels of anti-inflammatory cytokine (IL-10) were reduced in patients with insulin resistance.

An epidemiologic study (case control) on 591 patients with stroke (472 ischemic stroke, 83 hemorrhagic stroke, and 36 unknown subtype) revealed that increased levels of pro-inflammatory cytokines (IL-6 and TNF-alpha), c-reactive protein, and fibrinogen were associated with the risk of recurrent ischemic stroke; however, another pro-inflammatory cytokine, IL-18, was not associated with the risk of recurrent of ischemic stroke.[38] Furthermore, none of the markers of inflammation was associated with recurrence of hemorrhagic stroke.

In addition to cytokines, toxic chemicals, such as complements and adhesion molecules are released during inflammation. Activation of these molecules contribute to the progression of ischemic/perfusion injury in the brain.[39,40]

Using a mouse model of ischemic reperfusion injury, it was demonstrated that deficiency of protease-activated receptor-4 (PAR-4) caused 80% reduction of infarct volume, significant improvement in neurologic and motor functions, and reduction in blood–brain barrier disruption and brain edema compared with wild-type mice. These protective effects of PAR-4 deficiency are partially mediated through inhibition of platelet activation and reduction of microvascular inflammation (infiltration of leukocytes).[41]

Prostaglandins (PGs) are also released during inflammation. PGE2 accumulates at the site of injury in the brain after ischemic injury in rodent models. Both microsomal prostaglandin E synthase-1 (mPGES-1) and cyclooxygenase-2 (COX-2) participate in the production of PGE2; therefore, their levels may increase following ischemic injury. Indeed, coinduction of mPGES-1 and COX-2 activities were found after brain ischemia in mice.[42] Using mPGES-1 knockout mice, it was demonstrated that ischemic injury in the brain was less severe and that PGE2 production was not detected in knockout mice compared to that in wild-type mice. Intraperitoneal injection of either COX-2 inhibitor or PGE2 receptor (EP3) antagonist reduced progression of damage in the brain after ischemic injury. It was further observed that glutamate induced mPGES-1 in cultured hippocampus slices and that glutamate-induced toxicity was less severe compared with wild type mice. These results suggest that the progression of damage in the brain after ischemic injury is mediated via excessive production of PGE2 and accumulation of extracellular glutamate. Using a mouse model of ischemia/reperfusion, it was demonstrated that treatment with PGE2 type 1 receptor (EP1R) antagonist (SC5108) reduced damage to neurons after ischemia/reperfusion injury. EP1R-deficient mice showed similar protective effects in the brain after ischemia/reperfusion injury.[43] These results suggest that EP1R causes neuronal death by inhibiting pro-survival protein kinase AKT. Using a mouse model of ischemia, it was found that administration of COX-2 inhibitor and PGE2 receptor (EP4) agonist (1-902688) after stroke showed reduced neuronal death and infarct volume compared with control animal treated with vehicle. These results suggest that selective activation of EP-4 receptors could be of neuroprotective value after ischemic injury to the brain.[44] It was demonstrated that activation of PGE2 EP3 receptor contributed to the progression of ischemic injury and that administration of PGE2 EP3 receptor antagonist reduced ischemia-induced brain damage.[45]

Elevated levels of peroxisome proliferator-activated receptor-gamma (PPAR-gamma) appear to provide neuroprotection after ischemia/reperfusion injury. 15-Deoxy-12,14-prostaglandin J2 (15-PGJ2) forms as a metabolic product of PGD2 and acts as an endogenous agonist for 15-PGJ2. Using a rodent model of ischemia, it was demonstrated that administration of 15-PGJ2 improved survival of neurons, brain edema, and infarct volume after ischemic/reperfusion injury.[46] It has been reported that prostaglandin F2alpha (PGF2) and its receptor (FP) play an important role in the progression of brain damage after ischemia/reperfusion injury.[47] Using a mouse stroke model, it was shown that administration of FP antagonist (AL-8810) reduced neurological dysfunctions and infarct volume after ischemia. Similar results were obtained in FP receptor knockout mice.[48] These results further suggest that PGF2alpha plays an important role in the progression of brain damage after ischemia.

INCREASED GLUTAMATE RELEASE

Elevated levels of extracellular glutamate and aspartate play an important role in the progression of brain damage and neuronal death after ischemia/reperfusion injury in rats. Administration of inhibitors of all five phospholipases significantly reduced release of glutamate and aspartate into the extracellular fluid in the brain after ischemia. In addition, an inhibitor protein kinase C (PKC) also attenuated the release of glutamate and aspartate.[49] These results suggest that activation of phospholipases and PKC play an important role in the progression of brain damage after ischemia/reperfusion injury. Reuptake of released glutamate is necessary for preventing its accumulation that may cause neuronal death. Glia glutamate transporters (GLT-1 and GLAST) and neuronal glutamate transporter (EAAC1) are responsible for glutamate reuptake. Therefore, a reduction in the levels of these glutamate transporters may allow accumulation of glutamate into the extracellular fluid in the brain. It has been demonstrated that the levels of GLT-1 and EAAC1 are decreased after focal cerebral ischemia in rats.[50] In addition, pre-treatment with antagonist of group III metabotropic glutamate receptor prevented neuronal loss after ischemia/reperfusion injury in rats.[51] Another study showed that pre-treatment with ceftriaxone, an agonist of GLT-1, produced a significant reduction in neurological deficits and brain infarct volume by increasing the reuptake of extracellular glutamate.[52]

Since changes in the extracellular levels of glutamate are directly linked to the alterations in the intracellular levels of calcium, and since NO play an important role in the progression of brain damage after ischemia/reperfusion injury, inhibitors of calcium release from intracellular stores and NO may provide neuroprotection after ischemia/reperfusion injury. Indeed, it has been demonstrated that administration of dantrolene, an inhibitor of calcium, release[53] and lubeluzole, an inhibitor of NO production,[54] significantly reduced glutamate accumulation and reduced neuronal loss after global cerebral ischemia in rats.

HOW TO REDUCE OXIDATIVE STRESS OPTIMALLY

Oxidative stress in the body occurs when the antioxidant system fails to provide adequate protection against damage produced by free radicals (reactive oxygen species and reactive nitrogen species). Increased oxidative stress in the body is reduced by upregulating antioxidant enzymes as well as by existing levels of dietary and endogenous antioxidant chemicals, because they work by different mechanisms. For example, antioxidant enzymes reduce free radicals by catalysis, whereas dietary and endogenous antioxidant chemicals reduce free radicals by directly scavenging them.

In response to ROS, a nuclear transcriptional factor, Nrf2 (nuclear factor-erythroid 2-related factor 2) is translocated from the cytoplasm to the nucleus where it binds with ARE which increases the levels of antioxidant enzymes (gamma-glutamyl-cysteine ligase, glutathione peroxidase, glutathione reductase, and heme oxygen-ase-1) and phase 2 detoxifying enzymes (NAD(P)H: quinine oxidoreductase 1 and glutathione-S-transferase) in order to reduce oxidative damage.[55–57] In response to increased oxidative stress, existing levels of dietary and endogenous antioxidant chemical levels cannot be elevated without supplementation.

FACTORS REGULATING RESPONSE OF NRF2

Antioxidant enzymes are elevated by activation of Nrf2 which depends upon ROS-dependent and -independent mechanisms. In addition, elevated levels of antioxidant enzymes are also dependent upon the binding ability of Nrf2 with ARE in the nucleus. These studies are described here.

ROS-Dependent Regulation of NRF2

Normally, Nrf2 is associated with Kelch-like ECH associated protein 1 (Keap1) protein which acts as an inhibitor of Nrf2 (INrf2).[58] INrf2 protein serves as an adaptor to link Nrf2 to the ubiquitin ligase CuI-Rbx1 complex for degradation by proteasomes and maintains the steady levels of Nrf2 in the cytoplasm. INrf2 acts as a sensor for ROS/electrophilic stress. In response to increased ROS, Nrf2 dissociates itself from iNrf2-CuI-Rbx1 complex and translocates into the nucleus where it binds with ARE that increases antioxidant genes. It has been demonstrated that Nrf2 regulates INrf2 levels by controlling its transcription, whereas INrf2 regulates Nrf2 levels by controlling its degradation by proteasome.[59]

ROS-Independent Regulation of NRF2

Antioxidants such as vitamin E, genistein (a flavonoid),[60] allicin, a major organo-sulfur compound found in garlic,[61] sulforaphane, a organosulfur compound, found in cruciferous vegetables,[62] kavalactones (methysticin, kavain, and yangonin),[63] and dietary restriction[64] activate Nrf2 without stimulation by ROS.

Reduced Binding of NRF2 with ARE

Age-related decline in antioxidant enzymes in the liver of older rats compared to that in younger rats was due to reduction in the binding ability of Nrf2 with ARE; however, treatment with alpha-lipoic acid restored this defect, increased the levels of antioxidant enzymes, and restored the loss of glutathione from the liver of older rats.[65]

DIFFERENTIAL RESPONSE OF Nrf2 TO ROS STIMULATION DURING ACUTE AND CHRONIC OXIDATIVE STRESS

It appears that Nrf2 responds to ROS generated during acute and chronic oxidative stress differently. For example, acute oxidative stress during strenuous exercise translocates Nrf2 from the cytoplasm to the nucleus where it binds with ARE to upregulate antioxidant genes. However, during chronic oxidative stress commonly observed in older individuals and in neurodegenerative diseases, such as Parkinson's disease and Alzheimer's disease, Nrf2/ARE pathway becomes unresponsive to ROS. A reduction in the binding ability of Nrf2 with ARE was demonstrated in older rats.[65] The reasons for the Nrf2/ARE pathway to become unresponsive to ROS during chronic oxidative stress are unknown.

Nrf2 IN ISCHEMIC/REPERFUSION INJURY

No studies have been performed directly on changes in Nrf2 responses after ischemic/reperfusion injury in the brain. Since increased oxidative stress, inflammation, and glutamate release are involved in the acute and chronic phases of this form of brain injury, attenuation of these biochemical defects appear to be one of the rational choices for reducing the progression of brain damage after ischemic/reperfusion injury.

The following groups of selected nontoxic agents in combination may be useful in reducing oxidative stress optimally:

1. *Agents that can reduce oxidative stress by directly scavenging free radicals*: Some examples are dietary antioxidants, such as vitamin A, beta-carotene, vitamin C, and vitamin E, and endogenous antioxidants, such as glutathione, alpha-lipoic acid, and coenzyme Q_{10}.
2. *Agents that can reduce oxidative stress by activating Nrf2-regulated antioxidant genes without ROS stimulation*: Some examples are organosulfur compound sulforaphane found in cruciferous vegetables, kavalactones, found in Kava shrubs, and Puerarin, a major flavonoid from the root of *Pueraria lobata*,[62,63,66] genistein, and vitamin E[60] and coenzyme Q_{10}[67] activate Nrf2 without ROS stimulation.
3. *Agents that can reduce oxidative stress directly by scavenging free radicals as well as indirectly by activating Nrf2/ARE pathway*: Some examples are vitamin E,[60] alpha-lipoic acid,[65] curcumin,[68] resveratrol,[69,70] omega-3-fatty acids,[71,72] and NAC.[73]
4. *Agents reducing oxidative stress by ROS-dependent mechanism*: They include L-carnitine which generates transient ROS.[74]

A combination of selected agents from the above groups may reduce oxidative stress optimally and thereby may reduce the progression of acute and chronic phase of ischemic/reperfusion injury, and in combination with standard therapy, may improve the management of this form of brain injury.

How to Reduce Chronic Inflammation and Glutamate

Some individual antioxidants from the above groups have been shown to reduce chronic inflammation[75–82] and prevent the release[83] and toxicity[84,85] of glutamate.

A combination of selected agents from the above groups may reduce chronic inflammation and release of glutamate and its toxicity optimally and thereby may reduce the progression of acute and chronic phase of ischemic/reperfusion injury, and in combination with standard therapy, may improve the management of this form of brain injury.

Based on the studies discussed above, it is unlikely that the use of a single antioxidant or polyphenolic compound would increase the levels of antioxidant enzymes as well as dietary and endogenous antioxidants. Therefore, the use of a single agent would not reduce oxidative stress, inflammation, and glutamate optimally and thus may not have adequate effect in reducing the progression of brain injury following cerebral insufficiency and preventing the risk of developing neurological deficits in humans. Unfortunately, most studies have been performed with a single antioxidant or polyphenolic compound. These studies are described here.

PROTECTION OF BRAIN INJURY BY ANTIOXIDANTS IN ANIMAL MODELS

ALPHA-LIPOIC ACID AND N-ACETYLCYSTEINE

Pretreatment with alpha-lipoic acid increased survival and reduced brain damage after ischemia/reperfusion injury in rats.[86] As expected, reestablishment of circulation after ischemia caused focal infarct in the prefrontal cortex area of rats. Treatment with alpha-lipoic acid before introducing ischemia produced a dose-dependent decrease in infarct volume; however, it failed to reduce infarct volume when administered immediately before reperfusion.[87] This effect of alpha-lipoic acid was related to an increase in the levels of SOD2. Pretreatment with N-acetylcysteine (NAC) reduced ischemia/reperfusion injury in rats. Intraperitoneal injection of NAC at the time of reperfusion reduced the infarcts area and volume and improved neurological functions and glutathione levels. The protective effect of NAC was observed even when it was injected 6 h after reperfusion. The neuroprotective effects of NAC was mediated through reduction in the levels of pro-inflammatory cytokine (TNF-alpha and IL-1beta), inducible nitric oxide synthase (iNOS). NAC treatment also reduced activation of macrophage/microglia and neuronal death. These results suggest that NAC treatment protected the brain even after the onset of ischemia/reperfusion injury in rats.[88] The neuroprotective effects of NAC are mediated through downregulation of NF-kappaB.[89] Intravenous injection of cross-linked nanozymes (cl-nanozymes) with SOD1 or catalase decreased brain damage and improved sensorimotor functions in an animal model of ischemia/reperfusion injury.[90]

VITAMIN E, L-CARNITINE, LYCOPENE, AND VITAMIN D

Ischemia/reperfusion injury increased the levels of MDA and reduced activities of antioxidant enzymes (SOD and catalase), but no change in glutathione levels in rats. Pretreatment with alpha-tocopherol, lecithin, or combination of the two restored the levels of MDA and catalase activity to normal levels.[91] It is interesting to observe that lecithin also acts as an antioxidant similar to alpha-tocopherol and that both lecithin and alpha-tocopherol produce neuroprotection by reducing oxidative stress.

Pretreatment with alpha-tocopherol, L-carnitine, or a combination of the two reduced neuronal loss and the levels of a marker of oxidative stress (MDA) and increased SOD activity after ischemia/reperfusion injury in rats. The neuroprotective effect of L-carnitine was comparable to that of alpha-tocopherol. The neuroprotective effects of the combination of L-carnitine and alpha-tocopherol were similar to those produced by the individual agents.[92]

It has been reported that pretreatment with lycopene provided neuroprotection by increasing SOD activity and inhibiting apoptosis in Mongolian gerbils.[93]

Pretreatment with a combination of Vitamin D_3 and dehydroascorbic acid was most effective in providing neuroprotection compared to the individual agents.[94]

POLYPHENOLIC COMPOUNDS IN ANIMAL MODELS

HERBS

It has been shown that administration of rosmarinic acid reduced neuronal loss and brain edema by inhibiting NF-kB activation after ischemia/reperfusion injury in rats.[95] Injection of ethanol extract of the root of *Pongamia pinnata* decreased markers of oxidative stress, neuronal loss, infiltration of inflammatory cells, and improved learning ability and cognitive function after ischemia/reperfusion injury in rats.[96] Similar observations were made in an animal model of ischemia/reperfusion injury after treatment with methanol extract of Ocimum sanctum.[97]

RESVERATROL

Treatment with resveratrol improved neurological functions and reduced infarct volume after cerebral ischemia in rats.[98] Furthermore, this treatment also reduced the release of glutamate and aspartate and increased the levels of inhibitory neurotransmitters, GABA (gamma-aminobutyric acid), glycine, and taurine. Pretreatment with resveratrol reduced infarct volume and brain edema and improved neurological functions after ischemia/reperfusion injury in rats. Resveratrol treatment decreased the levels of MDA, restored the SOD activity, upregulated the protein and mRNA expression of Nrf2 and HO-1 (heme oxygenase), and downregulated the levels of Caspase-3.[99]

CURCUMIN, QUERCETIN, GENISTEIN, *GINKGO BILOBA*, AND GREEN TEA EXTRACT

Curcumin also protected the brain after ischemia/reperfusion injury by upregulating Nrf2 and HO-1 in rats.[100] Quercetin reduced brain damage after ischemia/reperfusion injury by elevating the levels of brain-derived nerve neurotrophic factor (BDNF) and p-Akt-proteins and decreasing the levels of Caspase-3.[101] Genistein protected the brain from transient global cerebral ischemia by reducing oxidative stress.[102] *Ginkgo biloba*[103] and green tea[104] extracts reduced brain damage after ischemia reperfusion injury by reducing markers of oxidative damage.

OTHER PROTECTIVE AGENTS

Preischemic treadmill training significantly inhibited the release of glutamate, while it increased the release of GABA during the acute phase of ischemia/reperfusion injury. Since excessive release of glutamate contribute to the neuronal death, pre-ischemic treadmill training improved neurological functions, reduced infarct volume after ischemia/reperfusion injury by inhibiting the release of glutamate, and increased the release of GABA in rats.[105,106]

PROTECTION OF BRAIN INJURY BY ANTIOXIDANTS IN HUMANS

There are no effective micronutrient therapies for reducing brain damage in patients with ischemia/reperfusion injury. Despite extensive evidence for the role of increased oxidative stress, inflammation, and glutamate release in the progression of brain damage during and after ischemia/reperfusion injury, no studies to reduce these biochemical defects optimally have been performed in humans. A few studies with the synthetic antioxidants in patients with acute ischemic stroke have produced some short-term beneficial effects on neurological functions.

EBSELEN

Ebselen is a seleno-organic compound (2-phenyl-1,2-benzisoselenazole-3 (2H)-one) which scavenges peroxynitrite and inhibit enzymes, such as lipooxygenase, NO synthase, NADPH oxidase, protein kinase Cand H+/K+-ATPase. It appears that administration of ebselen soon after acute ischemic stroke can improve neurological functions.[107]

A clinical study on 302 patients with acute ischemic stroke revealed that oral administration of ebselen (N = 151 patients) improved neurological functions when started within 24 h of the onset of stroke; however, it was ineffective when administered after 24 h in comparison to placebo controls (149 patients). The significant improvement in neurological functions was observed at 1 month after treatment with ebselen, but not after 3 months of treatment.[108]

EDARAVONE

A review of three trials involving 496 patients with acute ischemic stroke has described the effectiveness of edaravone, a synthetic free radical scavenger, in reducing brain damage. It was concluded that the number of patients with marked improvement in neurological functions increased in groups receiving standard care plus edaravone compared to the group who received only standard treatment.[109] The mechanisms of neuroprotection by edaravone may involve inhibition of protein oxidation and DNA adduct formation (8-OHdG) at the penumbra area during the early period after reperfusion, and reduction in the activation of microglia, expression of inducible nitric oxide synthase (iNOS), and 3-nitrotyrosine during the late phase of injury.[110]

OTHER PROTECTIVE AGENTS

An oral administration of aspirin within 48 h and tissue plasminogen activator within 3 h of ischemic stroke has shown some benefit. Synthetic free radical scavenger

NXY-059 has been useful if administered within 6 h of onset of ischemic stroke.[111] A clinical study on 90 patients with ischemic cerebrovascular disease showed that acupuncture can enhance functional recovery and increase the quality of life among survivors.[112]

PROBLEMS OF USING A SINGLE MICRONUTRIENT DURING ISCHEMIA/REPERFUSION INJURY

The use of single agents, such as alpha-lipoic acid, NAC, vitamin E, resveratrol, curcumin, quercetin, genistein, and *Ginkgo biloba* has produced some benefits in animal models of cerebral insufficiency. The use of single agents is unlikely to increase the levels of antioxidant enzymes through the Nrf2/ARE pathway as well as dietary and endogenous antioxidants. Therefore such studies are not sufficient to draw any conclusion regarding the value of micronutrients in reducing the progression of brain damage following ischemic/reperfusion injury.

Previous studies in other chronic diseases, such as beta-carotene in male heavy smokers for reducing the risk of lung cancer, vitamin E in Alzheimer's disease (AD) for improving cognitive function, and vitamin E in Parkinson's disease (PD) for improving the symptoms and as expected, produced inconsistent results varying from no effect in PD,[113] to modest beneficial[114] or no effect effects in AD,[115] and harmful effects in heavy male smokers.[116] This is due to the fact that patients with the above diseases have a high internal oxidative environment in which an individual antioxidant is oxidized and then acts as a pro-oxidant rather than as an antioxidant.

The fact that the patients with ischemia/reperfusion injury have a high internal oxidative environment suggests that administration of individual agents with antioxidant activity would result in oxidation of these agents. It is well known that an oxidized antioxidant acts as a pro-oxidant that may not produce beneficial clinical outcomes. On the contrary, an oxidized antioxidant is likely to increase the risk of developing neurological deficits after long-term consumption. Because of the failure to obtain consistent beneficial effects with individual agents in other neurodegenerative diseases, I recommend a preparation of micronutrients containing dietary and endogenous antioxidants, vitamin D, B vitamins with high doses of vitamin B_3, resveratrol, curcumin, and omega-3 fatty acids for reducing the progression of brain injury in patients with ischemia/reperfusion injury and reduce the risk of developing neurological deficits. This preparation of micronutrients would reduce oxidative stress, inflammation, and glutamate optimally. Additional rationales for using multiple micronutrients are described here.

RATIONALE FOR USING MULTIPLE MICRONUTRIENTS IN REDUCING BRAIN DAMAGE AFTER ISCHEMIC/REPERFUSION INJURY

The references for this section are described in a review.[117] The mechanisms of action of micronutrients and herbs in the proposed formulation are in part different; their distribution in various organs and cells, their affinity to various types of free radicals, and their biological half lives are different. Beta-carotene (BC) is more effective in quenching oxygen radicals than most other antioxidants. BC can perform certain biological functions that cannot be produced by its metabolite vitamin A and vice versa. It has been reported that BC treatment enhances the expression of the connexin gene which codes for a gap junction protein in mammalian fibroblasts in culture, whereas vitamin A treatment does not produce such an effect. Vitamin A can induce differentiation in certain normal and cancer cells, whereas BC and other carotenoids do not. Thus, BC and vitamin A have, in part, different biological functions in the body. The gradient of oxygen pressure varies within cells. Some antioxidants, such as vitamin E, are more effective as quenchers of free radicals in reduced oxygen pressure, whereas BC and vitamin A are more effective in higher atmospheric pressures. Vitamin C is necessary to protect cellular components in aqueous environments, whereas carotenoids and vitamins A and E protect cellular components in lipid environments. Vitamin C also plays an important role in maintaining cellular levels of vitamin E by recycling vitamin E radical (oxidized) to the reduced (antioxidant) form.

The form of vitamin E used in a preparation of micronutrients is also important. It has been established that D-alpha-tocopheryl succinate (vitamin E succinate) is the most effective form of vitamin both *in vitro* and *in vivo*. This form of vitamin E is more soluble than alpha-tocopherol and enters cells more readily; and therefore, it is expected that vitamin E succinate would cross the blood–brain barrier in greater amounts than alpha-tocopherol. However, this idea has not yet been tested in animals or humans. We have reported that an oral ingestion of vitamin E succinate (800 IU/day) in humans increased plasma levels of not only alpha-tocopherol but also of vitamin E succinate, suggesting that a portion of this form of vitamin E can be absorbed from the intestinal tract before hydrolysis to alpha-tocopherol, provided that the plasma pool of alpha-tocopherol is saturated. This observation is important because the conventional assumption based on the studies in rodents has been that esterified forms of vitamin E, such as alpha-tocopheryl succinate, alpha-tocopheryl nicotinate, and alpha-tocopheryl acetate, can be absorbed from the intestinal tract only after they are hydrolyzed to alpha-tocopherol. Our preliminary data showed that this assumption may not be true for the absorption of vitamin E succinate in humans provided that the plasma pool of alpha-tocopherol is saturated.

An endogenous antioxidant, glutathione, is effective in catabolizing H_2O_2 and anions. However, oral supplementation with glutathione failed to significantly increase plasma levels of glutathione in human subjects, suggesting that this tripeptide is completely hydrolyzed in the GI tract. Therefore, I propose to utilize N-acetylcysteine and alpha-lipoic acid that increase the cellular levels of glutathione by different mechanisms in a multiple micronutrient preparation.

Another endogenous antioxidant, coenzyme Q_{10}, may have some potential value in the prevention of cerebrovascular insufficiency. Since coenzyme Q_{10} is needed for the generation of ATP by mitochondria, it is essential to add this antioxidant in multiple micronutrient preparation. A study has shown that coenzyme Q_{10} scavenges peroxy radicals faster than alpha-tocopherol, and like vitamin C, can regenerate vitamin E in a redox cycle. However, it is a weaker antioxidant than alpha-tocopherol. Coenzyme Q_{10} administration has been shown to improve clinical symptoms in patients with mitochondrial encephalomyopathies.[118]

Nicotinamide (vitamin B_3), a precursor of NAD^+ attenuated glutamate-induced toxicity and preserved cellular levels of NAD^+ to support the activity of SIRT1. It is also a competitive inhibitor of histone deacetylase activity and restored memory deficits in AD transgenic mice. These preclinical data suggest that oral supplementation with nicotinamide may be safe and useful in preventing memory deficits among survivors of ischemia/reperfusion injury. Since memory loss may occur as a late effect of ischemia/reperfusion injury, addition of this form of vitamin B to a preparation of micronutrients may be needed.

Selenium is a cofactor of glutathione peroxidase, and Se-glutathione peroxidase acts as an antioxidant by increasing the intracellular level of glutathione. Therefore, selenium should be added to a multiple micronutrient preparation for the prevention of ischemia/reperfusion injury.

In addition to dietary and endogenous antioxidants, B vitamins, especially high doses of vitamin B_3 (nicotinamide), should be added to a multiple micronutrient preparation. B vitamins are also essential for normal health. Curcumin and resveratrol are added because they have shown some beneficial effects in animal models of ischemia/reperfusion injury. Omega-3 fatty acids were also added because they appear to produce some benefits in animal models of dementia.

Release of glutamate was blocked by vitamin E.[83] Both vitamin E[119] and coenzyme Q_{10}[85] also protect against glutamate-induced neurotoxicity in cell culture models.

REDUCING BRAIN DAMAGE AFTER
ISCHEMIA/REPERFUSION INJURY

The ischemic/reperfusion injury can be divided into two phases: acute phase and chronic phase. This form of brain injury occurs soon after restoring the blood circulation to the brain. During the acute phase of reperfusion injury, excessive amounts of free radicals derived from oxygen and nitrogen, toxic products of chronic inflammation (pro-inflammatory cytokines, PGE2, complements, and adhesion molecules), and glutamate are released which cause neuronal death, brain edema, increase in infarct volume, and disruption in brain–blood barrier. During the chronic phase of reperfusion injury, increased oxidative stress, chronic inflammation, and glutamate release also participate in the development of neurological deficits, such as cognitive dysfunction and abnormal behavior among survivors. Therefore, attenuation of these biochemical defects in combination with standard therapy may reduce the progression of brain damage during the acute phase as well as reduce the risk of developing neurological deficits during the chronic phase of ischemic/reperfusion injury.

RECOMMENDED MICRONUTRIENTS FOR
REDUCING BRAIN DAMAGE DURING ACUTE
PHASE OF ISCHEMIC/REPERFUSION INJURY

A preparation of multiple micronutrients for the acute phase of ischemic/reperfusion injury may include vitamin A (retinyl palmitate), vitamin E (both D-alpha-tocopherol and D-alpha-TS), natural mixed carotenoids, vitamin C (calcium ascorbate), coenzyme Q_{10}, R-alpha-lipoic acid, n-acetylcysteine, L-carnitine, vitamin D, all B-vitamins with high doses of vitamin B_3, selenium, omega-3 fatty acids, curcumin, and resveratrol.

No iron, copper, or manganese would be included, because these trace minerals are known to interact with vitamin C to produce free radicals. These trace minerals are absorbed from the intestinal tract more in the presence of antioxidants than in their absence that could result in increased body stores of free forms of these minerals. Increased iron stores have been linked to increased risk of several chronic diseases.[120] No heavy metals such as zirconium and molybdenum were added because of their potential neurotoxicity after long-term consumption.

The recommended micronutrient supplements should be taken orally and divided into two doses, half in the morning and the other half in the evening with meal. This is because the biological half lives of micronutrients are highly variable which can create high levels of fluctuations in the tissue levels of micronutrients if they are consumed once a day. A two-fold difference in the levels of certain micronutrients such as alpha-tocopheryl succinate can cause a marked difference in the expression of gene profiles.[121] In order to maintain relatively consistent levels of micronutrients in the brain, the proposed micronutrients should be taken twice a day.

This preparation can be administered before and soon after the onset of reperfusion injury. The above treatment with micronutrients should be continued for 4–6 weeks after which the formulation for chronic phase of ischemic/reperfusion injury should be adopted for the entire lifespan in order to reduce the risk of developing neurological deficits following ischemia/reperfusion injury.

The efficacy of proposed micronutrient formulation in individuals with cerebrovascular insufficiency should be tested by well-designed clinical studies. It is expected that the proposed recommendations would reduce initial damage to the brain during acute phase of reperfusion injury.

TOXICITY OF MICRONUTRIENTS

Antioxidants and B vitamins used in proposed micronutrient preparation are considered safe. Antioxidants at doses higher than those that are recommended for the proposed micronutrient preparation have been consumed by the US population for decades without significant toxicity. However, a few of them could produce harmful effects at certain high doses in some individuals when consumed daily for a long period of time. For example, vitamin A at doses of 10,000 IU or more per day can cause birth defects in pregnant women, and beta-carotene at doses of 50 mg or more can produce bronzing of the skin that is reversible on discontinuation. Vitamin C as ascorbic acid at high doses (10 g or more per day) can cause diarrhea in some individuals. Vitamin E at high doses (2000 IU or more per day) can induce clotting defects after long-term consumption. Vitamin B_6 at high doses (50 mg or more per day) may produce peripheral neuropathy, and selenium at doses of 400 mcg or more per day can cause skin and liver toxicity after long-term consumption. Coenzyme Q_{10} has no known toxicity, and recommended daily doses are 30–400 mg. N-acetylcysteine doses of 250–1500 mg and alpha-lipoic acid doses of 600 mg are used in humans without toxicity at these doses. All ingredients present in the proposed micronutrient preparations are safe and come under the category of "Food Supplement," and therefore, do not require FDA approval for their use.

RECOMMENDED MICRONUTRIENTS FOR REDUCING BRAIN DAMAGE DURING CHRONIC PHASE OF ISCHEMIC/REPERFUSION INJURY

A separate preparation of micronutrients for the chronic phase of ischemic/reperfusion injury containing lower doses of antioxidants and polyphenolic compounds than those found in the preparation for the acute phase, in combination with standard therapy, is recommended.

The efficacy of proposed micronutrient formulations, in combination with standard therapy, should be tested by well-designed clinical studies. It is expected that the proposed recommendations, in combination with standard therapy, would reduce the risk of developing neurological deficits after ischemic/reperfusion brain injury more than those produced by standard therapy alone.

DIET AND LIFESTYLE RECOMMENDATIONS FOR PATIENTS WITH ISCHEMIA/REPERFUSION INJURY

A balanced diet is necessary, in addition to supplementation with a preparation of multiple micronutrients, for reducing the risk of long-term adverse effects on brain functions, as well as improving the efficacy of standard therapy in the management of acute- and long-term consequences of ischemia/reperfusion injury. I recommend a balanced diet containing low fat and plenty of fruits and vegetables. Lifestyle recommendations include daily moderate exercise, reduced stress, no tobacco smoking, and reduced intake of caffeine.

CONCLUSIONS

Cerebrovascular insufficiency, a form of cerebrovascular disease, caused by poor blood supply to the brain can lead to transient ischemic stroke (mini-stroke) or stroke. Insufficient blood supply to the brain can occur by formation of clot (thrombosis) in the carotid artery that supplies blood to the brain, release of clot from another part of the body and lodged in the carotid artery, or by stenosis of the carotid artery. There are two major zones of ischemic injury referred to as core ischemic zones (necrosis of neurons and glia cells) and ischemic penumbra (surrounding ischemic area containing potentially viable neurons). The damage in the core ischemic zone is irreversible, whereas cells in the ischemic penumbra can regain function if the blood circulation is restored before they become dead. When blood circulation to the brain is restored, reperfusion injury occurs that can aggravate damage caused by ischemia.

Laboratory and human studies have revealed that increased oxidative stress, acute and chronic inflammation, and glutamate release occur after cerebral ischemia/reperfusion. These biochemical defects play an important role in the progression of brain damage after ischemic/reperfusion injury. Therefore, attenuation of the above biochemical defects appear to be one of the rational choices for reducing the progression of brain damage after ischemic/reperfusion injury. In order to reduce oxidative stress, inflammation, and glutamate optimally, it is essential to increase the levels of antioxidant enzymes as well as dietary and endogenous antioxidants. The levels of antioxidant enzymes are increased by ROS-dependent and -independent mechanisms of activation of the Nrf2/ARE pathway, whereas the levels of dietary and endogenous antioxidants can be increased by supplementation. This cannot be achieved by the use of one or two antioxidants in clinical studies. Unfortunately, most studies in animals and humans have been performed with one or two antioxidants. They include alpha-lipoic acid, N-acetylcysteine, vitamin E, L-carnitine, lycopene, vitamin D, synthetic antioxidants (Edaravone and Ebselen), and polyphenolic compounds, such as resveratrol, curcumin, and quercetin), and aspirin.

I have proposed separate micronutrient formulations for the acute phase and chronic phase of cerebral ischemic/reperfusion injury. The micronutrient preparation for the acute phase include vitamin A (retinyl palmitate), vitamin E (both D-alpha-tocopherol and D-alpha-TS), natural mixed carotenoids, vitamin C (calcium ascorbate), coenzyme Q_{10}, R-alpha-lipoic acid, n-acetylcysteine, L-carnitine, vitamin D, all B vitamins with high doses of vitamin B_3, selenium, omega-3 fatty acids, curcumin, and resveratrol. This preparation can be used in combination with standard therapy.

A separate preparation of micronutrients for the chronic phase of ischemic/reperfusion injury containing lower doses of antioxidants and polyphenolic compounds than those found in the preparation for the acute phase is recommended. This preparation can be used in combination with standard therapy.

The efficacy of proposed micronutrient formulations, in combination with standard therapy, should be tested by well-designed clinical studies. It is expected that the proposed micronutrient recommendations, in combination with standard therapy, would reduce the progression of brain damage during the acute phase and the risk of developing neurological deficits during the chronic phase of ischemic/reperfusion brain injury more than those produced by standard therapy alone.

REFERENCES

1. Qureshi AI, Chaudhry SA, Majidi S, Grigoryan M, Rodriguez GJ, Suri MF. Population-based estimates of neuroendovascular procedures: Results of a state-wide study. *Neuroepidemiology.* 2012; 39(2): 125–130.
2. Heron M. Deaths: Leading causes for 2008. *Nat Vital Stat Rep.* Jun 6 2012; 60(6): 1–94.
3. Lee LK, Bateman BT, Wang S, Schumacher HC, Pile-Spellman J, Saposnik G. Trends in the hospitalization of ischemic stroke in the United States, 1998–2007. *Int J Stroke.* Apr 2012; 7(3): 195–201.
4. Brinjikji W, Rabinstein AA, Cloft HJ. Hospitalization costs for acute ischemic stroke patients treated with intravenous thrombolysis in the United States are substantially higher than medicare payments. *Stroke.* Apr 2012; 43(4): 1131–1133.
5. Allen CL, Bayraktutan U. Oxidative stress and its role in the pathogenesis of ischaemic stroke. *Int J Stroke.* Dec 2009; 4(6): 461–470.
6. Lee WC, Wong HY, Chai YY et al. Lipid peroxidation dysregulation in ischemic stroke: Plasma 4-HNE as a potential biomarker? *Biochem Biophys Res Commun.* Sep 7 2012; 425(4): 842–847.

7. Ciancarelli I, Di Massimo C, De Amicis D, Carolei A, Tozzi Ciancarelli MG. Evidence of redox unbalance in post-acute ischemic stroke patients. *Curr Neurovasc Res.* May 2012; 9(2): 85–90.

8. Il'yasova D, Scarbrough P, Spasojevic I. Urinary biomarkers of oxidative status. *Clin Chim Acta.* Oct 9 2012; 413(19–20): 1446–1453.

9. Manzanero S, Santro T, Arumugam TV. Neuronal oxidative stress in acute ischemic stroke: Sources and contribution to cell injury. *Neurochem Int.* Apr 2013; 62(5): 712–718.

10. Ozkul A, Akyol A, Yenisey C, Arpaci E, Kiylioglu N, Tataroglu C. Oxidative stress in acute ischemic stroke. *J Clin Neurosci.* Nov 2007; 14(11): 1062–1066.

11. Leinonen JS, Ahonen JP, Lonnrot K et al. Low plasma antioxidant activity is associated with high lesion volume and neurological impairment in stroke. *Stroke.* Jan 2000; 31(1): 33–39.

12. Seet RC, Lee CY, Chan BP et al. Oxidative damage in ischemic stroke revealed using multiple biomarkers. *Stroke.* Aug 2011; 42(8): 2326–2329.

13. Vasiljevic B, Maglajlic-Djukic S, Gojnic M, Stankovic S. The role of oxidative stress in perinatal hypoxic–ischemic brain injury. *Srp Arh Celok Lek.* Jan–Feb 2012; 140(1–2): 35–41.

14. Radermacher KA, Wingler K, Langhauser F et al. Neuroprotection after stroke by targeting NOX4 as a source of oxidative stress. *Antioxid Redox Signal.* Apr 20 2013; 18(12): 1418–1427.

15. Tang XN, Cairns B, Kim JY, Yenari MA. NADPH oxidase in stroke and cerebrovascular disease. *Neurolog Res.* May 2012; 34(4): 338–345.

16. Dominguez C, Delgado P, Vilches A et al. Oxidative stress after thrombolysis-induced reperfusion in human stroke. *Stroke.* Apr 2010; 41(4): 653–660.

17. Kondo T, Reaume AG, Huang TT et al. Reduction of CuZn-superoxide dismutase activity exacerbates neuronal cell injury and edema formation after transient focal cerebral ischemia. *J Neurosci.* Jun 1 1997; 17(11): 4180–4189.

18. Kinouchi H, Epstein CJ, Mizui T, Carlson E, Chen SF, Chan PH. Attenuation of focal cerebral ischemic injury in transgenic mice overexpressing CuZn superoxide dismutase. *Proc Natl Acad Sci USA.* Dec 15 1991; 88(24): 11,158–11,162.

19. Shah ZA, Li RC, Thimmulappa RK et al. Role of reactive oxygen species in modulation of Nrf2 following ischemic reperfusion injury. *Neuroscience.* Jun 15 2007; 147(1): 53–59.

20. Hu SQ, Ye JS, Zong YY et al. S-nitrosylation of mixed lineage kinase 3 contributes to its activation after cerebral ischemia. *J Biol Chem.* Jan 20 2012; 287(4): 2364–2377.

21. Qi SH, Hao LY, Yue J, Zong YY, Zhang GY. Exogenous nitric oxide negatively regulates the S-nitrosylation p38 mitogen-activated protein kinase activation during cerebral ischaemia and reperfusion. *Neuropathol Appl Neurobiol.* Apr 2013; 39(3): 284–297.

22. Liu DH, Yuan FG, Hu SQ et al. Endogenous nitric oxide induces activation of apoptosis signal-regulating kinase 1 via S-nitrosylation in rat hippocampus during cerebral ischemia-reperfusion. *Neuroscience.* Jan 15 2013; 229: 36–48.

23. Gu Y, Dee CM, Shen J. Interaction of free radicals, matrix metalloproteinases, and caveolin-1 impacts blood–brain barrier permeability. *Front Biosci.* 2011; 3: 1216–1231.

24. Chiquete E, Ruiz-Sandoval JL, Murillo-Bonilla LM et al. Serum uric acid and outcome after acute ischemic stroke: PREMIER study. *Cerebrovasc Dis.* 2013; 35(2): 168–174.

25. Ryu WS, Kim CK, Kim BJ, Lee SH. Serum uric acid levels and cerebral microbleeds in patients with acute ischemic stroke. *PloS One.* 2013; 8(1): e55210.

26. Basso M, Ratan RR. Transglutaminase is a therapeutic target for oxidative stress, excitotoxicity and stroke: A new epigenetic kid on the CNS block. *J Cereb Blood Flow Metab.* Jun 2013; 33(6): 809–818.

27. Pluta R, Furmaga-Jablonska W, Maciejewski R, Ulamek-Koziol M, Jablonski M. Brain ischemia activates beta- and gamma-secretase cleavage of amyloid precursor protein: Significance in sporadic Alzheimer's disease. *Mol Neurobiol.* Feb 2013; 47(1): 425–434.

28. Suzuki S, Tanaka K, Suzuki N. Ambivalent aspects of interleukin-6 in cerebral ischemia: Inflammatory versus neurotrophic aspects. *J Cereb Blood Flow Metab.* Mar 2009; 29(3): 464–479.

29. Ito M, Kondo T, Shichita T, Yoshimura A. Post-ischemic innate immunity and its application for novel therapeutic strategy targeting brain inflammation. *Nihon Rinsho.* Jul 2013; 71(7): 1291–1301.

30. Shichita T, Ago T, Kamouchi M, Kitazono T, Yoshimura A, Ooboshi H. Novel therapeutic strategies targeting innate immune responses and early inflammation after stroke. *J Neurochem.* Nov 2012; 123 Suppl 2: 29–38.

31. Shichita T, Hasegawa E, Kimura A et al. Peroxiredoxin family proteins are key initiators of post-ischemic inflammation in the brain. *Nat Med.* Jun 2012; 18(6): 911–917.

32. Yang QW, Lu FL, Zhou Y et al. HMBG1 mediates ischemia-reperfusion injury by TRIF-adaptor independent Toll-like receptor 4 signaling. *J Cereb Blood Flow Metab.* Feb 2011; 31(2): 593–605.

33. Gelderblom M, Weymar A, Bernreuther C et al. Neutralization of the IL-17 axis diminishes neutrophil invasion and protects from ischemic stroke. *Blood.* Nov 1 2012; 120(18): 3793–3802.

34. Hendryk S, Czuba Z, Jedrzejewska-Szypulka H, Bazowski P, Dolezych H, Krol W. Increase in activity of neutrophils and proinflammatory mediators in rats following acute and prolonged focal cerebral ischemia and reperfusion. *Acta Neurochir Suppl.* 2010; 106: 29–35.

35. Lindsberg PJ, Strbian D, Karjalainen-Lindsberg ML. Mast cells as early responders in the regulation of acute blood–brain barrier changes after cerebral ischemia and hemorrhage. *J Cereb Blood Flow Metab.* Apr 2010; 30(4): 689–702.

36. Choe CU, Lardong K, Gelderblom M et al. CD38 exacerbates focal cytokine production, postischemic inflammation and brain injury after focal cerebral ischemia. *PloS One.* 2011; 6(5): e19046.

37. Ozkul A, Ayhan M, Akyol A, Turgut ET, Kadikoylu G, Yenisey C. The effect of insulin resistance on inflammatory response and oxidative stress in acute cerebral ischemia. *Neuro Endocrinol Lett.* 2013; 34(1): 52–57.

38. Welsh P, Lowe GD, Chalmers J et al. Associations of proinflammatory cytokines with the risk of recurrent stroke. *Stroke.* Aug 2008; 39(8): 2226–2230.

39. D'Ambrosio AL, Pinsky DJ, Connolly ES. The role of the complement cascade in ischemia/reperfusion injury: Implications for neuroprotection. *Mol Med.* Jun 2001; 7(6): 367–382.

40. Sughrue ME, Mehra A, Connolly ES, Jr., D'Ambrosio AL. Anti-adhesion molecule strategies as potential neuroprotective agents in cerebral ischemia: A critical review of the literature. *Inflamm Res.* Oct 2004; 53(10): 497–508.

41. Mao Y, Zhang M, Tuma RF, Kunapuli SP. Deficiency of PAR4 attenuates cerebral ischemia/reperfusion injury in mice. *J Cereb Blood Flow Metab.* May 2010; 30(5): 1044–1052.

42. Ikeda-Matsuo Y. The role of prostaglandin E2 in stroke-reperfusion injury. *Yakugaku Zasshi.* 2013; 133(9): 947–954.

43. Shimamura M, Zhou P, Casolla B et al. Prostaglandin E2 type 1 receptors contribute to neuronal apoptosis after transient forebrain ischemia. *J Cereb Blood Flow Metab.* Aug 2013; 33(8): 1207–1214.

44. Akram A, Gibson CL, Grubb BD. Neuroprotection mediated by the EP(4) receptor avoids the detrimental side effects of COX-2 inhibitors following ischaemic injury. *Neuropharmacology.* Feb 2013; 65: 165–172.

45. Ikeda-Matsuo Y, Tanji H, Narumiya S, Sasaki Y. Inhibition of prostaglandin E2 EP3 receptors improves stroke injury via anti-inflammatory and anti-apoptotic mechanisms. *J Neuroimmunol.* Sep 15 2011; 238(1–2): 34–43.
46. Xu F, Li J, Ni W, Shen YW, Zhang XP. Peroxisome proliferator-activated receptor-gamma agonist 15d-prostaglandin J2 mediates neuronal autophagy after cerebral ischemia-reperfusion injury. *PloS One.* 2013; 8(1): e55080.
47. Saleem S, Ahmad AS, Maruyama T, Narumiya S, Dore S. PGF(2alpha) FP receptor contributes to brain damage following transient focal brain ischemia. *Neurotox Res.* Jan 2009; 15(1): 62–70.
48. Kim YT, Moon SK, Maruyama T, Narumiya S, Dore S. Prostaglandin FP receptor inhibitor reduces ischemic brain damage and neurotoxicity. *Neurobiol Dis.* Oct 2012; 48(1): 58–65.
49. Phillis JW, O'Regan MH. Mechanisms of glutamate and aspartate release in the ischemic rat cerebral cortex. *Brain Res.* Aug 19 1996; 730(1–2): 150–164.
50. Rao VL, Bowen KK, Dempsey RJ. Transient focal cerebral ischemia down-regulates glutamate transporters GLT-1 and EAAC1 expression in rat brain. *Neurochem Res.* May 2001; 26(5): 497–502.
51. Chen JC, Hsu-Chou H, Lu JL et al. Downregulation of the glial glutamate transporter GLT-1 in rat hippocampus and striatum and its modulation by a group III metabotropic glutamate receptor antagonist following transient global forebrain ischemia. *Neuropharmacology.* Oct 2005; 49(5): 703–714.
52. Verma R, Mishra V, Sasmal D, Raghubir R. Pharmacological evaluation of glutamate transporter 1 (GLT-1) mediated neuroprotection following cerebral ischemia/reperfusion injury. *Eur J Pharmacol.* Jul 25 2010; 638(1–3): 65–71.
53. Nakayama R, Yano T, Ushijima K, Abe E, Terasaki H. Effects of dantrolene on extracellular glutamate concentration and neuronal death in the rat hippocampal CA1 region subjected to transient ischemia. *Anesthesiology.* Mar 2002; 96(3): 705–710.
54. Koinig H, Vornik V, Rueda C, Zornow MH. Lubeluzole inhibits accumulation of extracellular glutamate in the hippocampus during transient global cerebral ischemia. *Brain Res.* Apr 20 2001; 898(2): 297–302.
55. Itoh K, Chiba T, Takahashi S et al. An Nrf2/small Maf heterodimer mediates the induction of phase II detoxifying enzyme genes through antioxidant response elements. *Biochem Biophys Res Commun.* Jul 18 1997; 236(2): 313–322.
56. Hayes JD, Chanas SA, Henderson CJ et al. The Nrf2 transcription factor contributes both to the basal expression of glutathione S-transferases in mouse liver and to their induction by the chemopreventive synthetic antioxidants, butylated hydroxyanisole and ethoxyquin. *Biochem Soc Trans.* Feb 2000; 28(2): 33–41.
57. Chan K, Han XD, Kan YW. An important function of Nrf2 in combating oxidative stress: Detoxification of acetaminophen. *Proc Natl Acad Sci USA.* Apr 10 2001; 98(8): 4611–4616.
58. Williamson TP, Johnson DA, Johnson JA. Activation of the Nrf2/ARE pathway by siRNA knockdown of Keap1 reduces oxidative stress and provides partial protection from MPTP-mediated neurotoxicity. *Neurotoxicology.* Jun 2012; 33(3): 272–279.
59. Niture SK, Kaspar JW, Shen J, Jaiswal AK. Nrf2 signaling and cell survival. *Toxicol Appl Pharmacol.* Apr 1 2010; 244(1): 37–42.
60. Xi YD, Yu HL, Ding J et al. Flavonoids protect cerebrovascular endothelial cells through Nrf2 and PI3K from beta-amyloid peptide-induced oxidative damage. *Curr Neurovasc Res.* Feb 2012; 9(1): 32–41.
61. Li XH, Li CY, Lu JM, Tian RB, Wei J. Allicin ameliorates cognitive deficits ageing-induced learning and memory deficits through enhancing of Nrf2 antioxidant signaling pathways. *Neurosci Lett.* Apr 11 2012; 514(1): 46–50.

62. Bergstrom P, Andersson HC, Gao Y et al. Repeated transient sulforaphane stimulation in astrocytes leads to prolonged Nrf2-mediated gene expression and protection from superoxide-induced damage. *Neuropharmacology.* Feb–Mar 2011; 60(2–3): 343–353.

63. Wruck CJ, Gotz ME, Herdegen T, Varoga D, Brandenburg LO, Pufe T. Kavalactones protect neural cells against amyloid beta peptide-induced neurotoxicity via extracellular signal-regulated kinase 1/2-dependent nuclear factor erythroid 2-related factor 2 activation. *Mol Pharmacol.* Jun 2008; 73(6): 1785–1795.

64. Hine CM, Mitchell JR. NRF2 and the phase II response in acute stress resistance induced by dietary restriction. *J Clin Exp Pathol.* Jun 19 2012; S4(4).

65. Suh JH, Shenvi SV, Dixon BM et al. Decline in transcriptional activity of Nrf2 causes age-related loss of glutathione synthesis, which is reversible with lipoic acid. *Proc Natl Acad Sci USA.* Mar 9 2004; 101(10): 3381–3386.

66. Zou Y, Hong B, Fan L et al. Protective effect of puerarin against beta-amyloid-induced oxidative stress in neuronal cultures from rat hippocampus: Involvement of the GSK-3beta/Nrf2 signaling pathway. *Free Radic Res.* Jan 2013; 47(1): 55–63.

67. Choi HK, Pokharel YR, Lim SC et al. Inhibition of liver fibrosis by solubilized coenzyme Q_{10}: Role of Nrf2 activation in inhibiting transforming growth factor-beta1 expression. *Toxicol Appl Pharmacol.* Nov 1 2009; 240(3): 377–384.

68. Trujillo J, Chirino YI, Molina-Jijon E, Anderica-Romero AC, Tapia E, Pedraza-Chaverri J. Renoprotective effect of the antioxidant curcumin: Recent findings. *Redox Biol.* 2013; 1(1): 448–456.

69. Steele ML, Fuller S, Patel M, Kersaitis C, Ooi L, Munch G. Effect of Nrf2 activators on release of glutathione, cysteinylglycine and homocysteine by human U373 astroglial cells. *Redox Biol.* 2013; 1(1): 441–445.

70. Kode A, Rajendrasozhan S, Caito S, Yang SR, Megson IL, Rahman I. Resveratrol induces glutathione synthesis by activation of Nrf2 and protects against cigarette smoke-mediated oxidative stress in human lung epithelial cells. *Am J Physiol Lung Cell Mol Physiol.* Mar 2008; 294(3): L478–L488.

71. Gao L, Wang J, Sekhar KR et al. Novel n-3 fatty acid oxidation products activate Nrf2 by destabilizing the association between Keap1 and Cullin3. *J Biol Chem.* Jan 26 2007; 282(4): 2529–2537.

72. Saw CL, Yang AY, Guo Y, Kong AN. Astaxanthin and omega-3 fatty acids individually and in combination protect against oxidative stress via the Nrf2-ARE pathway. *Food Chem Toxicol.* Dec 2013; 62: 869–875.

73. Ji L, Liu R, Zhang XD et al. N-acetylcysteine attenuates phosgene-induced acute lung injury via upregulation of Nrf2 expression. *Inhal Toxicol.* Jun 2010; 22(7): 535–542.

74. Zambrano S, Blanca AJ, Ruiz-Armenta MV et al. The renoprotective effect of L-carnitine in hypertensive rats is mediated by modulation of oxidative stress-related gene expression. *Eur J Nutr.* Sep 2013; 52(6): 1649–1659.

75. Abate A, Yang G, Dennery PA, Oberle S, Schroder H. Synergistic inhibition of cyclo-oxygenase-2 expression by vitamin E and aspirin. *Free Radic Biol Med.* Dec 2000; 29(11): 1135–1142.

76. Devaraj S, Tang R, Adams-Huet B et al. Effect of high-dose alpha-tocopherol supplementation on biomarkers of oxidative stress and inflammation and carotid atherosclerosis in patients with coronary artery disease. *Am J Clin Nutr.* Nov 2007; 86(5): 1392–1398.

77. Fu Y, Zheng S, Lin J, Ryerse J, Chen A. Curcumin protects the rat liver from CCl4-caused injury and fibrogenesis by attenuating oxidative stress and suppressing inflammation. *Mol Pharmacol.* Feb 2008; 73(2): 399–409.

78. Lee HS, Jung KK, Cho JY et al. Neuroprotective effect of curcumin is mainly mediated by blockade of microglial cell activation. *Pharmazie.* Dec 2007; 62(12): 937–942.

79. Peairs AT, Rankin JW. Inflammatory response to a high-fat, low-carbohydrate weight loss diet: Effect of antioxidants. *Obesity (Silver Spring).* May 1 2008.
80. Rahman S, Bhatia K, Khan AQ et al. Topically applied vitamin E prevents massive cutaneous inflammatory and oxidative stress responses induced by double application of 12-O-tetradecanoylphorbol-13-acetate (TPA) in mice. *Chem Biol Interact.* Apr 15 2008; 172(3): 195–205.
81. Suzuki YJ, Aggarwal BB, Packer L. Alpha-lipoic acid is a potent inhibitor of NF-kappa B activation in human T cells. *Biochem Biophys Res Commun.* Dec 30 1992; 189(3): 1709–1715.
82. Zhu J, Yong W, Wu X et al. Anti-inflammatory effect of resveratrol on TNF-alpha-induced MCP-1 expression in adipocytes. *Biochem Biophys Res Commun.* May 2 2008; 369(2): 471–477.
83. Barger SW, Goodwin ME, Porter MM, Beggs ML. Glutamate release from activated microglia requires the oxidative burst and lipid peroxidation. *J Neurochem.* Jun 2007; 101(5): 1205–1213.
84. Schubert D, Kimura H, Maher P. Growth factors and vitamin E modify neuronal glutamate toxicity. *Proc Natl Acad Sci USA.* Sep 1 1992; 89(17): 8264–8267.
85. Sandhu JK, Pandey S, Ribecco-Lutkiewicz M et al. Molecular mechanisms of glutamate neurotoxicity in mixed cultures of NT2-derived neurons and astrocytes: Protective effects of coenzyme Q_{10}. *J Neurosci Res.* Jun 15 2003; 72(6): 691–703.
86. Panigrahi M, Sadguna Y, Shivakumar BR et al. alpha-Lipoic acid protects against reperfusion injury following cerebral ischemia in rats. *Brain Res.* Apr 22 1996; 717(1–2): 184–188.
87. Connell BJ, Saleh M, Khan BV, Saleh TM. Lipoic acid protects against reperfusion injury in the early stages of cerebral ischemia. *Brain Res.* Feb 23 2011; 1375: 128–136.
88. Khan M, Sekhon B, Jatana M et al. Administration of N-acetylcysteine after focal cerebral ischemia protects brain and reduces inflammation in a rat model of experimental stroke. *J Neurosci Res.* May 15 2004; 76(4): 519–527.
89. Shen WH, Zhang CY, Zhang GY. Antioxidants attenuate reperfusion injury after global brain ischemia through inhibiting nuclear factor-kappa B activity in rats. *Acta Parmacol Sin.* Nov 2003; 24(11): 1125–1130.
90. Manickam DS, Brynskikh AM, Kopanic JL et al. Well-defined cross-linked antioxidant nanozymes for treatment of ischemic brain injury. *J Control Rel.* Sep 28 2012; 162(3): 636–645.
91. Aabdallah DM, Eid NI. Possible neuroprotective effects of lecithin and alpha-tocopherol alone or in combination against ischemia/reperfusion insult in rat brain. *J Biochem Mol Toxicol.* 2004; 18(5): 273–278.
92. Onem G, Aral E, Enli Y et al. Neuroprotective effects of L-carnitine and vitamin E alone or in combination against ischemia-reperfusion injury in rats. *J Surg Res.* Mar 2006; 131(1): 124–130.
93. Fujita K, Yoshimoto N, Kato T et al. Lycopene inhibits ischemia/reperfusion-induced neuronal apoptosis in gerbil hippocampal tissue. *Neurochem Res.* Mar 2013; 38(3): 461–469.
94. Ekici F, Ozyurt B, Erdogan H. The combination of vitamin D3 and dehydroascorbic acid administration attenuates brain damage in focal ischemia. *Neurol Sci.* Jun 2009; 30(3): 207–212.
95. Luan H, Gdowski MJ, Newlands SD, Gdowski GT. Convergence of vestibular and neck proprioceptive sensory signals in the cerebellar interpositus. *J Neurosci.* Jan 16 2013; 33(3): 1198–1210a.
96. Raghavendra M, Trigunayat A, Singh RK, Mitra S, Goel RK, Acharya SB. Effect of ethanolic extract of root of Pongamia pinnata (L) pierre on oxidative stress, behavioral and histopathological alterations induced by cerebral ischemia—Reperfusion and long-term hypoperfusion in rats. *Indian J Exp Biol.* Oct 2007; 45(10): 868–876.

97. Yanpallewar SU, Rai S, Kumar M, Acharya SB. Evaluation of antioxidant and neuroprotective effect of Ocimum sanctum on transient cerebral ischemia and long-term cerebral hypoperfusion. *Pharmacol Biochem Behav.* Sep 2004; 79(1): 155–164.

98. Li C, Yan Z, Yang J et al. Neuroprotective effects of resveratrol on ischemic injury mediated by modulating the release of neurotransmitter and neuromodulator in rats. *Neurochem Int.* Feb 2010; 56(3): 495–500.

99. Ren J, Fan C, Chen N, Huang J, Yang Q. Resveratrol pretreatment attenuates cerebral ischemic injury by upregulating expression of transcription factor Nrf2 and HO-1 in rats. *Neurochem Res.* Dec 2011; 36(12): 2352–2362.

100. Yang C, Zhang X, Fan H, Liu Y. Curcumin upregulates transcription factor Nrf2, HO-1 expression and protects rat brains against focal ischemia. *Brain Res.* Jul 28 2009; 1282: 133–141.

101. Yao RQ, Qi DS, Yu HL, Liu J, Yang LH, Wu XX. Quercetin attenuates cell apoptosis in focal cerebral ischemia rat brain via activation of BDNF-TrkB-PI3K/Akt signaling pathway. *Neurochem Res.* Dec 2012; 37(12): 2777–2786.

102. Liang HW, Qiu SF, Shen J et al. Genistein attenuates oxidative stress and neuronal damage following transient global cerebral ischemia in rat hippocampus. *Neurosci Lett.* Jun 13 2008; 438(1): 116–120.

103. Urikova A, Babusikova E, Dobrota D et al. Impact of Ginkgo Biloba Extract EGb 761 on ischemia/reperfusion-induced oxidative stress products formation in rat forebrain. *Cell Mol Neurobiol.* Oct–Nov 2006; 26(7–8): 1343–1353.

104. Hong JT, Ryu SR, Kim HJ et al. Neuroprotective effect of green tea extract in experimental ischemia-reperfusion brain injury. *Brain Res Bull.* Dec 2000; 53(6): 743–749.

105. Jia J, Hu YS, Wu Y et al. Pre-ischemic treadmill training affects glutamate and gamma aminobutyric acid levels in the striatal dialysate of a rat model of cerebral ischemia. *Life Sci.* Apr 10 2009; 84(15–16): 505–511.

106. Jia J, Hu YS, Wu Y et al. Treadmill pre-training suppresses the release of glutamate resulting from cerebral ischemia in rats. *Exp Brain Res.* Jul 2010; 204(2): 173–179.

107. Parnham M, Sies H. Ebselen: Prospective therapy for cerebral ischaemia. *Expert Opin Investig Drugs.* Mar 2000; 9(3): 607–619.

108. Yamaguchi T, Sano K, Takakura K et al. Ebselen in acute ischemic stroke: A placebo-controlled, double-blind clinical trial. Ebselen Study Group. *Stroke.* Jan 1998; 29(1): 12–17.

109. Feng S, Yang Q, Liu M et al. Edaravone for acute ischaemic stroke. *Cochrane Database Syst Rev.* 2011; (12): CD007230.

110. Zhang N, Komine-Kobayashi M, Tanaka R, Liu M, Mizuno Y, Urabe T. Edaravone reduces early accumulation of oxidative products and sequential inflammatory responses after transient focal ischemia in mice brain. *Stroke.* Oct 2005; 36(10): 2220–2225.

111. Ly JV, Zavala JA, Donnan GA. Neuroprotection and thrombolysis: Combination therapy in acute ischaemic stroke. *Expert Opin Pharmacother.* Aug 2006; 7(12): 1571–1581.

112. Zhang FH. Effects of acupuncture at 7–9 am and 3–5 pm on plasma thromboxane and prostaglandin in patients with ischemic cerebrovascular disease. *J Tradit Chin Med.* Mar 2010; 30(1): 9–12.

113. Shoulson I. DATATOP: A decade of neuroprotective inquiry. Parkinson Study Group. Deprenyl and tocopherol antioxidative therapy of parkinsonism. *Ann Neurol.* Sep 1998; 44(3 Suppl 1): S160–S166.

114. Martin P, Leibovich SJ. Inflammatory cells during wound repair: The good, the bad, and the ugly. *Trends Cell Biol.* Nov 2005; 15(11): 599–607.

115. Colle D, Hartwig JM, Soares FA, Farina M. Probucol modulates oxidative stress and excitotoxicity in Huntington's disease models in vitro. *Brain Res Bull.* Mar 10 2012; 87(4–5): 397–405.

116. Albanes D, Heinonen OP, Huttunen JK et al. Effects of alpha-tocopherol and beta-carotene supplements on cancer incidence in the Alpha-Tocopherol Beta-Carotene Cancer Prevention Study. *Am J Clin Nutr.* Dec 1995; 62(6 Suppl): 1427S–1430S.

117. Kumar B, Andreatta C, Koustas WT, Cole WC, Edwards-Prasad J, Prasad KN. Mevastatin induces degeneration and decreases viability of cAMP-induced differentiated neuroblastoma cells in culture by inhibiting proteasome activity, and mevalonic acid lactone prevents these effects. *J Neurosci Res.* Jun 1 2002; 68(5): 627–635.

118. Chen RS, Huang CC, Chu NS. Coenzyme Q_{10} treatment in mitochondrial encephalomyopathies. Short-term double-blind, crossover study. *Eur Neurol.* 1997; 37(4): 212–218.

119. Behl C, Davis J, Cole GM, Schubert D. Vitamin E protects nerve cells from amyloid beta protein toxicity. *Biochem Biophys Res Commun.* Jul 31 1992; 186(2): 944–950.

120. Olanow CW, Arendash GW. Metals and free radicals in neurodegeneration. *Curr Opin Neurol.* Dec 1994; 7(6): 548–558.

121. Prasad KN, Kumar B, Yan XD, Hanson AJ, Cole WC. Alpha-tocopheryl succinate, the most effective form of vitamin E for adjuvant cancer treatment: A review. *J Am Coll Nutr.* Apr 2003; 22(2): 108–117.

10 Recommended Dietary Allowances/Dietary Reference Intakes/ Tolerable Upper Intake Level of Selected Micronutrients

INTRODUCTION

The changes in the nutritional guidelines have evolved significantly since World War II due to a rapid expansion of knowledge in nutrition and health. The nutritional guidelines referred to as Recommended Dietary Allowances (RDAs) were first established in 1941. The Food and Nutrition Board of the USA subsequently revised the guidelines every 5–10 years.

RDA (DIETARY REFERENCE INTAKE)

RDA refers to the value of the daily dietary intake level of a nutrient considered sufficient to meet the requirements of 97–98% of healthy individuals of different ages and gender. Because of rapid growth of research on the role of nutrients in human health, the Food and Nutrition Board of the Institute of Medicine (IOM) of the USA, in collaboration with Health Canada, updated the values of RDAs and renamed them as dietary reference intakes (DRIs) in 1998. Since then, the DRI values are used by both the USA and Canada. The DRI values of selected nutrients are listed in Tables 10.1 through 10.21. The DRI values are not currently used in nutrition labeling, but the RDA values of nutrients continue to be used for this purpose. The DRI values for carotenoids, alpha-lipoic acid, N-acetylcysteine, coenzyme Q_{10} and L-carnitine have not been determined. The values in Tables 10.1–10.21 are adapted and summarized from the tables of the Dietary Reference Intakes (DRI) published by http://www .nap.edu.

TABLE 10.1
DRIs of Antioxidants

Antioxidant Type	Age	RDA/AI (µg/d)	UL (µg/d)
Vitamin A			
	Infants		
	0–6 mo	400[a]	600
	7–12 mo	500[a]	600
	Children		
	1–3 y	300	600
	4–8 y	400	900
	Males		
	9–13 y	600	1700
	14–18 y	900	2800
	19 y and over	900	3000
	Females		
	9–13 y	600	1700
	14–18 y	700	2800
	19 y and over	700	3000
	Pregnancy		
	≤18 y	750	2800
	19–50 y	770	3000
	Lactation		
	≤18 y	1200	2800
	19–50 y	1300	3000

Note: The values are adapted and summarized from the DRI table published by http://www.nap.edu. RDA refers to recommended dietary allowance; AI, adequate intakes; UL, tolerable upper intake value. 1 µg of retinol equals 1 µg of RAE (retinol activity equivalent), 1 IU (international unit) of retinol equals 0.3 µg of retinol, and 2 µg of beta-carotene equals 1 µg of retinol.

[a] AI.

ADEQUATE INTAKE

Adequate intake (AI) refers to the value of a nutrient for which no RDA has been established, but the value established may be sufficient for everyone in the demographic group.

TABLE 10.2
DRIs of Antioxidants

Antioxidant Type	Age	RDA/AI (mg/d)	UL (mg/d)
Vitamin C			
	Infants		
	0–6 mo	40[a]	ND
	7–12 mo	50[a]	ND
	Children		
	1–3 y	15	400
	4–8 y	25	650
	Males		
	9–13 y	45	1200
	14–18 y	75	1800
	19 y and over	90	2000
	Females		
	9–13 y	45	1200
	14–18 y	65	1800
	19 y and over	75	2000

Note: The values are adapted and summarized from the DRI table published by http://www.nap.edu. RDA refers to recommended dietary allowance; AI, adequate intakes; UL, tolerable upper intake value; ND, not determined.

[a] AI.

TOLERABLE UPPER INTAKE LEVEL

The tolerable upper intake level (UL) is the maximum level of daily nutrient intake that is likely to pose no risk of adverse health effects. The UL value represents the total intake of a nutrient from food, water, and supplements.

RDA, AI, or UL values of nutrients are expected to be adequate for individuals for normal growth and survival; however, the values of micronutrients needed for the prevention or improved management of human diseases are not known at this time. The data on doses obtained from the use of a single micronutrient in the prevention or treatment of human diseases should not be extrapolated to the doses of the same micronutrient present in a multiple micronutrient preparation. Generally, whenever a single micronutrient is used in the laboratory or clinical studies, high doses of a micronutrient are needed to observe any biological effects. Low doses of the same micronutrient may be needed when used in combination with multiple micronutrients for the same effects.

TABLE 10.3
DRIs of Antioxidants

Antioxidant Type	Age	RDA/AI (mg/d)	UL (mg/d)
Vitamin E			
	Infants		
	0–6 mo	4[a]	ND
	7–12 mo	5[a]	ND
	Children		
	1–3 y	6	200
	4–8 y	7	300
	Males		
	9–13 y	11	600
	14–18 y	15	800
	19 y and over	15	1000
	Females		
	9–13 y	11	600
	14–18 y	15	800
	19 y and over	15	1000
	Pregnancy		
	≤18 y	15	800
	19–50 y	15	1000
	Lactation		
	≤18 y	19	800
	19–50 y	19	1000

Note: The values are adapted and summarized from the DRI table published by http://www.nap.edu. RDA refers to recommended dietary allowance; AI, adequate intakes; UL, tolerable upper intake value; ND, not determined. 1 IU of vitamin E equals 0.66 mg of D-alpha-tocopherol and 0.45 mg of DL-alpha-tocopherol.

[a] AI.

TABLE 10.4
DRIs of Vitamins

Vitamin Type	Age	RDA/AI (µg/d)	UL (µg/d)
Vitamin D			
	Infants		
	0–12 mo	5[a]	25
	Children		
	1–8 y	5[a]	50
	Males		
	9–50 y	5[a]	50
	50–70 y	10[a]	50
	>70 y	15[a]	50
	Females		
	9–50 y	5[a]	50
	50–70 y	10[a]	50
	>70 y	15[a]	50
	Pregnancy		
	≤18–50 y	5[a]	50
	Lactation		
	≤18–50 y	5[a]	50

Note: The values are adapted and summarized from the DRI table published by http://www.nap.edu. RDA refers to recommended dietary allowance; AI, adequate intakes; UL, tolerable upper intake value. 1 µg of cholecalciferol equals 40 IU of vitamin D.

[a] AI.

TABLE 10.5
DRIs of Vitamins

Vitamin Type	Age	RDA/AI (mg/d)	UL (mg/d)
Vitamin B$_1$ (Thiamin)			
	Infants		
	0–6 mo	0.2[a]	ND
	7–12 mo	0.3[a]	ND
	Children		
	1–3 y	0.5	ND
	4–8 y	0.6	ND
	Males		
	9–13 y	0.9	ND
	14 y and over	1.2	ND
	Females		
	9–13 y	0.9	ND
	14–18 y	1.0	ND
	19 y and over	1.1	ND
	Pregnancy		
	≤18–50 y	1.4	ND
	Lactation		
	≤18–50 y	1.4	ND

Note: The values are adapted and summarized from the DRI table published by http://www.nap.edu. RDA refers to recommended dietary allowance; AI, adequate intakes; UL, tolerable upper intake value; ND, not determined.

[a] AI.

TABLE 10.6
DRIs of Vitamins

Vitamin Type	Age	RDA/AI (mg/d)	UL (mg/d)
Vitamin B$_2$ (Riboflavin)			
	Infants		
	0–6 mo	0.3[a]	ND
	7–12 mo	0.4[a]	ND
	Children		
	1–3 y	0.5	ND
	4–8 y	0.6	ND
	Males		
	9–13 y	0.9	ND
	14 y and over	1.3	ND
	Females		
	9–13 y	0.9	ND
	14–18 y	1.0	ND
	19 y and over	1.1	ND
	Pregnancy		
	≤18–50 y	1.4	ND
	Lactation		
	≤18–50 y	1.6	ND

Note: The values are adapted and summarized from the DRI table published by http://www.nap.edu. RDA refers to recommended dietary allowance; AI, adequate intakes; UL, tolerable upper intake value; ND, not determined.

[a] AI.

TABLE 10.7
DRIs of Vitamins

Vitamin Type	Age	RDA/AI (mg/d)	UL (mg/d)
Vitamin B$_6$			
	Infants		
	0–6 mo	0.1[a]	ND
	7–12 mo	0.3[a]	ND
	Children		
	1–3 y	0.5	30
	4–8 y	0.6	40
	Males		
	9–13 y	1.0	60
	14–50 y	1.3	80
	50–70 y and over	1.7	100
	Females		
	9–13 y	1.0	60
	14–18 y	1.2	80
	19–30 y	1.3	100
	50 y and over	1.5	100
	Pregnancy		
	≤18 y	1.9	80
	19–50 y	1.9	100
	Lactation		
	≤18 y	2.0	80
	19–50 y	2.0	100

Note: The values are adapted and summarized from the DRI table published by http://www.nap.edu. RDA refers to recommended dietary allowance; AI, adequate intakes; UL, tolerable upper intake value; ND, not determined.

[a] AI.

TABLE 10.8
DRIs of Vitamins

Vitamin Type	Age	RDA/AI (µg/d)	UL (µg/d)
Vitamin B_{12} (Cobalamin)			
	Infants		
	0–6 mo	0.4[a]	ND
	7–12 mo	0.5[a]	ND
	Children		
	1–3 y	0.9	ND
	4–8 y	1.2	ND
	Males		
	9–13 y	1.08	ND
	14 y and over	2.4	ND
	Females		
	9–13 y	1.8	ND
	14 y and over	2.4	ND
	Pregnancy		
	≤18–50 y	2.6	ND
	Lactation		
	≤18–50 y	2.8	ND

Note: The values are adapted and summarized from the DRI table published by
http://www.nap.edu. RDA refers to recommended dietary allowance; AI,
adequate intakes; UL, tolerable upper intake value; ND, not determined.

[a] AI.

TABLE 10.9
DRIs of Vitamins

Vitamin Type	Age	RDA/AI (mg/d)	UL (mg/d)
Pantothenic acid			
	Infants		
	0–6 mo	1.7[a]	ND
	7–12 mo	1.8[a]	ND
	Children		
	1–3 y	2[a]	ND
	4–8 y	2[a]	ND
	Males		
	9–13 y	4[a]	ND
	14 y and over	5[a]	ND
	Females		
	9–13 y	4[a]	ND
	14 y and over	5[a]	ND
	Pregnancy		
	≤18–50 y	6[a]	ND
	Lactation		
	≤18–50 y	7[a]	ND

Note: The values are adapted and summarized from the DRI table published by http://www.nap.edu. RDA refers to recommended dietary allowance; AI, adequate intakes; UL, tolerable upper intake value; ND, not determined.

[a] AI.

TABLE 10.10
DRIs of Vitamins

Vitamin Type	Age	RDA/AI (mg/d)	UL (mg/d)
Niacin	**Infants**		
	0–6 mo	2[a]	ND
	7–12 mo	0.4[a]	ND
	Children		
	1–3 y	6.0	10
	4–8 y	8.0	15
	Males		
	9–13 y	12	20
	14–50 y	16	30
	50–70 y and over	16	35
	Females		
	9–13 y	12	20
	14–18 y	14	30
	19 y and over	14	35
	Pregnancy		
	≤18 y	18	30
	19–50 y	18	35
	Lactation		
	≤18 y	17	30
	19–50 y	17	35

Note: The values are adapted and summarized from the DRI table published by http://www.nap.edu. RDA refers to recommended dietary allowance; AI, adequate intakes; UL, tolerable upper intake value; ND, not determined.

[a] AI.

TABLE 10.11
DRIs of Vitamins

Vitamin Type	Age	RDA/AI (µg/d)	UL (µg/d)
Folate			
	Infants		
	0–6 mo	65[a]	ND
	7–12 mo	80[a]	ND
	Children		
	1–3 y	150	300
	4–8 y	200	400
	Males		
	9–13 y	300	600
	14–18 y	400	800
	19 y and over	400	1000
	Females		
	9–13 y	300	600
	14–18 y	400	800
	19 y and over	400	1000
	Pregnancy		
	≤18 y	600	800
	19–50 y	600	1000
	Lactation		
	≤18 y	500	800
	19–50 y	500	1000

Note: The values are adapted and summarized from the DRI table published by http://www.nap.edu. RDA refers to recommended dietary allowance; AI, adequate intakes; UL, tolerable upper intake value; ND, not determined.

[a] AI.

TABLE 10.12
DRIs of Micronutrients

Micronutrient Type	Age	RDA/AI (µg/d)	UL (µg/d)
Biotin			
	Infants		
	0–6 mo	0.5[a]	ND
	7–12 mo	0.6[a]	ND
	Children		
	1–3 y	8[a]	ND
	4–8 y	12[a]	ND
	Males		
	9–13 y	20	ND
	14–18 y	25	ND
	19 y and over	30	ND
	Females		
	9–13 y	20	ND
	14–18 y	25	ND
	19 y and over	30	ND
	Pregnancy		
	≤18 y	30[a]	ND
	19–50 y	30[a]	ND
	Lactation		
	≤18 y	35[a]	ND
	19–50 y	35[a]	ND

Note: The values are adapted and summarized from the DRI table published by http://www.nap.edu. RDA refers to recommended dietary allowance; AI, adequate intakes; UL, tolerable upper intake value; ND, not determined.

[a] AI.

TABLE 10.13
DRIs of Minerals

Mineral Type	Age	RDA/AI (mg/d)	UL (mg/d)
Calcium			
	Infants		
	0–6 mo	210[a]	ND
	7–12 mo	270[a]	ND
	Children		
	1–3 y	500[a]	2500
	4–8 y	800[a]	2500
	Males		
	9–18 y	1300[a]	2500
	19–50 y	1000[a]	2500
	51 y and over	1200[a]	2500
	Females		
	9–18 y	1300[a]	2500
	19–50 y	1000[a]	2500
	51 y and over	1200[a]	2500
	Pregnancy		
	≤18 y	1300[a]	2500
	19–50 y	1000[a]	2500
	Lactation		
	≤18 y	1300[a]	2500
	19–50 y	1000[a]	2500

Note: The values are adapted and summarized from the DRI table published by http://www.nap.edu. RDA refers to recommended dietary allowance; AI, adequate intakes; UL, tolerable upper intake value; ND, not determined.

[a] AI.

TABLE 10.14
DRIs of Minerals

Mineral Type	Age	RDA/AI (mg/d)	UL (mg/d)
Magnesium			
	Infants		
	0–6 mo	30[a]	ND
	7–12 mo	75[a]	ND
	Children		
	1–3 y	80	65
	4–8 y	130	110
	Males		
	9–13 y	240	350
	14–18 y	410	350
	19–30 y	400	350
	31 y and over	420	350
	Females		
	9–13 y	240	350
	14–18 y	360	350
	31 y and over	320	350
	Pregnancy		
	≤18 y	400	350
	19–30 y	350	350
	31–50 y	360	350
	Lactation		
	≤18 y	360	350
	31–50 y	320	350

Note: The values are adapted and summarized from the DRI table published by http://www.nap.edu. RDA refers to recommended dietary allowance; AI, adequate intakes; UL, tolerable upper intake value; ND, not determined.

[a] AI.

TABLE 10.15
DRIs of Minerals

Mineral Type	Age	RDA/AI (mg/d)	UL (mg/d)
Manganese			
	Infants		
	0–6 mo	0.003[a]	ND
	7–12 mo	0.6[a]	ND
	Children		
	1–3 y	1.2[a]	2
	4–8 y	1.5[a]	3
	Males		
	9–13 y	1.9[a]	6
	14–18 y	2.2[a]	9
	19 y and over	2.3[a]	11
	Females		
	9–13 y	1.6[a]	6
	14–18 y	1.6[a]	9
	19 y and over	1.8[a]	11
	Pregnancy		
	≤18 y	2.0[a]	9
	19–50 y	2.0[a]	11
	Lactation		
	≤18 y	2.6[a]	9
	19–50 y	2.6[a]	11

Note: The values are adapted and summarized from the DRI table published by http://www.nap.edu. RDA refers to recommended dietary allowance; AI, adequate intakes; UL, tolerable upper intake value; ND, not determined.

[a] AI.

TABLE 10.16
DRIs of Minerals

Mineral Type	Age	RDA/AI (μg/d)	UL (μg/d)
Chromium			
	Infants		
	0–6 mo	0.2[a]	ND
	7–12 mo	5.5[a]	ND
	Children		
	1–3 y	11[a]	ND
	4–8 y	15[a]	ND
	Males		
	9–13 y	25[a]	ND
	14–50 y	35[a]	ND
	51 y and over	30[a]	ND
	Females		
	9–13 y	21[a]	ND
	14–18 y	24[a]	ND
	19–50 y	25[a]	ND
	Pregnancy		
	≤18 y	29[a]	ND
	19–50 y	30[a]	ND
	Lactation		
	≤18 y	44[a]	ND
	19–50 y	45[a]	ND

Note: The values are adapted and summarized from the DRI table published by http://www.nap.edu. RDA refers to recommended dietary allowance; AI, adequate intakes; UL, tolerable upper intake value; ND, not determined.

[a] AI.

TABLE 10.17
DRIs of Minerals

Mineral Type	Age	RDA/AI (µg/d)	UL (µg/d)
Copper			
	Infants		
	0–6 mo	200[a]	ND
	7–12 mo	220[a]	ND
	Children		
	1–3 y	340	1000
	4–8 y	440	3000
	Males		
	9–13 y	700	5000
	14–18 y	890	8000
	19 y and over	900	10,000
	Females		
	9–13 y	700	5000
	14–18 y	890	8000
	19 y and over	900	10,000
	Pregnancy		
	≤18 y	1000	8000
	19–50 y	1000	10,000
	Lactation		
	≤18 y	1300	8000
	19–50 y	1300	10,000

Note: The values are adapted and summarized from the DRI table published by http://www.nap.edu. RDA refers to recommended dietary allowance; AI, adequate intakes; UL, tolerable upper intake value; ND, not determined.

[a] AI.

TABLE 10.18
DRIs of Minerals

Mineral Type	Age	RDA/AI (mg/d)	UL (mg/d)
Iron			
	Infants		
	0–6 mo	0.27[a]	40
	7–12 mo	11	40
	Children		
	1–3 y	7	40
	4–8 y	10	40
	Males		
	9–13 y	8	40
	14–18 y	11	45
	19 y and over	8	45
	Females		
	9–13 y	8	40
	14–18 y	15	45
	19–50 y	18	45
	50 y and over	8	45
	Pregnancy		
	≤18–50 y	27	45
	Lactation		
	≤18 y	10	45
	19–50 y	9	45

Note: The values are adapted and summarized from the DRI table published by http://www.nap.edu. RDA refers to recommended dietary allowance; AI, adequate intakes; UL, tolerable upper intake value; ND, not determined.

[a] AI.

TABLE 10.19
DRIs of Minerals

Mineral Type	Age	RDA/AI (µg/d)	UL (µg/d)
Selenium			
	Infants		
	0–6 mo	15[a]	45
	7–12 mo	20[a]	60
	Children		
	1–3 y	20	90
	4–8 y	30	150
	Males		
	9–13 y	40	280
	14 y and over	55	400
	Females		
	9–13 y	40	280
	14 y and over	55	400
	Pregnancy		
	≤18–50 y	60	400
	Lactation		
	≤18–50 y	70	400

Note: The values are adapted and summarized from the DRI table published by http://www.nap.edu. RDA refers to recommended dietary allowance; AI, adequate intakes; UL, tolerable upper intake value; ND, not determined.

[a] AI.

TABLE 10.20
DRIs of Minerals

Mineral Type	Age	RDA/AI (mg/d)	UL (mg/d)
Phosphorus			
	Infants		
	0–6 mo	100[a]	ND
	7–12 mo	275[a]	ND
	Children		
	1–3 y	460	3000
	4–8 y	500	3000
	Males		
	9–18 y	1250	4000
	19–70 y	700	4000
	>70 y	700	3000
	Females		
	9–18 y	1250	4000
	19–70 y	700	4000
	>70 y	700	3000
	Pregnancy		
	≤18 y	1250	3500
	19–50 y	700	3500
	Lactation		
	≤18 y	1250	4000
	19–50 y	700	4000

Note: The values are adapted and summarized from the DRI table published by http://www.nap.edu. RDA refers to recommended dietary allowance; AI, adequate intakes; UL, tolerable upper intake value; ND, not determined.

[a] AI.

TABLE 10.21
DRIs of Minerals

Mineral Type	Age	RDA/AI (mg/d)	UL (mg/d)
Zinc			
	Infants		
	0–6 mo	2[a]	4
	7–12 mo	3	5
	Children		
	1–3 y	3	7
	4–8 y	5	12
	Males		
	9–13 y	8	23
	14–18 y	11	34
	19 y and over	11	40
	Females		
	9–13 y	8	23
	14–18 y	9	34
	19 y and over	8	40
	Pregnancy		
	≤18 y	12	34
	19–50 y	11	40
	Lactation		
	≤18 y	13	34
	19–50 y	12	40

Note: The values are adapted and summarized from the DRI table published by http://www.nap.edu. RDA refers to recommended dietary allowance; AI, adequate intakes; UL, tolerable upper intake value; ND, not determined.

[a] AI.

CONCLUSIONS

The initial nutritional guidelines, RDAs, have been replaced by DRIs and are currently used by the USA and Canada. The DRI values of nutrients are sufficient for the growth and development of the 97–98% of the healthy individuals. The DRI values for carotenoids, alpha-lipoic acid, N-acetylcysteine, coenzyme Q_{10}, and L-carnitine have not been determined. The optimal values needed for prevention or improved management of human diseases are not known. Studies are in progress to establish these values.

Index

Page numbers followed by t indicate tables.